OXFORD MEDICAL PUBLICATIONS

Oxford Handbook of
Clinical and
Healthcare
Research

T0355063

Published and forthcoming Oxford Handbooks

Oxford Handbook of
Clinical and Healthcare Research

Editors

Sumantra (Shumone) Ray

Senior Medical Advisor/Clinician Scientist, Medical Research Council (Human Nutrition Research) and Chair of the UK Need for Nutrition Education/Innovation Programme (NNEdPro), Cambridge University Hospitals/School of Clinical Medicine; Fellow of Wolfson College, University of Cambridge, UK

Sue Fitzpatrick

Director at Redtree People and Sue Fitzpatrick Training; Former Head of Education and Training, The Institute of Clinical Research, UK

Associate Editors

Rajna Golubic

Gates Scholar, Medical Research Council and University of Cambridge (Epidemiology Unit and St. John's College) and Trust Doctor at the West Suffolk Hospital, UK

Susan Fisher

Former Research Manager, Medical Research Council (Human Nutrition Research), Cambridge, UK

Editorial Assistance

Sarah Gibbings

Research Assistant/Coordinator, Medical Research Council (Human Nutrition Research), Cambridge, UK

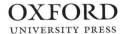

OXFORD
UNIVERSITY PRESS

OXFORD
UNIVERSITY PRESS

Great Clarendon Street, Oxford, OX2 6DP,
United Kingdom

Oxford University Press is a department of the University of Oxford.
It furthers the University's objective of excellence in research, scholarship,
and education by publishing worldwide. Oxford is a registered trade mark of
Oxford University Press in the UK and in certain other countries

First Edition published in 2016
Reprinted 2016

Impression: 2

Published in the United States of America by Oxford University Press
198 Madison Avenue, New York, NY 10016, United States of America

British Library Cataloguing in Publication Data
Data available

Library of Congress Control Number: 2015941607

ISBN 978–0–19–960847–8

Printed and bound in China by
C&C Offset Printing Co., Ltd.

Foreword

Research is important: without it we cannot develop new knowledge on why people get ill, what is the best treatment when they become ill, or how best to prevent illness in the future. Research data is used to support clinical decision-making, devising policy and making personal lifestyle decisions. However, to provide a sound basis research must be robustly designed, conducted and reported. In today's world, research data is being put under increasing scrutiny. It is becoming more common for research findings to be challenged. Policy makers, health professionals and the public expect research to be conducted transparently, including making research findings widely available in an appropriate format.

This *Oxford Handbook of Clinical and Healthcare Research* provides a practical guide for doctors, nurses, pharmacists, dieticians/nutritionists and other health professionals as well as students/trainees involved in all forms of clinical, translational, and public health research. It is timely with the recent publication of the EU Clinical Trial Regulation that will be applied in May 2016. This legislation will take the form of a regulation to ensure a greater level of harmonization of the rules of conducting clinical trials in Europe and a requirement for transparency. This handbook will provide you with the tools you need to conduct robust research studies, to collect valid and reproducible data and to do so in a manner that is open to scrutiny whilst protecting the research participants from harm. The initial chapters cover basic statistical concepts and study design, including discussion of how to evaluate evidence. Later in the book there is a more in depth look at clinical trials design, how to write a trial protocol and a description of the drug development pathway.

The book will introduce you to Good Clinical Practice (GCP). Although GCP is often seen as a bureaucratic burden, what it set outs to achieve is:

- To produce valid research data, and
- To protect the rights, dignity and well-being of participants.

Many specific aspects of GCP are picked up in the book, including study monitoring, accountabilities of research staff and sponsors, IMP accountability and consent. GCP is not presented here as a recipe to follow by the letter. Rather readers are encouraged to develop processes that deliver what is needed for your study. It is through the development of a risk-based approach to GCP that efforts can be focused on managing significant risks posed to participants and to data validity. One size does not fit all.

Perhaps not surprisingly, conducting research in the UK (as well as more widely) can involve a multitude of regulatory requirements. Many of these are covered here, including the need for research ethics committee approval and some of the processes used by the Health Research Authority, as well as an overview of the Human Tissue Authority and Clinical Trial Authorisation by the Medicines and Healthcare products Regulatory Authority. Beyond the law, Research Governance defines specific responsibilities of individuals and organizations, and requires appropriate lines of management and communication to ensure high standards are maintained throughout the research process. Again, the handbook provides an understanding of who should be accountable for what, including how tasks should be delegated to members of the research team. You can find out about safety reporting requirements and what to do if the protocol is not followed.

The handbook also provides some details of how to conduct various complex, study-related tasks. For example, how do you capture your data? Accurate collection of data is central to delivering sound science. It sounds simple enough, but if you are reliant on a team to collect and collate data, how do you ensure that they are all doing things in the same way? How can you be sure that the data collected by one person are equivalent those collected by another? How are you going to ensure that your research data remain confidential? Equally, when conducting a blinded drug trial, how do you ensure that all of your control group are indeed receiving placebo/control treatment, in light of the fact that control and test drug look identical? If your trial is taking place over a number of sites, how do you ensure that each site has the correct blinded control/intervention medication, and that it is stored correctly and used within its shelf life? How do you make sure that all participants on the trial are randomized in the agreed ratio, and are allocated to the correct blinded medication? Answers to all these questions are provided.

You will also learn what you need to know about managing your study: ensuring that you can complete on time and within budget. Guidance is provided on how to use document control to ensure everyone is using the correct version of protocols, consent forms or other documents. You are also given information on archiving research records; an often forgotten element that will require active management and possibly funding after your study has ended.

At the end of the day, you would want to generate new, robust knowledge about human health and disease, and to ensure that this knowledge is made available to other experts, policy makers, prescribers, patients and the general public so that they can consider it and use in their decision-making. Publication is an important element of disseminating research findings and guidance is given on how to go about publishing your findings to ensure you maximise impact. We are now in an era where not disseminating your research outputs, positive or negative, is simply not acceptable.

The handbook covers research fraud and misconduct. A culture that supports quality research must consider the potential for fraud. High impact publications can, and are, being challenged. This should not be considered an insult, but rather an opportunity to demonstrate the quality of what you do. With appropriate Quality Assurance in place, as described here, such anxieties can be easily dispelled!

Finally, you will be expected to make your good quality research datasets available to others, to input into meta-analyses, to undergo further scrutiny and re-analysis thereby maximizing their use and potentially helping to inform policy development. Many funders and publishers are asking that you consider sharing data through Open Access publication, DNA sequence information and tissue samples to optimize their use. The ethical imperative to share and maximize use should not, however, undermine research participants' right to confidentiality.

Starting research for the first time can be daunting. A good researcher will develop a multitude of skills and expertise over time. This Handbook is a very good place to start. Using the start-up toolkit at the end of this handbook, and you should find getting your study underway significantly easier than you might first think.

Dr Rachel Smith
BSc, MSc, PhD
Head of Training and Communications
Regulatory Support Centre, UK Medical Research Council

Professor Chim C Lang
BMSc, MB ChB, MD, FRCP (Edin & Lond), FACC
Professor of Cardiology, Clinical Pharmacology and Medicine
Ninewells Hospital and Medical School, University of Dundee
Chair of Medical Academics (Scotland), British Medical Association

Preface

This book was commissioned to integrate guidance on how to conduct both clinical as well as healthcare-related research. There are a multitude of texts on clinical research alone and also stand-alone books on broader healthcare-related research methods. In our handbook we have tried to combine both of these skill-sets as seamlessly as possible, whilst pointing out where the main differences lie. Since starting this handbook there have been a number of significant changes to the clinical research landscape as well as the drug development process, both in Europe and also globally. In clinical trials, much more emphasis is now placed on patient outcomes as well as demonstrating efficacy, whilst the ever widening scope of healthcare-related research ranges from quantitative analyses of 'big data' across populations to in-depth qualitative and educational/behavioural studies in individuals. The common denominator unifying both clinical and wider healthcare-related research is the need to ensure high quality data and the ability to readily translate findings for the benefit if patients and the public. This joint mission has resulted in convergence of the disciplines that underpin clinical and healthcare research.

The handbook is split broadly into three sections. Let us consider each section in turn, through the story of five fictitious but fairly typical examples of students/trainees, each about to undertake research as part of their degrees/training: Adam (Master's Student in Nursing), Betty (Pre-Registration Pharmacist), Jing (Medical Doctor in Academic Training), Khaled (Physiotherapist in Research Training), and Vidya (Nutrition and Dietetics Graduate on a PhD Programme). All five meet at a Research Symposium and stumble upon this handbook as a recommended resource.

The first section deals with basic research methods. The chapters start from the conceptual point of why we conduct research and the bedrock of quantitative and qualitative know-how required as a first step towards the investigation of any research question. This section also outlines how evidence-based medicine and critical appraisal are utilized in an applied research setting. Adam, Betty, Jing, Khaled, and Vidya all find this section equally beneficial. Adam, who is undertaking a qualitative piece of educational research draws mostly from the chapter written specifically in this area. Vidya finds the basics of statistics and epidemiology most relevant to strengthen concepts. Jing uses the critical appraisal section for weekly journal clubs.

The second section deals with general research process. The chapters deal with the regulatory environment, ethical, and safety requirements when conducting a research project. The management of clinical research is discussed and we take the reader through the life cycle of a research project from concept to fruition and publication. All five characters in our story use the material from this section as a toolkit to help navigate their individual research journeys.

The third section also concentrates on research process but the exacting requirements of clinical trials in investigational products are detailed and where there are significant differences in healthcare research these are discussed. Khaled finds this section useful to delineate where the similarities and differences lie in the methods and compliance measures required for his trials of non-pharmaceutical treatments. Betty and Jing both find that this section is particularly relevant to their aspirations of becoming a research pharmacist, and clinical trialist, respectively. Vidya finds this section useful to help decide that her research would be of a dietary rather than nutraceutical nature. Adam uses this section for continuing professional development.

No matter whether the users of this handbook are students, trainees or professionals, like our five fictitious characters, we are sure that this will prove a useful resource both to the uninitiated as well as those looking to read across horizontally between methodologies.

Throughout the book we provide examples wherever possible, key references and signposting to other useful resources, including weblinks which can be accessed for updates in this continuously moving field of clinical and healthcare research.

We hope that this handbook will serve as a faithful companion to all those undertaking clinical and healthcare research both across professions as well as across the globe and we look forward to shaping future editions to the evolving needs of a professionally diverse audience.

Acknowledgements

We would like to give heartfelt thanks to our many expert contributors for their breadth and depth of knowledge which has culminated in this comprehensive handbook. We also express huge gratitude to the co-editors, Rajna and Sue, and assistant editor, Sarah, who together with the Oxford University Press team, including Michael and Fiona, have tried to keep us on the straight and narrow.

It has been a very long journey from concept to completion but we sincerely hope we have produced a useful pocket reference for any healthcare professional who wishes to conduct meaningful research.

Finally we would like to thank Minha and Jim, our partners and family (including Nikitah who entered the world during the compilation of this handbook!) for their inordinate patience and support in the production process!

Contents

Contributors

Pauline Allen
eCRF/CRF Design Manager,
Syna Qua non Ltd, Diss Business
Park, UK

Suzanna Almoosawi
Research Associate, Newcastle
University,
Human Nutrition, Research
Centre and Institute of Health &
Society, Medical School, Newcastle
University, UK

Sarah Casey
Health, Safety and Quality
Manager, Medical Research
Council,
Human Nutrition Research,
Elsie Widdowson Laboratory,
Cambridge, UK

Darren Cole
Manager of Data Operations
Medical Research Council,
Human Nutrition Research,
Elsie Widdowson Laboratory,
Cambridge, UK

Nicky Dodsworth
VP, Quality Assurance, Risk &
Research, Premier Research,
Wokingham, UK

Nina Downes
Director, Diamond Clinical, High
Wycombe, UK

Joan Gandy
Lead Scientific Advisor
UK Need for Nutrition
Education/Innovation Programme
(NNEdPro), Cambridge, UK

Helen Glenny
Clinical Research Consultant,
Welwyn Garden City, UK

Chris Graf
Associate Editorial Director
Wiley-Blackwell UK

Karen Grover
eCRF/CRF Design Manager,
Syna Qua non Ltd, Diss Business
Park, UK

Lyn Haynes
Senior Lecturer
Canterbury Christchurch
University, Canterbury, UK

Janice Hedgecock
Director, Greatspur Clinical
Development, Norwich, UK

Babara Hepworth Jones
Head, Process and Training
Country Clinical Operations UK,
Roache Product Ltd, Welwyn
Garden City, UK

Helen Hill
Research Fellow, University
of Liverpool, Department of
Women's and Children's Health,
Institute of Translational Medicine,
Liverpool, UK

Liz Hooper
Archivist and Records Management
Consultant, Phlex Global,
Amersham, UK

Sheri Hubby
Senior Director, US Quality
Assurance, Risk & Compliance,
Premier Research, Fort Myers,
Florida, USA

Golam Kabir
Researcher, University of Dundee
Medical School, Dundee, UK

Priya Kalia
Research Associate,
Biomaterials, Biomimetics,
Biophotonics Division, Dental
Institute, King's College
London, UK

Eric Klaver
Director, FourPlus Clinical,
Amsterdam, The Netherlands

Chim Lang
Professor of Cardiology,
Division of Cardiovascular and
Diabetes Medicine, Ninewells
Hospital and Medical School
Dundee, UK

Celia Laur
Researcher in Applied Health
Sciences,
University of Waterloo,
Onatario, Canada

Sue Miles
Head of Clinical Trials,
Brecon Pharmaceuticals Ltd,
Hay-on-Wye, UK

Polly Page
Group leader: Nutrition, Surveys
and Studies Medical Research
Council, Human Nutrition
Research, Elsie Widdowson
Laboratory, Cambridge, UK

Richard Parker
Statistician, University of
Edinburgh, Edinburgh, UK

Minha Rajput Ray
Lead Medical Advisor,
UK Need for Nutrition
Education/Innovation Programme
(NNEdPro), Cambridge, UK

Alan Robertson
Specialty Registrar/Clinical
Research Fellow, Division of
Cardiovascular and Diabetes
Medicine, Ninewells Hospital and
Medical School
Dundee, UK

David Talbot
Director, Diamond Clinical, High
Wycombe, UK

Ben Thompson
Postgraduate, British College of
Osteopathic Medicine, London, UK

Ruzan Udumyan
Epidemiologist at Clinical
Epidemiology and Biostatistics,
School of Medical Sciences,
Örebro University, Sweden

Cheryl Whitehead
Independent Pharmaceutical
Professional, High Wycombe, UK

Lou Whelan
Managing Editor
The Journal Office,
UK

Symbols and abbreviations

ABPI	Association of the British Pharmaceutical Industry
ACE	angiotensin converting enzyme
ACLS	Aerobics Center Longitudinal Study
ADME	absorption distribution metabolism and excretion
ADR	adverse drug reaction
AE	adverse event
AIP	application integrity policy
ALCOA	attribute, legible, contemporaneous, original, accurate
AMI	acute myocardial infarction
AMRC	Association of Medical Research Charities
ANOVA	analysis of variance
API	active pharmaceutical ingredient
AR	attributable risk
AR	adverse reaction
ARIC	Atherosclerosis Risk in Communities Study
ARSAC	Administration of Radioactive Substances Advisory Committee
AUC-ROC	area under the curve receiver operating characteristic
AV	audio visual
BLA	biologics licence applications
BMA	British Medical Association
BMI	body mass index
BMJ	British Medical Journal
C of A	certificate of analysis
CA	competent authority
CAPA	corrective and preventative action
CAT	computerized tomography scan
CD	compact disk
CDF	career development fellowships
CDP	clinical development plan
CFR	Code of Federal Registers
CGSDI	clinical governance support and development indicator
CHAIN	Contact Help Advice and Information Network
CHARM	Candesartan in Heart Failure: Assessment of Reduction in Mortality and Morbidity
CHMP	Committee for Human Medicinal Products
CHRE	Council for Healthcare Regulatory Excellence

CI	chief investigator
CI	confidence interval
CI	cumulative incidence
CINAHL	Cumulative Index to Nursing and Allied Health Literature
Cmax	maximum concentration of the treatment in the body
CONSORT	Consolidated Standards of Reporting Trials
COPE	Committee on Publication Ethics
CPMP	Committee for Proprietary Medicinal Products
CRA	clinical research associate
CRC	clinical research coordinator
CRF	case record form
CRO	Contract Research Organization
CSR	clinical study report
CT	clinical trial
CTA	clinical trial administrator
CTA	Clinical Trial Agreement
CTA	Clinical Trial Authorization
CTIMP	clinical trials in investigational medicinal products
CTMS	clinical trial management systems
DARE	Database of Abstracts of Reviews of Effects
DCF	data clarification form
DI	designated individual
DIA	Drug Information Association
DM	doctorate in medicine (superspeciality)
DNA	deoxyribonucleic acid
DPA	Data Protection Act
DQLI	Dermatology Quality Life Index
DrPH	doctorate in public health
DSUR	development safety update report
E6	ICH efficacy guideline number six
EBG	evidence-based guideline
EBID	evidence-based individual decision-making
EMB	evidence-based medicine
EC	Ethics Committee
ECG	electro cardio graph
eCRF	electronic case record form
EDC	electronic data capture
eDCT	electronic data capture tools
EEA	European Economic Area

EHR	electronic health records
EIC	editor in chief
EMA	European Medicines Agency
EMBASE	Excerpta Medica dataBASE
EMWA	European Medical Writers Association
EPAR	European Public Assessment Report
EPIC	European Prospective Investigation into Cancer and Nutrition
EPSRC	Engineering and Physical Sciences Research Council
ESC	European Society of Cardiology
eTMF	electronic trial master files
EU	European Union
EudraCT	European Union Drug Regulating Authorities Clinical Trials Database
EVDB	EudraVigilance Database
FD	financial disclosure
FDA	Food and Drug Administration
FOI	freedom of information
FTP	free transfer protocol
GCP	good clinical practice
GCP RMA	Good Clinical Practice Records Managers Association
GLP	good laboratory practice
GMC	General Medical Council
GMP	good manufacturing practice
GP	general practitioner
GSK	Glaxo Smith Klein
GxP	good (clinical, laboratory, manufacturing pharma covigilance) practice
HF	heart failure
HF-ACTION	heart failure: a controlled trial investigating outcomes of exercise training
HIPAA	Health Insurance Portability and Accountancy Act
HIV	human immunodeficiency virus
HOD	head of department
HSC	health and social care
HT Act	Human Tissue Act
HTA	Human Tissue Authority
HFEA	Human Fertilisation and Embryology Authority
IB	investigator brochure
IC	informed consent

ICF	informed consent forms
ICH GCP	International Conference on Harmonisation of Good Clinical Practice
ICMJE	International Committee of Medical Journal Editors
ID	identification
IDMC	Independent Data Monitoring Committee
IEC	Independent Ethics Committee
IMP	investigational medicinal products
IMPD	Investigational Medicinal Product Dossier
IMRAD	introduction, methods, results and discussion
INTERHEART	a global case-control study of risk factors for acute myocardial infarction
IOM3	Institute of Materials, Mining and Metallurgy
IOP	intraocular pressure
IP	investigational product
IR	incidence rate
IRAS	Integrated Research Application System
IRB	institutional review board
ISF	investigator site file
ISI	Inter Service Intelligence
ISO	International Organization for Standardization
IT	information technology
IV	intravenous
IVRS	interactive voice recognition system
IWRS	interactive web response system
JAMA	Journal of American Medical Association
JUPITER	Justification for the Use of Statins in Primary Prevention: an Intervention Trial Evaluating Rosuvastatin
LH	licence holder
LR	likelihood ratio
MAA	marketing authorization approval
MAH	marketing authorization holder
MA (IMP)	MHRA Register of Holders of Manufacturers Authorisations for Investigational Medicinal Products
MCRN	Medicines for Children Research Network
MD	doctor of medicine (post-graduation)
ME	myalgic encephalopathy
MEDLINE	Medical Literature Analysis and Retrieval System Online
MCT	Mental Capacity Act
MHRA	Medicines and Healthcare Products Regulatory Agency

MI	myocardial infarction
MODEPHARMA	medication services for clinical trials
MPhil	master of philosophy
MRC	Medical Research Council
MRes	master of research
MRI	magnetic resonance imaging
MS	member state
MSc	master of science
MTD	maximum tolerated dose
NCR	no carbon required
NDA	new drug application
NeLH	National Electronic Library for Health
NHANES	National Health and Nutrition Examination Survey
NHS	National Health Service
NICE	National Institute for Health and Care Excellence
NIH	National Institute of Health
NIHR	National Institute for Health Research
NIMP	non investigational medicinal product
NMAP	network mapper
NNT	number needed to treat
NOAEL	no observable adverse effect level
NPL	National Physics Laboratory
NRES	National Research Ethics Service
NVivo	NVivo qualitative data analysis software
OMNI	organizing medical networked information
ORI	odds ratio
ORI	Office of Research Integrity
P	probability
PASS	post-authorization safety studies
PD	pharmacodynamics
PD	persons designated
PDF	portable document format
PGx	pharmacogenetics
PhD	doctor of philosophy
PHS	Public Health Service
PI	principal investigator
PIS	patient information sheet
PK	pharmacokinetic
PLoS	Public Library of Science
PM	project manager

PREDIMED	study assessing the efficacy of the Mediterranean diet in the prevention of cardiovascular diseases
PRISMA	preferred reporting items for systematic reviews and meta-analyses
PSUR	periodic safety update report
PV	predicted value
QA	quality assurance
QALY	quality adjusted life years
QC	quality control
QoL	quality of life
QP	qualified person
R&D	research and development
RAE	research assessment exercise
RCT	randomized controlled trial
RE	regional editor
REC	Research Ethics Committee
REF	Research Excellence Framework
RGF	Research Governance Framework
RNA	ribonucleic acid
RR	relative risk
RSI	reference safety information
RSM	Royal Society of Medicine
SaaS	Software as a Service
SAE	serious adverse events
SBA	summary basis of approval
SD	standard deviation
SDV	source data verification
SE	standard error
SE	subject editor
SF 36	short form health survey
SFDA	State Food and Drug Administration (China)
SHSCW	Specialist Health Services Commission for Wales
SI	statutory instrument
SIGN	Scottish Intercollegiate Guidelines Network
SMART	specific, measurable, achievable, realistic and time bound
SMO	Site Management Organization
SmPC	summary of medicinal product characteristics
SOP	standard operating procedures
SPA	special protocol assessments
SPOKE	structure processes outputs knowledge exchange

SPSS	statistical package for the social sciences
SQUIRE	Standards for Quality Improvement Reporting Excellence
STROB	STrengthening the Reporting of OBservational studies in epidemiology
SUSAR	suspected unexpected serious adverse reactions
TCES	Tissue and Cell Engineering Society
TIMI	Thrombolysis in Myocardial Infarction
TLF	tables, listings and figures
TMF	trial master file
TSB	Technology Strategy Board
UKRIO	United Kingdom Research Integrity Office
UKSB	United Kingdom Society for Biomaterials
USB	universal serial bus
USM	urgent safety measures
VPN	virtual private networks
WHI	Women's Health Initiative
WHO	World Health Organization
WI	work instructions
WISDOM	WISDOM Centre for Clinical Governance
WISE	Women in Science, Engineering and Construction
WMA	World Medical Association

Chapter 1

Research: why and how?

The importance of research

What is research?

Research is broadly defined as a systematic investigation with the aim of advancing existing knowledge. It is a process of rigorous reasoning which is based on theories, methods, and findings. It relies on the application of the scientific method and uses inquiries, observations, and experiments to answer questions about the causes of different phenomena. Importantly, scientific research does not give absolute answers but provides probable answers based on the evidence. The main purpose of research is to inform action.

Medical research: overview of recent history

Over the last two centuries medical research has resulted in significant drug discoveries that have improved people's lives, such as penicillin and other antibiotics, vaccines for various infectious diseases, aspirin, beta-blockers, insulin, etc. Furthermore, the explosion of medical technology has led to the introduction of new diagnostic procedures such as X-rays, electrocardiography, defibrillation, medical ultrasonography, magnetic resonance, etc., which substantially improved detection of diseases. The modern era of surgery has made a great impact on human health after the introduction of organ transplantation, open-heart surgery, and joint replacement.

Before the 1950s conclusions about human diseases were made based on the study of anatomy, physiology, and pathology, using case studies or case series as the main method. Statistical techniques were not used in medicine prior to then. Statisticians who made a marked contribution to the application of statistics in medicine include:

- Ronald Fisher—father of modern statistics
- Austin Bradford Hill—wrote a series of articles published in the *Lancet* about the use of statistics in medical research, and a commentary in the *British Medical Journal* in which he proposed statistics as part of the medical curriculum.

The role and importance of research in everyday clinical practice

In their everyday work, healthcare professionals rely on common sense a great deal. However, there are various explanations for observed clinical phenomena and they do not necessarily take into account external factors. There are numerous guidelines that clinicians have to follow in order to deliver the best possible care for the patient. One example is the National Institute for Health and Care Excellence (NICE) guidance which contains recommendations on the most effective way to diagnose, treat, and prevent diseases. The three main areas in which NICE publishes guidelines are health technologies, clinical practice, and health promotion and ill-health avoidance. This guidance is developed according to the best available evidence from the medical literature which is based on the findings of clinical and healthcare research and evaluation of efficacy and cost-effectiveness of different circumstances.

To identify the best research on a specific clinical or healthcare-related question, a systematic literature search has to be conducted. Databases such as MEDLINE, EMBASE, the Cochrane Database of Systematic Reviews, the Database of Abstracts of Reviews of Effects (DARE), and many others contain medical articles. Furthermore, the European Clinical Trials Database (EudraCT) is a database of clinical trials but it does not contain articles. MEDLINE is the most commonly used database. Although there is an overlap in the literature between these databases, each of them contains a predominant type of articles. For example, the Cochrane Database of Systematic Reviews contains systematic reviews and meta-analyses on various clinical topics. In addition, the Cumulative Index to Nursing and Allied Health Literature (CINAHL) covers nursing and allied health. To be able to find articles of interest in these databases, healthcare professionals need to acquire literature search and critical appraisal skills (Chapter 6). This can enable them to judge the quality of the evidence and decide what they are going to apply in a particular clinical situation.

The initiative to perform systematic literature reviews on medical topics has contributed to the development of the concept of evidence-based medicine (EBM, see Chapter 5). EBM assumes applying the best evidence that can be found in the medical literature to the patient with a problem, resulting in the best possible care. The first work on a quality-related systematic review on a topic in medicine was published by Archie Cochrane in the 1970s and focused on therapies in perinatal care. He also advocated the use of EBM in clinical practice and provided a rationale for that in his seminal book, *Effectiveness and Efficiency*. The famous eponymous Cochrane Collaboration conducts systematic reviews of randomized trials with the aim of providing high-quality evidence for healthcare decision making.

Fundamental reasons for doing research

There are several reasons why medical professionals conduct research. The commonly cited reasons are:

- To answer important questions and solve problems
- To serve society
- Intellectual curiosity
- To achieve a qualification
- To aid decision making

Goals of research

There are three main goals of scientific research.

Description

Description starts with observation and aims to define and classify subjects and phenomena and their relationships. By collecting information about a large group of people, a researcher can describe the characteristics of interest and compare them according to selected variables. For example, consider the following clinical research questions. Do people who are physically active on a regular basis have a lower body-fat percentage compared to those who are inactive? Does a particular headache have a different distribution and intensity than migraine? Having collected data, researchers make a systematic and precise description of what they found. A good description provides a basis for prediction. In a description of their observations, researchers use operational definitions which are precise and applicable to specific situations in order to facilitate the collection of standardized data. On the other hand, conceptual (or theoretical) definition pertains to the meaning in terms of the existing theories. For example, obesity is conceptually defined as excess body fat whereas operationally it refers to individuals whose body-mass index is greater than 30 kg/m^2.

Prediction

Predictions are made in the form of hypotheses that are established on existing theories and concepts. They play a major role in scientific research and clinical practice. Predictions provide an answer to the question of whether performing a certain action will affect the outcome of interest that is central in diagnostic reasoning. For example, a patient with a breast lump may have a benign lesion but may also have any form of carcinoma. A clinician uses histological analysis and other diagnostic tools and procedures to confirm the possible diagnosis.

Explanation

Explanation is focused on finding the causes for the observed phenomena and represents the most difficult goal of research. In order to infer a causal relationship, other possible causes have to be systematically eliminated. Since human diseases have multiple determinants, medical researchers often have to rely on theories from various disciplines, ranging from pathophysiology to sociology. A given cause may be necessary, sufficient, neither, or both. To assess whether a relationship between the cause and effect exists, researchers use considerations (often called criteria). The most widely used criteria in medicine are Bradford Hill's criteria of causation (Box 1.1), and they have to be met for an association to be deemed causal. An observed statistically significant correlation between the variables does not mean causal association. Causation as well as the relationship between a clinical question and study design will be presented in detail in Chapter 3.

Box 1.1 Bradford Hill's proposed criteria for causation

- Strength of association
- Consistency—similar findings in different settings
- Specificity in the causes
- Biological plausibility
- Temporality—cause precedes an effect in time
- Dose–response relationship
- Coherence—does not conflict with the current knowledge about the association of interest
- Experimental evidence
- Analogy—a phenomenon from one area can be applied to another area

The scientific method: how do we know something is true or really works?

The scientific method: general considerations

In order for research to be considered scientific, it must be conducted in accordance with the scientific method. This method comprises a group of techniques used for investigating phenomena, acquiring new knowledge, or correcting and integrating previous knowledge. It dates back to Aristotle (384–322 BC) who pioneered empirical research. However, the scientific method in its current form was revised by the philosophers and scientists during the Enlightenment.

Key characteristics of scientific method include:

Open system of thought

Research is unprejudiced and based on an open system of thought. Researchers reject authority as the ultimate basis of truth and rely on empirical evidence which is based on direct or indirect observation. Continual testing, review, and criticism of each others' work is an essential element in the development of scientific research, and represents the most important aspect which distinguishes researchers from practitioners and laypeople.

Objective considerations and logic

Researchers are committed to objectivity and to forming judgements based on facts that are unbiased by personal impressions. A careful logical analysis of the problem is necessary for adherence to the scientific method.

Rigorous and replicable methodology, available to everyone, which can become subject to scrutiny

Researchers use rigorous methods to investigate their questions of interest. The scientific method uses observation and measurement (quantitative or qualitative) to obtain data about the characteristics of interest and to analyse the findings. The methods published in scientific journals are available to other members of the scientific community and can be criticized.

Parsimony

To avoid inconsistency, ambiguity, and redundancy, the scientific method is based on the principle of parsimony which presupposes that the simplest explanation that fits the evidence is the best one; i.e. the best hypothesis is the one with the fewest new assumptions.

Formulation of general conclusions

The process of reasoning in the scientific method involves drawing general conclusions based on individual facts; this is referred to as inductive reasoning. However, the limitations of the conclusions must be acknowledged as well.

Thinking like a scientist: the steps of the scientific method

Obtaining knowledge through science represents a combination of empirical and rational approaches.

- An empirical approach assumes objective observation of events and experiences through the senses. It results in the collection of facts.
- A rational approach presupposes logical reasoning and results in a sound conclusion.

A scientist integrates the two approaches through the process of data collection (from empirical observations) and hypothesis testing (using a rational approach). A hypothesis is defined as a 'supposition arrived at from observation or reflection, that leads to refutable predictions'.

Since conducting clinical and healthcare research involves using the scientific method, it is important to know the steps involved. Although different sources list slightly different steps, they are all very similar.

Observation

The process of scientific research starts with the observation of the phenomenon of interest. It relates to collecting information about the variables we are planning to study. The possibility exists that a new observation will contradict a long-standing theory.

For example, we observed that women aged 30–40 are more physically active than men in the same age group.

Questioning

Formulating an answerable and meaningful research question is critical because everything that follows is performed to answer the research question. The purpose of the research question is to identify the problem in specific terms.

For example, do women spend more time than men at moderate to vigorous physical activity? The variable which is to be measured here is time spent at moderate to vigorous physical activity, expressed in minutes or hours per day.

Hypothesis testing

Formulation of a hypothesis is based on prior knowledge and involves deductive reasoning, i.e. inference from general to specific. Hypothesis testing can result in acceptance or rejection of the hypothesis. It is important to bear in mind that once the hypothesis has been formulated it should not be changed even if the findings are not consistent with expectations. A valid and reliable method has to be used to measure the parameters of interest and a sample size has to be big enough for the study to have statistical power.

Using the physical activity example, the hypothesis would state women and men significantly differ in the amount of time spent at moderate to vigorous physical activity. To test this hypothesis we would have to calculate a required sample size (based on the statistical test and the level of significance) and assess time spent at moderate to vigorous physical activity using an objective method (e.g. a movement sensor). Once the measurements are completed, data have to be collected and analysed.

Conclusion

A conclusion is the final step of the scientific method and represents the summary of the results and whether they support or contradict the hypothesis. Inductive reasoning is used at this stage to generalize the findings if they are generalizable. A conclusion also involves comments about the success and effectiveness of the methods used and directions for the future research.

How do we know that something works?

To answer the question of whether or not something really works, we should consider the strength of evidence. In clinical and healthcare research, we are concerned with the effectiveness of interventions, which could be various modes of treatment (surgery, medications, or other treatment) for certain diseases, or interventions that target behavioural change, e.g. smoking cessation, increasing the level of physical activity, drinking alcohol in moderation, decreasing salt consumption, etc.

A formal evaluation of effectiveness of an intervention is not required if it apparently has an effect on the outcome. For example, no rigorous evaluation would be needed to assess the efficacy of thyroxin substitution in patients with congenital hypothyreosis. However, the majority of clinical and public health interventions are not obvious and need to be evaluated. The study design (Chapter 3) which is considered a gold standard in clinical research is the double-blinded randomized controlled trial (RCT). To be confident in the results of an RCT, its design, conduct, and analysis have to be rigorous and appropriate statistical tests have to be performed. Only then it can be inferred that the observed statistically significant difference in the outcome between the groups is indeed due to the effect of the intervention.

Box 1.2 Summary of the scientific method

Current considerations are summarized here:

- Identify the importance and possible impact of your research
- Identify what has been so far demonstrated by other colleagues
- Define a research question that is meaningful and researchable
- Develop a hypothesis and provide a rationale for it
- Define specific aims which are measurable and focused
- Choose an appropriate research design
- Analyse the data
- Draw conclusions
- Communicate the findings
- Evaluation of communication impact
- Transformation through changing policy and practice

Different types of research

Regulations driving clinical research are described in Chapter 9–11.

Several classifications of clinical and healthcare research are currently being used.

According to the type of data

Quantitative
- Uses the analysis of numerical data
- Involves large number of participants representative of the population of interest
- Aims at using statistics to explain the observations
- Uses various instruments to collect data (questionnaires, monitors, other tools)

Qualitative
- Data are in the form of words, pictures, and objects
- Involves small number of participants
- Aims at providing a complete and detailed description
- Researcher serves as data-gathering instrument

Both the qualitative and the quantitative research methods are governed by the scientific principles.

According to availability of data at the beginning of research

Primary
- Data does not exist at the beginning of the study and a researcher has to collect the data using appropriate methods

Secondary
- Secondary analysis of existing epidemiological data
- Synthesis of existing research
- Main method is a systematic review with or without meta-analysis (a statistical technique used to pool data from independent studies)

According to research setting

Public health
- Considers factors affecting health of a population

Clinical research
- Pertains to the assessment of safety and effectiveness of medications and diagnostic procedures and devices
- It is conducted on humans in four phases, ending with post-marketing surveillance

Pre-clinical research (microbiology, physiology, biochemistry, molecular biology, etc.)
- Research in basic science, precedes clinical trials
- Involves animal experiments, human tissue, or cell lines (the Human Tissue Act is addressed in Chapter 10)

According to study design

Further details of this classification are presented in Chapter 3.

Observational
- Does not involve interventions on the part of the investigator
- Descriptive (examine patterns of diseases and risk factors)

Case reports and case series
- Describe the experience of a single patient or a group of patients with a similar diagnosis
  - Routine data
  - Prevalence surveys
  - Clinical audit (Chapter 7)—uses research methods but does not necessarily constitute the scientific method of research
  - Advantages of descriptive studies: useful for hypothesis formulation
  - Disadvantages of descriptive studies: lack of comparison group, case reports cannot be used to test the presence of a statistical association

Analytic (examines the associations between risk factors and diseases)
- Cross-sectional
  - Exposure and outcome assessed at the same time
  - Prevalence of diseases and risk factors in a population
  - Advantages: relatively quick, easy, and inexpensive, can study multiple exposures and outcomes
  - Disadvantages: temporal sequence and causal association between exposure and outcome cannot be established
  - Examples: Health Survey for England (UK) and National Health and Nutrition Examination Survey (NHANES in the US) are both being conducted as a series of cross-sectional examination
- Case-control
  - Subjects are selected on the basis of having a disease (cases, controls)
  - Groups are compared with respect to the proportion of having a history of exposure
  - Advantages: relatively quick and inexpensive; suitable for the evaluation of the diseases with long latent periods and for rare diseases; can assess multiple risk factors for a single disease
  - Disadvantages: cannot directly calculate the incidence of disease unless the study is population-based; difficult to establish temporal sequence and causal association between exposure and outcome; prone to recall bias; inefficient for rare exposures
  - Example: INTERHEART study (a global case-control study of risk factors for acute myocardial infarction)
- Cohort
  - Can be prospective (disease has not occurred at the beginning of the study) and retrospective (disease has occurred at the time the study is initiated)
  - Subjects are selected on the basis of having the exposure and are followed up over time to assess the outcome
  - Direct measurement of disease incidence

- Advantages: can directly calculate the incidence of disease among exposed and non-exposed; can elucidate temporal relationship between exposure and outcome; bias in exposure assessment is minimized (prospective studies)
- Disadvantages: expensive and time-consuming (especially if prospective); inefficient for rare diseases; requires availability of adequate records (retrospective); losses to follow-up may substantially affect the validity of the results
- Examples: Nurses' Health Study, Health Professionals Follow-up Study, Atherosclerosis Risk in Communities Study (ARIC), European Prospective Investigation into Cancer and Nutrition (EPIC), Whitehall Study, Aerobics Center Longitudinal Study (ACLS)

Experimental
- Involves interventions
- Randomized clinical trials (Chapter 14)
    - Efficacy (explanatory) trials—tests the efficacy of a treatment (or an intervention) among highly selected participants and under controlled conditions
    - Effectiveness (pragmatic) trials—tests the efficacy of a treatment (or an intervention) under real conditions among participants who were not highly selected and provides useful information about the practice
- Are deemed to be the gold standard in clinical research
- Resembles a controlled experiment in the laboratory
- Subjects are enrolled on the basis of their exposure (treatment) status
- Random allocation of the treatment in a sufficiently large sample size
- Provides greater assurance about the validity of the findings than observational studies
- Advantages: provides the most direct epidemiologic evidence on which to judge whether an exposure prevents or causes a disease
- Disadvantages: ethical concerns; costs; feasibility; non-compliance
- Examples: Justification for the Use of Statins in Primary Prevention: An Intervention Trial Evaluating Rosuvastatin (JUPITER), Scandinavian *Simvastatin* Survival Study (4S), Women's Health Initiative (WHI) Clinical Trial of oestrogen plus progestin in post-menopausal women, Thrombolysis in Myocardial Infarction (TIMI) trial, Candesartan in Heart Failure: Assessment of Reduction in Mortality and Morbidity (CHARM), Effects of the Mediterranean Diet on the Primary Prevention of Cardiovascular Diseases (PREDIMED)

The most appropriate research strategy and the design of the study depend on two key factors: research question and available resources which include time, budget, equipment, and staff.

Hierarchy of evidence

Levels of evidence

Several grading systems for evidence are being used in guidelines and recommendations. One of the commonly used systems for grading the evidence is outlined below (from the *Oxford Handbook of Key Clinical Evidence*).

- Ia: systematic review or meta-analysis of RCTs
- Ib: at least one RCT
- IIa: at least one well-designed controlled study without randomization
- IIb: at least one well-designed quasi-experimental study, such as a cohort study
- III: well-designed non-experimental descriptive studies (comparative studies, correlation studies, case-control studies, case series, case reports)
- IV: expert committee reports, opinions formal consensus

Levels of recommendation

The levels of recommendation are based on the strength of evidence.

- A: based on hierarchy I evidence
- B: based on hierarchy II evidence or extrapolated from hierarchy I evidence
- C: based on hierarchy II evidence or extrapolated from hierarchy I or II evidence
- D: directly based on hierarchy IV evidence or extrapolated from hierarchy I, II, or III evidence

These are some examples from the European Society of Cardiology (ESC) guidelines for the pharmacological treatment indicated in patients with symptomatic heart failure (HF):

Level A: An ACE inhibitor is recommended, in addition to a beta-blocker, for all patients with an EF ≤ 40% to reduce the risk of HF hospitalization and the risk of premature death.

Level B: Ivabradine should be considered to reduce the risk of HF hospitalization in patients in sinus rhythm with an EF ≤ 35%, a heart rate remaining ≥ 70 bpm, and persisting symptoms despite treatment with an evidence-based dose of beta-blocker (or maximum tolerated dose below that), ACE inhibitor (or angiotensin receptor blocker), and a mineralocorticoid receptor antagonist (or angiotensin receptor blocker).

Level C: In terms of the treatment of hypertension in patients with symptomatic HF, a thiazide diuretic (or if the patient is treated with a thiazide diuretic, switching to a loop diuretic) is recommended when hypertension persists despite treatment with a combination of as many as possible of an ACE inhibitor (or angiotensin receptor blocker), beta-blocker, and mineralocorticoid receptor antagonist.

Final remarks

Research, management, education, and services constitute the four pillars of healthcare whereby research plays a pivotal role (Box 1.2 and Figure 1.1).
- Research is critical in order to develop, maintain, and improve services
- Research requires good management, and management approaches need to be founded through research
- Research skills require good education and teaching, which in turn can be evaluated using research methods
- We suggest the Be-'SPOKE' approach to conducting research relevant to clinical/healthcare practices is a problem-solving approach to research led by a clinical/healthcare driven hypothesis (Box 1.3)

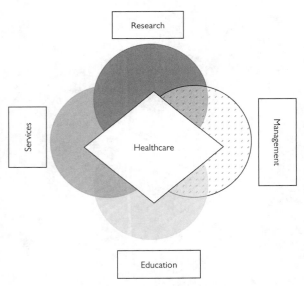

Figure 1.1 The pivotal role of research in clinical/healthcare practice.

Box 1.3 The Be-'SPOKE' approach to conducting research relevant to clinical/healthcare practices

Structures—Institutions
Processes—Governance
Outputs—Outcomes
Knowledge
Exchange } Translation for healthcare benefit

Further reading

Bradford Hill A. Statistics in medical curriculum? *BMJ* 1947;11:366.

Cochrane AL. *Effectiveness and Efficiency. Random Reflections on Health Services.* London: Royal Society of Medicine, 1971.

Harrison J, Kulkarni K, Baguneid M, et al. *Oxford Handbook of Key Clinical Evidence.* Oxford: Oxford University Press, 2009.

Hill AB. The environment and disease: association or causation? *Proc R Soc Med* 1965;58:295–300.

Jackson SL. *Research Methods, a Modular Approach.* Belmont: Thomson Wadsworth, 2008.

Porta M. *A Dictionary of Epidemiology.* 5th edn. Oxford: Oxford University Press, 2008.

Sackett DL, Rosenberg WM, Gray JA, et al. Evidence based medicine: what it is and what it isn't. *BMJ* 1996; 312(7023):71–2.

Ward H, Toledano MB. *Oxford Handbook of Epidemiology for Clinicians.* Oxford: Oxford University Press, 2012.

National Institute for Clinical Excellence. Guideline Development Methods: Reviewing and grading the evidence (updated 2012), available at: https://www.nice.org.uk/article/pmg6/chapter/6-Reviewing-the-evidence

European Clinical Trials Database (EudraCT), available at: https://eudract.ema.europa.eu/

Encyclopaedia Britannica, Aristotle, Philosophy of Science, available at: www.britannica.com/EBchecked/topic/34560/Aristotle/254718/The-unmoved-mover

Navigating research methods: basic concepts in biostatistics and epidemiology

Basic concepts in biostatistics

> **N.B.** Epidemiology and biostatistics are essential tools in clinical research
> (see the *Oxford Handbook of Medical Statistics* and the *Oxford Handbook
> of Epidemiology for Clinicians*). An understanding of the basic concepts
> in both disciplines as well as advantages and limitations of the methods
> applied are important both for investigators conducting clinical research
> and for clinicians interpreting clinical research reports.

Statistics is the branch of applied mathematics concerned with the collection and interpretation of quantitative data, the use of probability theory
to estimate population parameters, and the art of dealing with variation of
data in order to obtain reliable results and conclusions. **Biostatistics**, also
called medical statistics, is the application of statistics to the field of biological sciences, health, medicine, and medical practice.

Concepts and methods of biostatistics are used to **summarize** and **analyse data** from epidemiological research. Study data are expressed through
either **numerical or categorical** variables (Figure 2.1).

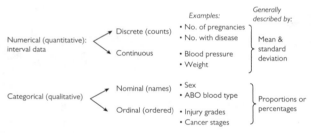

Figure 2.1 Types of clinical data.

Descriptive statistical methods

These are used to perform exploratory analysis and obtain informative
summaries of the data from a study. Descriptive statistics describe large
amounts of data in a manageable and/or sensible way by reducing lots of
data into simpler summaries. They form the basis of virtually every quantitative analysis of data. Techniques used for descriptive analysis include
organization and summarization of data into **summary measures, graphs,
and tables**. Three main characteristics of a single variable explored (uni-
variate analysis) in descriptive analysis include the **distribution**, the **central
tendency**, and the **dispersion** (spread, variability).

The frequency distribution

This is a summary of the frequency of individual values or ranges of values
for a variable, i.e. it shows numbers of times each possible outcome occurs
in the sample. For example, we describe sex distribution by listing the number or percentage of males and females. However, we cannot specify all

possible outcomes of continuous data as they are too numerous to list. A more sensible option for continuous variables is to group values into ranges and then determine frequencies thereafter.

Distribution shapes

In terms of distribution shapes, data can be characterized as having the normal (Gaussian) distribution, skewed distributions, and bimodal (with two peaks) distributions.

Why are they important? The information on distribution shapes may be relevant to the further statistical procedures we want to use. For example, many popular significance tests such as t-test and analysis of variance (ANOVA) are 'parametric' tests which require the data to have certain properties, including 'normality of distribution of the population'.

Normal distribution

In general, this is most applicable to continuous data. Graphically, normal distribution is described by a 'bell-shaped' curve. In a normal distribution, data are most likely to be at the mean. It can be fully described by two parameters such as the **mean** and the **standard deviation** (SD), and it has useful characteristics. For example, it is possible to obtain probability of any value by knowing how many SDs the value is away from the mean. Thus, it is useful to know that about 68% of the values under a normal distribution curve fall within one SD of the mean, about 95% fall within two SDs of the mean, and 99.7% of the distribution lies within three SDs of the mean (Figure 2.2). Total probability (area under the curve) = 1.

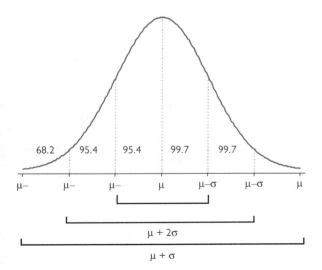

Figure 2.2 Normal distribution curve.

Examples of natural phenomena with normal distribution include height and blood pressure. However, normally we don't know the distribution shapes of the populations and we assess them from the samples. The simplest method of assessing normality is to look at the distribution shape using frequency distribution histogram. Visual appraisals must be followed by better methods such as tests for normality (e.g. the Kolmogorov–Smirnov test, or the Shapiro–Wilk and Anderson–Darling tests) and homogeneity of variance. Please refer to the *Oxford Handbook of Medical Statistics* for details of these tests.

Summary measures

These include measures of central tendency (they aim to characterize the centre of a sample measurements) such as median, mean, mode, and measures of variability such as range, interquartile range, standard deviation, and variance. The most useful measures of variability are variance and standard deviation (Box 2.1).

Box 2.1 Definitions of summary measures

Measures of central tendency

Mean is the sample average = sum of the values divided by the number in the sample.

Median is the middle observation after putting the data values in order (50th percentile).

Unlike mean, median is not affected by outliers.

Mode is the most frequent value in the sample.

Measures of dispersion

Variance is a measure of the dispersion of data points around their mean value = the average of the **squared** differences from the mean.

Standard deviation (SD) is the **square root** of the **variance**.

Good-quality graphs and tables

These are effective means of communicating data, and need to contain enough information to be easily and quickly understood without reference to the text. Compared to tables, graphs are more effective tools for simple, visual representation of the data and for displaying complex relationships. Tables are particularly good for displaying complex data with precision and are easier to prepare.

In summary, descriptive statistics are applied **to describe** main features of the data, to show the emerging patterns, and to summarize data in a meaningful way. Descriptive statistics do not allow us to draw conclusions beyond the data we have analysed or reach conclusions regarding any hypotheses we might have made.

However, in epidemiological research, a sample is often selected to be able to make inferences about the population from which the sample was drawn, which means that although *the analysis is based on the sample, the real focus is on what happens in the respective population.*

Inferential statistics

Inferential statistics is applied **to make inferences about a population from the sample data**, a process that is an essential aspect of epidemiological research. Inferential statistics as a method is also used to assess the strength of the evidence, to make comparisons and predictions, and to ask more questions and suggest future research.

The inferences are made based on the results of **estimation of parameter(s)** and **hypothesis testing**.

The measurements of the sample are called **statistics**, the measurements of the population are called **parameters** (represented by Greek letters), and we want to move from the sample statistics (e.g. mean ($\bar{x}$) and standard deviation (s)) to the population parameters (e.g. mean (μ) and standard deviation (σ); ($\bar{x}$ is a random variable, μ is constant)) (Box 2.2).

Box 2.2 Common terms in statistics

Population parameters are population-level properties/attributes of characteristic(s) of interest. Examples of parameters include averages, proportions, percentiles, and correlation coefficients.

The corresponding sample properties/attributes of characteristics are called **sample statistics**. Sample statistics approximate the corresponding population parameters but **are not equal** to them.

Statistical inference deals with the uncertainty issues which arise in approximating parameters by statistics.

Some sample statistics (mean, SD, shape of distribution) are good predictors of their corresponding population parameter, whereas others (mode, median) are not able to predict their population parameter. Instead of predicting a single value we predict a range of values (confidence intervals) in which the population mean is likely to be found. The appropriate range capturing a population mean depends on the shape of the distribution (e.g. a bimodal distribution is likely to need a larger range than a normal distribution).

Sampling

There are numerous sampling strategies used to select a sample from a given population. By selecting a random sample, each member of the population gets an equal chance of being selected for the sample, hence **random (or probability) sampling** removes selection bias, and provides known probability of being chosen needed for statistical estimations. There are four basic types of random sampling methods: simple random sampling, systematic sampling, stratified sampling (proportionate and disproportionate), cluster or multistage sampling.

Non-probability sampling

Procedures are less desirable as they are very prone to sampling biases, cannot measure how representative the sample is, and cannot calculate sampling error. However, they might be unavoidable in some circumstances. The examples of non-probability (non-random) sampling include voluntary response, judgement, snowball, convenience, quota, and purposive sampling (see the *Oxford Handbook of Medical Statistics*).

Sampling distribution

We can draw multiple samples from the same population and different samples are most likely to provide different means due to **sampling variation**. If we took many independent samples of the same size from a given population and computed a mean for each sample, then we will end up with many different means. The frequency distribution of all these means is called a **sampling distribution**. If we did that with a very large number of samples, the sampling distribution of the means would look like **normal distribution** (even if the distribution in the population is not normal) if the samples are large enough.

The variability of a sampling distribution is measured by its variance or SD. The SD of the sampling distribution is called the **standard error (SE) of the sample mean**, and it can be used to measure how precisely the population mean is estimated by the sample mean (Box 2.3).

> ## Box 2.3 Difference between standard deviation and standard error
> The **standard deviation of the population** (σ) measures the amount of variability in the population.
>
> The **standard deviation of the sample (s)** measures the amount of variability in the specific sample.
>
> **Standard error (SE)** measures the likely deviation of the sample mean from the population mean.

The mean of the sampling distribution will approximate the **population mean**. The smaller the SE, the more likely it is that sample mean is close to the population mean. For a sample of sample size n, SE can be estimated as the SD of the sample divided by the square root of the sample size (n).

The sampling distribution of the mean is a very important distribution. The uncertainty of the inferences (about the characteristics of a population based on the information from a representative sample) is based on the sampling distribution of the statistic. Sampling distribution is used to construct the confidence interval (CI) for the mean and for significance testing.

Confidence intervals

Confidence intervals are one of the valuable estimation tools in epidemiologic research showing the amount of SE in a study (narrow CI indicates little random error, i.e. 'good precision'). CI tells us that if the same population is sampled on numerous occasions using the same sampling method and interval estimates are computed for each sample, some of the resulting intervals would include the true population parameter and some would not. A 95% CI is the most commonly used CI and is a range of values from estimate (e.g. mean): −1.96SE to estimate +1.96SE. It is usually interpreted as a range of values that contains the true population parameter with probability 0.95. In other words, we expect that the 95% CI will include the true population value 95% of the time. Unfortunately, we do not know whether the CI obtained from a specific sample is one of the 95% or one of the 5%.

Significance tests

Significance tests are used **to test hypotheses**. In general, hypothesis is defined as 'a supposition or proposed explanation made on the basis of limited evidence as a starting point for further investigation' (Concise Oxford Dictionary definition). A statistical hypothesis is basically an assumption about a population parameter which may or may not be true (the best way to determine the truthfulness of the statistical hypothesis would be to examine the entire population, which is often not feasible).

Significance (or hypothesis) testing is a method for testing a hypothesis about a population parameter or a relationship between two variables using sample data. We begin by formulating the relevant null (often denoted H_0 (read 'H-nought')) and alternative (denoted H_1) hypotheses. The null hypothesis is a starting point, a statement being tested, which may be about the hypothesized value of the population parameter (e.g. the population mean), or that the effect of interest is zero (e.g. when comparing groups of subjects, or treatments). The alternative hypothesis is a statement that contradicts the null hypothesis (e.g. by stating that the population parameter is not equal to the value stated in the null hypothesis, or that the effect of interest is not zero).

We then use appropriate statistical tests to calculate the relevant **test statistic** (such as a t-statistic or a Chi-square statistic) in order to evaluate the **probability of obtaining the observed data (or more extreme data) if the null hypothesis were true**. This probability is usually called the **P value** (Box 2.4), which can be compared with the pre-specified significance level (denoted by α), and can help decide **whether or not the study results are likely to be due to chance alone (random sampling error)**. *By convention*, the α level of significance is often set at 0.05, which means that we consider the results to be statistically significant (i.e. unlikely to be due to chance) if the probability that the observed result could be due to chance is less than 5% ($p < 0.05$).

Two types of errors can result from a hypothesis test: type I error, when a null hypothesis is rejected when it is true, and type II error, when the alternative hypothesis is rejected (i.e. a study fails to reject the null hypothesis) when the alternative hypothesis is true (Table 2.1). The probability of committing a type I error is called the significance level or alpha, and is denoted by α. The probability of committing a type II error is called beta, and is often denoted by β. The probability of *not* committing a type II error—in other words, rejecting the null hypothesis when it should be—is called the power of the test (= $1-\beta$). The higher the power the better, if costs are feasible. The power can be increased by increasing the sample size, reducing the variance of the individual observations, increasing significance level α (e.g. from 0.01 to 0.05).

The choice of appropriate statistical test depends on type of data being analysed (continuous, nominal, etc.), the type of study design (whether the groups (if more than one) are independent or paired/matched), the distribution of the data (normally distributed or not), whether the data is continuous, and the number of groups.

Box 2.4 P value

Used to measure the strength of evidence in support of a null hypothesis. The P value is the probability of observing data as or more extreme than what we observed, **assuming the null hypothesis is true.**

If the P value is less than the significance level, we reject the null hypothesis.

Caution

- Interpretation of P value as probability that the null hypothesis is correct is wrong as the **probability of data given $H_0 \neq$ probability of H_0 given data**
- Statistical significance $\neq$ clinical significance (e.g. a result can be statistically significant but the observed effect not clinically appreciable due to its small size)
- P value is highly dependent on sample size
- P value < 0.05 does not prove H_0 is wrong, just unlikely
- Multiple tests can lead to 'significant' difference by chance alone (e.g. 20 tests on the same sample can yield one 'significant' difference by chance at the 5% level)
- There is a close link between two-sided P value and CI, as both are based on similar aspects of the theoretical distribution of the test statistic. However, CI is **more informative and preferable to P value** as it provides information not only on statistical significance of findings, but also precision of the estimate of interest. It provides an insight into the range of plausible low and high values, and is presented in the units of the variable of interest, which is helpful when interpreting the results

Conventional interpretation of P values

p > 0.10	result is not significant
0.05 < p < 0.10	result is marginally significant
0.01 < p < 0.05	result is significant
p < 0.01	result is highly significant

Table 2.1 Hypothesis testing

The result	The truth	
	H_0 is correct	H_a is correct
Accept H_0	Correct	Type II or β-error
Reject H_0	Type I or α-error	Correct $(1 - \beta)$

Table 2.2 Statistical tests

Type of data	One sample	Comparing groups		
		Number of groups	Independent groups	Paired/matched samples
Continuous and normal	Z-test. One-sample t-test	2	Student test	Paired t-test
		≥ 3	Analysis of variance (ANOVA)	Repeated measures ANOVA
Continuous and non-normal or ordinal	Kolmogorov–Smirnov test, sign test	2	Mann–Whitney U test, Median test	Sign test, Wilcoxon signed ranks test
		≥ 3	Kruskal–Wallis test, Median test, Jonckheere–Terpstra test	Friedman test, Quade test
Nominal	Z-test, Chi-square test	2	Chi-square test (2 × k), Fisher's exact test	McNemar's test
		≥ 3	Chi-square test (r × k), Fisher–Freeman–Halton	Cochran Q-test

Table 2.2 presents examples of tests used for statistical significance. Please refer to the *Oxford Handbook of Medical Statistics* for more comprehensive explanations of these statistical tests and further details of parametric and non-parametric tests.

Describing the relationship between two quantitative variables

Two statistical techniques are used: **correlation analysis** and **regression analysis**.

Correlation analysis is used to measure the strength of the association between two variables. This can be done by calculating the **correlation coefficient** (also just called the correlation). There are several types of correlation coefficients, and the choice of a suitable measure depends on variable types and the distribution of the two variables (if continuous). For example, **Pearson product–moment** correlation coefficient (the most widely used correlation tool) is used to measure the degree of the linear association between two random continuous and normally distributed variables. It can range between −1 and +1. The closer the values are to 1, the stronger is the linear association (−1 is a perfect negative linear correlation, 0 is no linear correlation, +1 is a perfect positive linear correlation). However, there could be nonlinear relationship between the variables.

When the two variables are continuous and non-normally distributed or ordinal, **Spearman's rank** correlation coefficient is preferred, which is calculated on ranks (not raw data), and tests for general association between two variables (not specifically linear relationship). Other types of correlation include **point bi-serial** correlation (a special case of the Pearson product-moment correlation used when one variable is continuous normal and one is dichotomous); **phi coefficient** (when both variables are dichotomous), **contingency coefficient** (for nominal variables).

When two variables are highly correlated, then one variable can be used to predict the other variable, and that's what the regression analysis is for. Hence, regression analysis is a statistical method used to predict or estimate the value of one variable (termed 'dependent variable', 'outcome', 'response', or 'regressand') given the value of one or multiple variables (called 'independent variable', 'predictor', 'explanatory variable', 'covariate', or 'regressor'). The relationship is expressed in the form of a regression equation: the model. We aim to produce better models to be able to generate more accurate predictions by adding more predictor variables and/or developing better predictor variables. Regression models with more than one predictor variable are called **multiple regression** models, whereas those with one predictor are called **simple regression** models. **Regression coefficients** represent **measures of association**; to interpret them as **measures of effect**, the modelled regression function should provide approximately unconfounded representation of the effects of interest. Regression models are used extensively in epidemiological research, in particular, **linear**, **logistic** and **Cox proportional hazards** regression. While the regressand and the regressor may be measured on any scale, the choice of a regression model depends on the nature of the regressand (Table 2.3).

Table 2.3 Types of generalized linear regression models

Model	Response	Distribution	Regression coefficient interpretation
Linear	Continuous	Normal (Gaussian)	Change in average response (Y) per unit change in predictor (X)
Logistic	Dichotomous	Binomial	Log odds ratio
Cox proportional hazards	Time (from a specified baseline) to the occurrence of an event of interest	Semi-parametric	Log relative hazard

Caution
- Correlation or association does not imply causation
- The magnitude of correlation depends on, for example, sampling (is it random and representative?), measurement of the variables (are they reliable, valid?)
- The correlation coefficient is a sample statistic, like a mean, and may not be representative of all individuals
- Correlation and regression analyses have distinct purposes

In summary, inferential statistics is concerned with making inferences or predictions about a population from observations and analyses of a representative sample. Correlation is used to quantify the strength of the relationship between two variables (tests for interdependence), whereas regression is used to estimate the value of one variable from other variable(s). To generalize results from a study to the source population, tests for statistical significance are applied which estimate the probability of obtained results being due only to random chance.

When analysing data, the correct statistical method should be used. Statistical methods rely on assumptions and it is important to check these.

Basic concepts in epidemiology

Introduction

Epidemiology is defined as 'the study of the distribution and determinants of *health-related states or events* in specified populations, and the *application of this study to the control of health problems*'. **Clinical epidemiology** is one of the sub-disciplines of epidemiology, first introduced in 1938 by John Paul as a 'new basic science for preventive medicine, concerned with circumstances … under which human disease is prone to develop'. Since the 1960s the focus of clinical epidemiology shifted from population health toward individual patient. In 1967 David Sackett defined clinical epidemiology as 'the application, by a physician who provides direct patient care, of epidemiologic and biostatistical methods to the study of diagnostic and therapeutic processes in order to effect an improvement in health'. In 1968 Alvan Feinstein defined clinical epidemiology and its 'territory' as 'the clinic-ostatistical study of diseased populations…'.

In summary, although the core methods and techniques are common for all sub-disciplines of epidemiology, the fundamental difference is that unlike other branches of epidemiology that aim to improve health of populations, clinical epidemiology aims to enhance, guide, aid, and inform clinical decision making, integrating **the best available evidence** in order to improve health of **individual patients**.

Given the rapidly growing body of research evidence available nowadays, identifying strong, **valid** (close to the truth), clinically **useful** (applicable) evidence to aid clinical decision making becomes highly important. The term **evidence-based medicine** is often used to stand for the translation of the results of clinical epidemiology into clinical practice, emphasizing patient-centred outcomes assessment and levels of evidence.

In clinical epidemiology, the study is normally conducted in a clinical setting using a **defined patient population**. The field of clinical epidemiology focuses on measurement of clinical phenomena. More specifically it accents the following areas: *abnormality, diagnosis, disease frequency, risk, prognosis, treatment/clinical care, prevention, cause*. This chapter presents a brief overview of areas that are central concerns of clinical epidemiology.

Definitions of normality and abnormality

'[T]he medical meaning of "normal" has been lost in the shuffle of statistics'.

Alvan Feinstein, 1977

Defining and distinguishing 'normal' from 'abnormal' is the first priority in any clinical consultation as whether or not any further investigation or treatment is needed depends on whether the patient's symptoms, signs, or diagnostic test results are normal or abnormal (Box 2.5). However, the classification is often difficult, crude, and subject to misclassification, particularly:
• in patients with 'subtle manifestations' of disease;
• due to the fact that most clinical variables are not dichotomous, i.e. do not break into normal and abnormal results but rather have a continuum of values reflecting smooth transition from low to high values with increasing levels of 'abnormality' (e.g. where do 'abnormal' values of blood pressure (interval data) begin or when should a large

Box 2.5 Disadvantages of statistical definition of normality

- There is no biological rationale for using threshold values to define abnormality for many variables and the risk of disease can be increased even within the 'statistically normal' range of values. For example, there is a continuous association between blood pressure and coronary heart disease.
- The relationship between the statistical definition of what is 'unusual', 'uncommon', and clinical disease is not straightforward. For example, for some measurements only highly extreme values, well beyond 95th percentile, are associated with symptomatic disease. Kidney failure is an example.
- For some measurements, extreme values are beneficial rather than abnormal. For example, high bone density lowers risk of fractures.

liver or a large prostate be considered abnormally large (ordinal data)). (*Probability of misclassification is very low for nominal data such as blood type, death, surgery*);
- because frequency distributions for 'normal' and 'abnormal' almost always overlap even when frequency distributions are different for people with and without disease.

How is 'abnormal' distinguished? The following criteria have been successfully used to define abnormal clinical findings: being **unusual (not common)**, **associated with disease, treatable**.

The first criterion classifies frequently occurring values as normal and those occurring infrequently as abnormal. This is a statistical definition with an arbitrary cut-off point to distinguish normal and abnormal values, which classifies all values beyond two standard deviations from the mean as abnormal. Assuming the observations under consideration approximate a normal (in the statistical sense) distribution, we would define 2.5% of observations in each tail of the distribution as abnormally low or high. However, most biologic measurements are not normally distributed, and therefore an approach which does not assume a statistically normal distribution is preferable and that is by using a fraction (percentile) of the actual distribution. For example, we can classify 5% of observations as abnormal using the 95th percentile point as the cut-off line between normal and abnormally high values.

The second approach, based on defining as abnormal observations that are associated with the risk of developing or having a disease, seems more logical. For example, increasing risk of mortality has been observed at a BMI of 29 (Box 2.6).

The third criterion used to distinguish between normal and abnormal is determined by evidence from randomized controlled trials (RCT), designed to detect the point at which treatment is beneficial. It should be noted that the definition of treatable levels or what is worth treating may change over time (blood pressure is an example), based on new evidence. According to this criterion, a measurement can be evaluated as abnormal if treatment at that level is associated with an improved outcome.

Box 2.6 **Abnormal as associated with disease: points to consider**

- The threshold distinguishing normal from abnormal can vary by disease, e.g. BMI in mortality vs cardiovascular disease.
- Distribution of clinical variables can change with age, sex, race, nutrition; and definition of normal/abnormal can vary by these variables. For example, the 'normal' range for creatinine in the blood has been defined as approximately 0.6–1.2 milligrams (mg) per decilitre (dl) in adult males and 0.5–1.1 mg per dl in adult females.
- Identifying a threshold value that neatly separates cases and non-cases is not easy, due to an overlap between distributions of clinical measurements for healthy and diseased people, which leads to two types of misclassification expressed in terms of sensitivity and specificity of a test.

Diagnosis and diagnostic tests/criteria

Doctors use various **diagnostic tests** (such as clinical information from patient's history, physical examination, imaging procedures, laboratory investigations (biochemical, genetic, microbiological, or physiological), or a constellation of different clinical findings) in order to diagnose any treatable disease.

So, what are the basic principles used to interpret diagnostic tests? The relationship between a test's result and true diagnosis yields four possible combinations of disease status and test result, as summarized in **Table 2.4**. In two of these combinations, the test results are correct (**true positive** and **true negative**), and in the other two situations results are wrong (**false positive** and **false negative**). To be able to identify these categories, we need an absolutely **accurate** method, often referred to as **gold standard**, or **criterion standard**, or **reference standard** of determining disease status, against which we can determine the accuracy of other tests. The gold standard can be a relatively simple test (e.g. an antibody test for HIV infection), or expensive and risky (e.g. biopsy). Sometimes follow-up time can be used as a gold standard; that is, to allow disease to reveal itself (screening for most cancers is an example).

However, the gold standard is not always feasible to use either because it is likely to be expensive or invasive, therefore simpler and cheaper tests are often used in routine clinical practice as proxies. Nevertheless, the use of simpler methods is justified when their validity and precision are known and the probability of misclassification is low.

Table 2.4 Relationship between true diagnosis and a diagnostic test

Test result	Disease present	Disease absent
Positive	True positive	False positive
Negative	False negative	True negative

The practical utility of a given test depends on its performance measures such as **sensitivity** and **specificity** which are used while deciding whether or not to use the test. An alternative approach to describe test performance is **likelihood ratio (LR)**. However, clinicians are more interested in a test's positive and negative predictive values as they answer the clinically important question, 'given the test result, what is the probability that a patient has (does not have) the disease?'

The predictive value (PV) depends on the sensitivity and specificity of the test and, most importantly, on the prevalence of the disease in the population being tested. Thus, when the prevalence is low, positive PV drops even with a high sensitivity and high specificity. The impact of prevalence on PV is more profound when sensitivity and specificity are low. Given the relationship between PV of a test and prevalence, it is better to apply diagnostic tests to patients with an increased probability of having the disease under question (Box 2.7).

Box 2.7 Relationship between sensitivity, specificity, and predictive value

$$\text{Positive predictive value} = \frac{\text{Sensitivity} \times \text{Prevalence}}{(\text{Sensitivity} \times \text{Prevalence}) + (1 - \text{Specificity}) \times (1 - \text{Prevalence})}$$

Derived from Bayes theorem of conditional probabilities.

Although tests that are both highly sensitive and specific are the desired ones, in practice, due to the trade-off between the two, clinicians often work with tests that are not both highly sensitive and specific. For this reason, clinicians often use a combination of multiple tests including patient's disease history, physical examination, and laboratory tests. These test combinations are called **clinical prediction** or **diagnostic decision-making rules** (sensitivity, specificity, and LRs are estimated for these rules as well) (Boxes 2.8 and 2.9).

Prognosis

> 'The physician who cannot inform his patient what would be the probable issue of his complaint, if allowed to follow its natural course, is not qualified to prescribe any rational treatment for its cure.'
>
> Hippocrates

Prognosis is the prediction of the probable clinical course and outcome of a disease. Disease consequences (i.e. outcomes in prognostic research) of interest may include recovery or disease recurrence, discomfort, disability, health-related quality of life, complications, death, etc. In general, important clinical outcomes can be summarized using the five Ds: death, disease, discomfort, disability, and dissatisfaction. A measurable patient characteristic, a condition, or a situation associated with the subsequent outcome of a disease is called a **prognostic factor**. Variables that are associated with an increased risk of the disease onset (**risk factors**) can be either similar or different from those related to worse prognosis (**prognostic factors**).

Box 2.8 Definitions used for diagnostic tests

Sensitivity

This is the probability of a positive test in the presence of disease. A very sensitive test is most helpful to the clinician when the test result is negative (i.e. to rule out a diagnosis).

Specificity

This is the probability of a negative test in the absence of disease. Highly specific tests are particularly useful when the test result is positive (i.e. to rule in a diagnosis).

N.B. there is a trade-off between sensitivity and specificity of a test: increasing one reduces the other.

Positive predictive value

This is the probability of disease when the test result is positive, e.g. BNP has high positive predictive value for heart failure.

Negative predictive value

This is the probability of not having the disease when the test result is negative, e.g. D-dimers have high negative predictive value for pulmonary embolism.

Likelihood ratios

These express how many times more (or less) likely a test result is to be found in diseased compared with non-diseased people.

Box 2.9 Issues related to evaluating diagnostic tests performance

- We need information on all four cells in the Table 2.4 to evaluate accuracy of the test. However, quite often the information on negative tests is not sufficient as people with negative results do not undergo further testing.
- The information on test performance can be misleading:
  - if test has been applied only to patients with the condition under question, i.e. we get no information on how the test would behave in the non-diseased
  - if a test's properties were estimated in a sample of patients different from those to whom it will be applied in clinical practice
- Specificity and sensitivity may not be accurately assessed:
  - if an improper gold standard has been used
  - if estimates were derived from studying a relatively small sample of patients.

For example, age is associated with both increased risk of experiencing acute myocardial infarction (AMI) and poor survival after it. Whereas, high blood pressure is a known risk factor for an AMI but a positive prognostic sign when present during the acute event. Clinical prediction rules, mentioned in this chapter, are also used to estimate the likely prognosis.

Sound knowledge of probable prognosis can help to determine the right treatment. The question is how information on prognosis is obtained, how it can be described, what biases can affect the description, and how to control them.

Given that clinical experience is often based on a set of patients that may not be representative of all patients with a particular disease and may not have adequate follow-up, properly designed epidemiological research is necessary to obtain reliable information on prognosis. Ideally, studies of prognosis should include all patients with the disease under study in a defined geographic region (feasible where national electronic medical records are available), or include an adequate description of study population, the setting, and the sampling methodology. The cohort of patients with the disease under study is followed forward in time (long enough to observe the end points of interest (can vary by disease)). Clinical outcomes are measured thereafter and prognostic factors are identified. 'Zero time', a specified time point in the course of disease (e.g. time of diagnosis), should be clearly defined and be the same for all patients in the study. Alternatively, prognosis can be studied using case-control design. However, outcome rates cannot be obtained from such studies.

Prognosis can be described as a **clinical course** (i.e. as evolution of a disease under direct medical treatment) or the **natural history** of disease (i.e. evolution of a disease without medical intervention). Often prognosis is expressed in terms of **rate** (i.e. proportion of people with an event of interest in a given time period). Commonly rates to describe prognosis include five-year survival, case fatality, disease-specific mortality, treatment response, remission, recurrence. However, despite convenience and simplicity of summarizing prognosis by a single rate, rates are not very informative in the sense that they do not reflect the clinical course of the disease. For example, different conditions with similar summary rates can in fact have very different clinical courses.

It is preferable to use **survival analysis** (also called **time-to-event analysis**) to describe prognosis in the cohort over time, which unlike summary rates mentioned in this chapter estimates the average likelihood of an outcome under question at any point in time. Survival analyses may include selected groups, for example, patients who survive the first day after AMI. **Kaplan–Meier analysis** is often used. While interpreting survival curves, several points must be considered. The precision of the estimates (points on the survival curve) depends on the number of patients on whom the estimate is based. For example, survival estimates toward the end of the follow-up may not be precise and may be affected by what happens to the remaining patients. In addition, the shape of the curve may create an impression that the event rate is higher at the beginning of follow-up than later on, when the slope flattens, although the slope can flatten due to the diminishing number of patients even if the event rate is relatively constant over time.

Studies aiming to identify prognostic factors compare prognosis in patients with different characteristics. Several survival curves are then displayed (according to these characteristics), and the effects of these factors, relative to one another, are summarized by a **hazard ratio**.

In the follow-up of cohorts to determine prognosis, initial selection strategy and incomplete follow-up are main sources of bias. Outcome ascertainment bias is possible for less clear-cut outcomes.

Treatment

Treatment is an intervention intended to improve the course of diagnosed disease. It may take any form, including counselling, drug prescriptions, surgery, etc., and might be applied at any point in the natural history of disease. The understanding of what treatment is useful for a particular condition is shaped over time based on information from various activities in medicine including case reports, knowledge of underlying biological mechanisms, epidemiologic studies of populations, clinical observations, folk medicine (herbal remedies), etc. Unlike some treatments, when effects are obvious without formal assessment (e.g. antibiotics for pneumonia), most interventions, especially those indicated for chronic diseases, require clinical research to establish their value.

Observational and experimental studies are the main methods used to evaluate the effects of treatments and the two differ with respect to feasibility and scientific strength. Observational studies of treatment are 'a type of prognosis studies, where treatment is the prognostic factor of interest'. The main advantage of observational studies is their feasibility. The main disadvantage is the possibility of misleading, biased conclusions due to systematic differences between treatment groups, other than the treatment itself.

Experimental studies are a type of cohort study where the conditions of the study are highly controlled and managed by investigators. The randomized, double-blind, controlled clinical trial is the gold standard of medical research where the key feature is **random assignment of treatment** (*not by physician or patient choice*), and whereby the experimental group receives the treatment under investigation, and the control group may receive placebo, or usual care or the current 'best available' treatment.

Clinical trials can be classified into **efficacy** and **effectiveness** trials. Efficacy trials show whether treatment can work under 'ideal' conditions such as patients' compliance to treatment, the best possible care, and the absence of 'extraneous effects' from other diseases. Effectiveness trials are designed to show whether treatment can work in ordinary clinical practice. These include circumstances when some patients will be non-compliant to assigned treatment, will change the treatment, and will drop out of the study (analysis is according to treatment assigned, called 'intention to treat').

Treatment effects are summarized using measures like relative risk reduction, absolute risk reduction, and number needed to treat.

Since these trials are conducted using highly selected groups of patients to increase homogeneity in order to strengthen internal validity, the main limitation of randomized controlled trials (RCT) is reduced generalizability (external validity); in other words, it may be difficult to generalize the results of clinical trials to ordinary clinical practice. To overcome this limitation, **large, simple trials** are conducted, whereby the inclusion criteria are less restricted and most patients with the condition of interest are eligible. The patients are **randomly allocated** to treatment groups, but their care is the same as usual otherwise, and the outcome of interest is usually death.

Treatment that has been shown to be effective on average may not be effective for an individual patient. Therefore, although the evidence from valid, rigorous clinical research provides the rationale for initiating a particular treatment, whether or not the treatment works in a patient is a better reason to continue or stop the treatment.

Guidance from clinical trials is not available for many medical interventions. The growing number of well-designed trials makes development of **evidence-based guidelines** possible (e.g. the National Institute for Health and Care Excellence (NICE) develops and provides clinical guidelines on the appropriate treatment of specific diseases (♒ www.nice.org.uk/#panel1) to the National Health Service of the UK).

Alternatives to randomized trials include comparisons of experimental and control patients across time and place, and before-and-after studies (uncontrolled trials), which despite being convenient, can produce biased results.

Prevention

Main types of preventative activities in clinical practice include behavioural interventions (i.e. counselling advocating lifestyle changes such as smoking cessation, increased physical activity, weight loss), immunizations, screening (i.e. identification of asymptomatic disease or risk factors), and chemoprevention (i.e. pharmacological interventions to prevent disease, e.g. statin use for hypercholesterolaemia).

Quite often screening tests are those used as diagnostic tests. However, when applied for screening the following need to be considered (not relevant for diagnosis): difference between prevalence and incidence screens and potential biases in screening studies such as lead-time, length-time, and compliance biases. Thus, after the first round of screening in the population (prevalence screen), the number of new cases identified will drop at subsequent screenings (incident screen), which also means that positive predictive value for screening test results will diminish after prevalence screen. Lead-time bias arises when early detection of a medical condition by screening creates a spurious impression of improved survival, when in fact early treatment is no more effective than treatment at the time of clinical presentation (i.e. when patient experiences symptoms and seeks medical care), and hence, screening gives more 'disease time', and not more survival time. Use of mortality rates instead of survival rates can help avoid lead-time bias. Length-time bias occurs when outcome seems better in the screened group simply because screening is more likely to detect cases that progress slowly from onset to symptoms and diagnosis (e.g. slow-growing tumours). Compliance bias occurs when outcome in screened groups is better due to compliance and not screening.

Prevention can be classified into primary (e.g. immunizations for infectious diseases), secondary (e.g. mammography to detect asymptomatic breast cancer), and tertiary (i.e. for reducing risks in patients with established disease, e.g. beta-blockers after MI to reduce mortality risk), depending on when in the course of disease the intervention took place.

Clinical research encourages the practice of prevention in ordinary clinical practice and informs of the effectiveness of various techniques in order to reduce risk of disease onset (primary prevention) and improve prognosis (tertiary prevention).

In order to decide what medical conditions to include in preventive care, the following should be considered:

- The burden of condition in terms of death, disease, disability, discomfort, dissatisfaction
- The understanding of the natural history of a condition
- Whether a condition is detectable at a latent stage
- The quality of the screening test in terms of sensitivity, specificity, safety, simplicity, the effects of false-positive results, cost
- The availability and quality (effectiveness, safety and cost-effectiveness) of intervention for primary prevention, and quality and effect of early treatment for secondary prevention
- Clinical, social, and ethical acceptability of the screening

Further reading

Aday LA, Cornelius LJ. *Designing and ConductingHealth Surveys: A Comprehensive Guide*. Oxford: John Wiley & Sons, 2006.

Davidoff F, Haynes B, Sackett D, et al. Evidence based medicine. *BMJ* 1995;310:1085–6.

Feinstein AR. Clinical epidemiology. I. The populational experiments of nature and of man in human illness. *Ann Intern Med* 1968;69:807–20.

Griffiths M. Evidence based medicine. Must be applied critically. *BMJ* 1995;311:257.

Guyatt G, Cairns J, Churchill D, et al. Evidence-based medicine. A new approach to teaching the practice of medicine. *JAMA* 1992;268:2420–5.

Hards, M. *Medical Statistics and Biostatistics defined*. ℘ www.medicalstatistician.com/index.php/medical-statistics-biostatistics-defined.html 2012

Last JM, Spasoff RA, Harris SS. *A dictionary of epidemiology*. Oxford: Oxford University Press, 2001.

Oxman AD, Sackett DL, Guyatt GH. Users' guides to the medical literature. I. How to get started. The Evidence-Based Medicine Working Group. *JAMA* 1993;270:2093–5.

Paul JR. President's Address Clinical Epidemiology. *J Clin Invest 1938*;17:539–41.

Sackett DL, Winkelstein W, Jr. The relationship between cigarette usage and aortic atherosclerosis. *Am J Epidemiol* 1967;86:264-70.

Navigating research methods: quantitative and clinical/epidemiological methods

Introduction

> 'Any science is as objective as its capability of measuring the events which it purports to be observing and relating. Epidemiology has not been exempt from the usual evolutionary development of this necessary aspect of its methodology'.

Abraham M Lilienfeld

Although initially, epidemiology borrowed study methods, techniques of measurement, and analyses from other disciplines, it has 'developed the study as art and science by means of innovative approaches to methodology and the elaboration of earlier techniques'.

The term 'quantitative methods' could be narrowed to mean statistical methods or treated more broadly in terms of the epidemiologic methods of study. This chapter will focus on the discussion of widely used methods of epidemiologic study (mainly analytic). More specifically, it will provide a brief overview of what questions can be answered using quantitative research methods, and what study types are used in epidemiological research, as well as the potential errors in epidemiological studies.

Epidemiology studies the frequency, distribution, and determinants of health states in specified human populations and translates research findings into practice in order to improve health. Epidemiological methods can be used to measure health and disease, to explore whether a factor is a cause, determinant risk factor, or predictor for a specified health problem, to evaluate diagnostic tests, and to study the effectiveness of intervention/treatment and clinical care. Clinical epidemiology, as one of the sub-disciplines of epidemiology, is more concerned with questions relevant to clinical practice. Therefore, methods of clinical epidemiology are used to obtain quantitative evidence on diagnosis, aetiology, and prognosis of disease, and on the effects of interventions.

Study types

Choosing the **appropriate study type** and **design** is a crucial step in any epidemiological research as the study type and design are major determinants of quality of scientific evidence produced by a study and consequently, its clinical value.

Design of an epidemiologic study starts with formulating the research question/hypothesis (this stage is referred to as **theoretical design**). A well-formulated research question will suggest the most appropriate study type/design to answer the question.

Epidemiological studies can be classified as either observational or experimental (Figure 3.1). The randomized, double-blind, controlled clinical trial is the 'gold standard' of medical research. However, a trial may be unethical, not feasible, or too expensive, making observational study designs preferable.

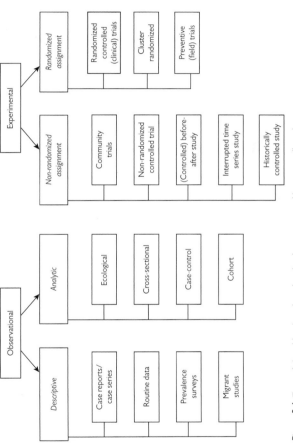

Figure 3.1 Types of clinical/epidemiological studies (primary research): not mutually exclusive.

Observational studies

The investigator measures but does not intervene. Observational studies can be further classified into descriptive and analytic studies. Descriptive studies are commonly used to explore patterns of disease occurrence and to study frequency distribution of disease or risk factors for disease by person, place, and time. Descriptive studies do not have a comparison group and are best suited to identify health problems and generate hypothesis about exposure–disease relationships.

Analytical studies

These are used to investigate associations between disease and exposure, in other words, **to explain disease occurrence**, identifying causes of disease or risk factors associated with increased risk of disease after taking into account the effect of potential confounders. They allow **testing hypothesis** about exposure–disease relationships.

In clinical epidemiology diagnostic and prognostic research can be classified as descriptive, aetiologic research as analytic (causal), and experimental research as either descriptive or analytic.

The classification of studies into descriptive vs analytic studies may involve some ambiguity; for example, ecological (correlation) studies can be classified as either, and cross-sectional studies can be both descriptive (e.g. prevalence surveys) and analytic (when used to look at exposure–disease association). In general, this distinction is not very important. It is important, however, to understand key features, theoretical and practical advantages and limitations of each type, to consider all potential sources of **bias** and **confounding**, and to strive to minimize them in order to get valid results and to make causal inferences. Hence, while **interpreting the results** of epidemiologic studies, the following possible explanations need to be considered: chance variation (random error), bias (systematic error), confounding or true association (Box 3.1).

Box 3.1 Sources of error in epidemiological studies

Potential errors can be classified into those related to studying sample **selection** and **measurement** of outcome, exposure, and covariates. These errors in turn can be either **random** or **systematic**.

Since epidemiological studies do not normally study a whole population but only a sample from it, random sampling error (**chance**) is inevitable. This can be assessed by statistical methods (confidence interval, p-value), and may be reduced by increasing sample size. Random measurement error (imprecision) can be due to biological variation and measuring error and can be reduced by taking repeated measurements.

Bias can mask the existing association or create a spurious association. Main types of bias include **selection bias** and **information (measurement) bias**. Selection bias occurs when selection and/or follow-up procedures lead to systematic differences between characteristics of those entering or remaining in a study and those not selected initially or lost to follow-up, and where those characteristics are related to exposure or outcome under study.

Information bias

Occurs when systematic error is introduced into measurements (e.g. systematically underestimating or overestimating true value) and/or the way information on exposure or disease is obtained from the study groups is systematically different. The examples of information bias include recall bias, interviewer bias, and observer bias.

Confounding

Occurs when a third factor, a potential confounding variable, is a risk factor for disease even among the unexposed and is associated with exposure (in source population or among controls, in case-control study) and is not in the causal pathway between disease and exposure. A confounding factor may mask an actual association or falsely demonstrate an apparent association between the study variables where no real association between them exists. Methods to control confounding include restriction, matching, randomization, stratification, and statistical adjustment.

Main features of analytical observational studies

Ecological studies

These compare the prevalence of exposure and occurrence of disease in populations, not individuals, hence the unit of observation is the population. The comparisons may be between populations in different places at the same time, or in a time series, by comparing the same population (in one place) at different times. Time-series comparisons, especially if the time period is short, may reduce some of the socio-economic confounding which is a potential problem in ecological studies. These studies are good for hypothesis generation or initial investigation of causal hypothesis.

Advantages

Easy, cheap, and quick to conduct if routine data are readily available; useful to explore relatively new hypothesis; useful when interested in the effect from ecological variables; when adequate measurement of individual-level variables is not possible or individual-level study is not possible; for example, to study the effect of geographical and temporal factors on disease incidence or the effect of a government policy change on health outcomes.

Disadvantages

Difficult to interpret associations in aetiological terms; the inference is limited with respect to individuals, due to high probability of **ecological fallacy** (when characteristics of individuals are wrongly inferred from grouped (aggregate) data); potential for systematic differences between places in disease coding and classification and the exposure measurement; usually rely on data collected for other purposes, which means data on different exposures or factors may not be available; difficult to control for confounding.

Cross-sectional analytical studies (a snapshot in time)

Measure the exposure and disease simultaneously at a single point in time or time interval (Figure 3.2). They can be used for studying exposure–disease association, diagnostic test evaluation, are useful for investigating exposures that do not change over time (e.g. sex, blood group), and for assessing the healthcare needs of populations. Repeated cross-sectional surveys can be useful for studying trends.

Sample selection

The sample should be selected to be representative of the whole population (probability sampling methods are preferable), and selected without knowledge of either their disease or exposure status in order to avoid **selection bias**.

Advantages

May study several outcomes; are efficient in terms of time and cost; can be analysed using methods for case-control studies yielding an odds ratio; are good for generating hypothesis for further cohort studies.

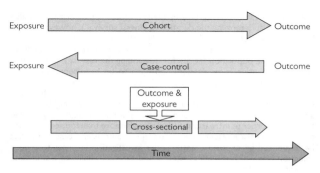

Figure 3.2 Direction of inquiry in analytical epidemiological studies.

Disadvantages
Difficult to interpret associations in causal terms; does not identify temporal relationship; not feasible for rare diseases; susceptible to survivor bias; does not produce incidence rate or relative risk.

Case-control studies

Are the most frequently conducted analytical epidemiological studies. Unlike cross-sectional studies, case-control studies involve time directionality (Figure 3.2) and are retrospective (meaning the investigator looks backward from the disease to identify a possible cause/determinant), except for nested case-control studies (when cases and controls are drawn from a cohort study).

The conduct of case-control study starts by selecting a sample of people with disease/condition of interest (**cases**), and a **suitable** disease-free sample at risk (**controls**). Predictor variables are measured afterwards. Hence, the study attempts to identify potential causes/determinants by comparing the **odds of past exposures** of interest in cases and controls. Controls allow estimating the expected exposure rate in cases if there was no association between exposure and disease.

Exposure status of cases and controls should be determined following the same protocol and concurrently for cases and controls in order to minimize the effects of short-term changes (e.g. seasonal changes). Exposure estimates are prone to **recall bias** (when cases may remember their past exposure more accurately or differently than controls do) and **interviewer bias** (when the interviewer interprets the exposure information differently for cases and controls), which can be minimized by 'blinding interviewers' to study hypothesis or disease status of subjects.

Selection of cases and controls

Cases should be selected after the diagnostic criteria and case definition are clearly established, and should be representative of all the cases in a specified population. Ideally, the study should include incident cases (as prevalence is influenced not only by the risk of developing disease but also by factors that determine the duration of illness 'survival'); however, prevalent cases may also be included, especially if the disease under study is rare. Cases can be **population-based** or **hospital-based**. **Controls** should be from the same base population (at risk for developing the disease), as the cases and selected using some random approach to be representative of the source population (i.e. exposure prevalence in controls and in the source population should be similar). Multiple controls, either from the same source (controls of similar type) or different sources (e.g. neighbourhood and hospital controls) can be used, especially when cases are very difficult to obtain in order to increase statistical power (more than four controls per case is usually not efficient). The inclusion of controls and cases **must not be influenced by exposure status** under investigation in order to reduce **selection bias** which can affect internal and external validity of a study and an estimated odds ratio (see Box 3.2 for measures).

Box 3.2 Measures used in epidemiological research

Measures of disease occurrence

Prevalence

Measures the amount of disease in a population at a defined point in time (a function of incidence and duration). It is calculated as number of people with disease at a specified point in time divided by total number of people in the population; useful for measuring the overall disease burden, assessing healthcare needs and planning health services; reported as proportion or percentage along with time point of an estimate; obtained from cross-sectional study (also known as survey).

Cumulative incidence (CI)

Measures the proportion of people who develop disease during a defined time period. It is calculated as number of new cases in a cohort during defined time period divided by total number 'at risk' at the beginning of the time period; reported as proportion along with time period of an estimate; the best observational study design to obtain CI is cohort and is estimated accurately only when all subjects are followed for the entire follow-up period; appropriate and common measure of outcome in clinical trials where it is called **experimental event rate** (for CI in the intervention group), and **control event rate** (for CI in the control group). CI measures **absolute risk**, which is the probability of occurrence of a particular event over a specified time period for an average individual population member. Hence, risk gives useful information at the individual level, for example, for predicting change in health status of an individual or assessing the prognosis of a patient, etc.

Incidence rate (IR)

Also called incidence density: measures how quickly new cases of disease are occurring and therefore, reflects the so-called underlying force of morbidity. Calculated as number of new cases of disease within a given time period divided by the total 'person time at risk' during time period;

Box 3.2 (*Contd.*)

reported using 'per 1000 or 10 000 or 100 000, etc. person years'. IR handles censoring (i.e. inability to follow study participants for an endpoint of interest due to loss to follow-up, end of study, other outcome occurring first (competing risk)); best observational study design to obtain IR is cohort. Rate has no useful interpretation at the individual level.

Odds

The ratio of the probability of event occurring to the probability of event not occurring. Calculated as probability divided by 1.0 minus probability; approximates a probability when the probability is less than about 10%. A risk of 30% can be expressed as odds of 3 to 7.

Effect measures

Difference measures

Give an indication of disease burden due to the exposure and of the potential benefit of a preventive intervention if disease can be attributed to the exposure.

Attributable risk (AR)

Measures the excess risk due to exposure to a particular factor. It is calculated by subtracting CI in unexposed from CI in exposed **risk difference**. AR can also be used to describe **rate difference**, which is calculated by subtracting IR in unexposed from IR in exposed. The term 'attributable risk' is appropriate to use only when it is reasonable to assume causal relationship between the exposure and the outcome. The synonymous terms used in clinical epidemiology are **absolute risk reduction** or **absolute risk increase** depending on whether the risk is reduced or increased in the treatment group.

Ratio measures

Give an indication of the strength of the association between the exposure and the outcome and can help us decide whether the exposure might actually cause the disease.

Relative risk (RR)

Also called risk ratio. Tell us how many times more likely is that someone exposed to the factor under study will develop an outcome of interest relative to someone not exposed (RR does not inform of the actual amount of disease occurrence). It is simply calculated by dividing the CI in exposed by the CI in unexposed. RR is also used to describe rate ratio (calculated by dividing IR of disease in exposed group by the IR of disease in unexposed group). If a disease is rare (risk less than about 10%), then the risk ratio and rate ratio are almost identical. RR can be calculated from cohort studies.

Relative risk reduction

Is often used to report results of *treatment trials* to measure the amount by which the treatment has reduced the RR and is calculated by subtracting the RR from 1.0. The term **relative risk increase** is used for studies with a positive association (RR > 1.0) with the treatment factor.

(*continued*)

Box 3.2 (*Contd.*)
Odds ratio (OR)
Is a way of comparing the probability of a certain event in two groups. Calculated as ratio of the odds of a disease in exposed to the odds of a disease in unexposed. OR is the measure of exposure–disease association calculated from *case-control* studies.

If a disease is rare, then odds ratio, risk ratio, and rate ratio are almost equal and can be interpreted as a relative risk. Attributable risk of disease associated with a particular exposure cannot be calculated in case-control studies. Instead, **attributable fraction** is calculated to assess the potential public health importance of the exposure.

Advantages
The best approach for investigating risk factors for rare diseases; applicable to common diseases; well suited to the study of diseases with long latency; suitable when randomization is unethical; may study several exposures; efficient with respect to cost and time; require relatively small sample size; yield odds ratio, which approximates relative risk when disease is rare.

Disadvantages
Susceptible to bias, especially selection bias and recall bias; potential survivor bias, interviewer bias; cannot establish temporal relationship; control for extraneous variables (confounders) may be incomplete; selection of appropriate control group may be difficult; cannot estimate disease incidence and therefore cannot calculate absolute risk, attributable risk, or relative risk.

Cohort studies

Cohort studies are considered a gold standard of observational studies as they provide stronger evidence towards causality. Cohort studies are longitudinal. The study begins with selecting a population sample free of disease under question, then it measures predictor variables and classifies according to exposure status (present or absent). Thereafter, the whole cohort is followed up to measure disease/outcome occurrence by exposure status (Figure 3.2).

In prognostic studies, cohort is a group of patients with a particular condition/ diagnosis followed for the outcome of interest.
Cohort studies can be classified into:
• prospective or retrospective (according to the timing of data collection).
• fixed, when cohort is established at enrolment and membership ages over time, or dynamic (also called open), when patients enter the study population throughout the study period when eligibility criteria are met (participants have different maximum observation times, and membership varies over time).
• population-based (e.g. birth cohorts) or special (often in occupational epidemiology).

Selection of the comparison population

The comparison population (unexposed) can be from the same study population (**internal**), which minimizes the differences between exposed and unexposed, or from another cohort (**external**), which is common in occupational epidemiology, or the general population.

Advantages

Can study rare exposures; investigate several diseases/outcomes at once; can be used where randomization is not possible or is unethical; temporal ambiguity is minimized (although still possible when there is a long pre-clinical phase before diagnosis, creating potential for reverse causality); produce reliable assessment of exposure (no recall bias); usually selection bias is not a major issue in terms of internal validity (although can affect external validity (generalizability)); avoids survivor bias; incidence rates, absolute risk, attributable risk are estimable; time-to-event analysis is possible.

Disadvantages

Most expensive among observational studies; take a long time (years) and increase potential for losses to follow-up (follow-up bias as well as non-response bias during data collection in cohort studies are similar to selection bias in case-control studies); potential for outcome ascertainment bias (which can be minimized by the use of objective measures, independent or 'blinded' observers); not suitable for rare diseases; not suitable for diseases with long induction; often requires large sample sizes and measuring exposure for all may not be feasible; control for extraneous variables (confounders) may be incomplete.

Costs as well as required time can be reduced by conducting a **retrospective (historical) cohort study**. In a retrospective cohort study, both the exposure and disease data have been collected before the actual study begins. This design is often used for the assessment of the association between cancer and occupational exposures. However, existing data may not include information that is important or all variables needed, or if data available, they may be inaccurate or incomplete; no control over nature and quality of measurements.

Cohort studies can be less expensive when **nested case-control design** is applied since, for example, expensive laboratory tests need to be done only for those who are later chosen as cases and controls. In addition, since cases and controls are both chosen from a defined cohort, where information on exposures and risk factors have been collected before outcome development, probability of recall bias is eliminated and exposure data are more likely to represent the pre-illness state. Other observational study designs (e.g. case-cohort, case-crossover) are not discussed here.

Experimental also called intervention studies

Are used to search for means to reduce a population's exposure to identified risk factors in order to prevent disease occurrence (primary prevention); to evaluate efficacy of preventive and therapeutic measures for a particular disease; to assess effectiveness of health services. Experimental studies can be designed as randomized controlled trials (preferred if possible); trials without comparison group (e.g. case report, case series); trials with histori-cal controls; or trials with simultaneous but non-randomized controls (e.g. community trials).

Randomized design

Common for **clinical trials** (Chapter 14) to assess a treatment (e.g. therapy vs no therapy, therapy vs placebo, or new therapy vs current therapy) for a specific disease, and for **field (preventive) trials** to assess interventions aimed at reducing harmful exposures. Unlike clinical trials, field trials select healthy participants who are at risk of developing disease. Another impor-tant element of randomized trials is 'blinding' (masking) of subjects, data collectors measuring outcome variables, and data analysts. The study is called 'single blind' if only subjects do not know which treatment they are receiving, and 'double blind' if neither the subjects nor the researchers are aware of the treatment. In 'unblinded' trials, the outcome of treatment may be influenced by practitioners' and patients' preferences for one or other intervention. Blinding is less important when the outcome measure is less dependent on subjective interpretation (e.g. death or 'biochemical parameter').

The steps involved in the conduct of randomized controlled trials include selection of eligible sample from the population; measurement of baseline variables; random allocation of intervention 'exposure', whereby each subject has an equal chance of being assigned to any group in the study; application of intervention; follow-up of the cohort; and measurement of outcome variables. The effect of an intervention is measured by comparing the outcome in the experimental group with that in a control group. Ethical considerations are essential in the design of these studies.

The purpose of randomization (works if sample size is adequately large) is to make groups as similar as possible except for the factor (intervention) under study; in other words, to control for known and unknown, measured and unmeasured confounders, and to remove the potential for bias in the choice of treatment ('confounding by indication').

Subtypes of randomized clinical trials include **parallel group design** (when patients are randomly allocated to one of the two treatments and are fol-lowed in parallel), **crossover design** (where each patient serves as his own control), and **factorial design** (when two treatments are tested simultane-ously as well as treatment synergy (i.e. combination)).

Advantages

Can produce the strongest causal evidence; the best and only possible design for evaluation of new drug; usually selection bias is not a major issue (although possible if allocation process is not properly concealed); able to control the effect of confounders.

Disadvantages

Expensive; may not be suitable for a particular research question due to ethical/safety issues (e.g. study of suspected treatment toxicities, or assign-ment to smoking vs no smoking groups); not suitable for rare outcomes and evaluation of life-long effects; generalizability is reduced due to sample selection criteria and 'unusually ideal' conditions compared to usual practice;

potential for outcome ascertainment bias; potential of non-compliance to experimental or control regimens, and losses to follow-up which dilute study results.

Community trials

Community trials are appropriate when intervention cannot be delivered and evaluated at the individual level (e.g. water fluoridation and dental care study). However, they can include only a small number of communities, random allocation of communities is usually not practicable, and therefore, it is difficult to make conclusions about effectiveness of such trials.

In summary, both randomized and non-randomized studies pose potential threats to internal (the extent to which the results of a study are correct for the study sample) and external (the extent to which the results of a study hold true in other settings) validity. 'Understanding what kind of study has been done is a prerequisite to thoughtful reading of research.'

Meta-analysis

An important quantitative technique used in healthcare and clinical research is meta-analysis (see the *Oxford Handbook of Medical Statistics*), a statistical technique which combines results of several independent studies in order to obtain a more precise estimate of a treatment effect or any other association of interest. A well-conducted meta-analysis needs to be carefully planned in advance which includes the following major steps:

• A detailed written protocol
• Definition of inclusion and exclusion criteria and a comprehensive literature search strategy
• Calculation of the overall (pooled) effect whereby the results from large studies are given greater weight than those from smaller studies
• There are two main statistical approaches in the calculation of the pooled effect: 1) *fixed-effects* meta-analysis which assumes that there is no between-study heterogeneity and the effect varies only due to chance, and 2) *random-effects* meta-analysis which assumes that there are real differences in the effect between the studies as well as variability due to chance
• Graphical display of the results in a standardized format (forest plot) which allows for a comparison between the studies and an examination of heterogeneity
• A thorough sensitivity analysis to examine robustness of the results to the changes of the assumptions, exclusion of the studies with small sample size, etc.

The following points should be considered in the interpretation of any meta-analysis: combinability of individual studies, robustness of the results to changes of the assumptions, and the possible contribution of the results to the process of decision making regarding patient management or formulating public health guidelines.

Further reading

Breslow NE, Day NE. *Statistical Methods in Cancer Research*. IARC Scientific Publications No. 32, 1980.

Euser AM, Zoccali C, Jager KJ, et al. Cohort studies: prospective versus retrospective. *Nephron Clin Pract* 2009;113:c214–c217.

Grimes DA, Schulz KF. An overview of clinical research: the lay of the land. *Lancet* 2002;359:57–61.

Grimes DA, Schulz KF. Compared to what? Finding controls for case-control studies. *Lancet* 2005;365:1429–33.

Grobbee DE, Hoes AW. *Clinical Epidemiology: Principles, Methods and Applications for Clinical Research*. London: Jones and Bartlett Publishers, 2009.

Lilienfeld AM. Advances in quantitative methods in epidemiology. *Public Health Rep* 1980;95:462–9.

McKee M, Britton A, Black N, et al. Methods in health services research. Interpreting the evidence: choosing between randomised and non-randomised studies. *BMJ* 1999;319:312–5.

Rothman KJ, Greenland S. *Objectives of Epidemiologic Study Design. Modern Epidemiology*. Philadelphia, PA: Lippincott-Raven, 1998.

Tu JV, Ko DT. Ecological studies and cardiovascular outcomes research. *Circulation* 2008;118:2588–93.

Navigating research methods: qualitative methods

Objectives

- To outline qualitative research methods using the example of educational research
- To demystify and position educational research within an accessible social research framework
- To explore and evaluate suitable methodological approaches
- To consider how to handle the products of the research
- To provide an overall insight of the value of educational research, in particular a mixed-methods approach, within the healthcare setting

What constitutes educational research?

Educational research is social research and the training of the majority of healthcare personnel is grounded in 'conventional scientific standards'. It is this juxtaposition that Gergen and Gergen suggest is a major detractor from the pursuit of social research after 'purer' scientific research.[7]

Nevertheless, social research does incorporate elements of the scientific approach that should put the healthcare researcher (referred to as 'the researcher' from this point on) within a research framework that is partially familiar to him or her.

The research process, regardless of the paradigm adopted, is multi-phased and Table 4.1 outlines these according to Bryman.[3]

Table 4.1 The phases of the research process (after Bryman)[3]

The research process
Formulating the research objectives
Choosing the research
Securing research participants
Collecting and analysing data
Interpreting data
Disseminating findings

Broom and Willis describe paradigms as the overarching philosophical, ideological stance, or world view that will form the assumptive platform from which new knowledge will be explored.[2] Thus, the researcher needs to start from his or her own standpoint and determine how this relates to the research philosophy. This requires consideration and exploration, particularly with regard to how these are grounded in the educational research paradigm. Epistemological considerations pertain to what should be regarded as acceptable knowledge (positivism vs 'interpretivism'). Johnson argues that 'critical theory' is the third research paradigm.[9]

Ontological considerations take into account whether the social entities 'have a reality external to social actors, or whether they can and should be considered social constructions built up from perceptions and actions of social actors'. The two ontological positions are objectivism and constructionism.[2]

Johnson raises the methodological question ('how can the researcher go about finding out whatever he or she believes can be known?') as the third critical consideration when embarking on research.[9] The *methodology*, or research strategy, refers to the kind of theoretical framework that will be used to shape the research. This framework will be important in defining the interpretation of data. This is not to say that *theory* should be used to define the data, but as a theoretical framework the methodology is useful in helping the researcher make sense of the data in context with the social world. The methodology should be used as a guideline, allowing the researcher to be creative in interpreting the data.

Underpinning any research is the acquisition of data to deconstruct 'the situation' in order to address, change, and improve that situation. What approaches should the researcher adopt? Johnson suggests considering two critical questions when embarking on a research project:[9]
- How does one address the challenges/dilemmas (the situations) associated with research in one paradigm or in mixed paradigms?
- How does knowledge of the researcher's philosophical stance help the researcher in researching?

In order to deconstruct the range of representations of paradigms, methods, approaches, and methodologies for the researchers new to healthcare education, these will be presented in tabulated and diagrammatic forms in an overview of these complex relationships in Figure 4.1, and detailed in the next section.

Bryman explains 'interpretivism' as subsuming the views of others who have been influenced by different intellectual traditions.[3]

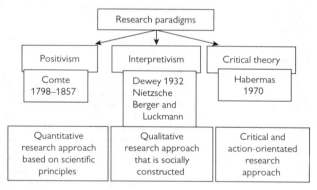

Figure 4.1 An overview of the relationship between the research paradigms, research approaches, and research methodologies.

Evaluating the research paradigms, approaches, and methodologies

In this section, a number of research approaches will be compared and contrasted in order to justify the use to a mixed-method multidisciplinary approach to social educational research.

Table 4.2 combines a summary of Newby's approach to methods and research design.[15]

In unfolding these perspectives on social reality, Greenfield (1975) defined the realism of the positivist/objectivist school (quantitative) as being external from the individual as 'the world exists and is knowable as it really is. Organizations are real entities with a life of their own'. As individuals are mere players within society, the researcher treats the individual and society as separate entities. By comparison, she described the idealistic and subjectivist (qualitative) thus: 'the world exists but different people construe it in very different ways. Organizations are invented social reality'. Individuals are the basis of the social structure and cannot be treated as separate entities, so personal accounts are a key tool in gaining a better understanding of a given situation.

The disciplinary backgrounds may differ in approach and perspective, but the search for an explanation and/or solution remains the central point of departure.

Robson's work[16] informs the researcher as to the worldview that underpins the selection of the adopted research paradigm; that is, quantitative or qualitative. Healthcare researchers seek to explore the underlying causes of a situation that are part of the real world 'where the social dimension is important and approaches which take serious note of this aspect have a clear attraction'. His point of departure infers a scientific attitude implying that the research is carried out within a systematic, sceptical, and ethical manner that permeates the research.

Healthcare is carried out in the real world and is inseparable from social which is why the 'qualitivist' paradigm,[16] with its social constructivist research approach, is most likely to facilitate the exploration of the root causes of the topic at the core of the research.

Essentially, the divide is between purist (scientific method/qualitative) and pragmatic researchers. Robson grounds this assumption by purporting the view that a pragmatic approach would blend the quantitative and qualitative traditions. He labels this approach a 'multi-strategy research design',[16] reflecting Tritter[17] who called it 'mixed methods and multi-disciplinary research'.

Tritter[17] emphasizes the importance of the ability to triangulate evidence using the mixed-methods research method that enables a more holistic approach to research in healthcare settings. Cook[5] supports this view because only through consulting multiple sources of evidence can understanding of a given situation deepen. He further supports the value of a mixed-methods research approach by stating that 'we need carefully planned, theory building, programmatic research reflecting a variety of paradigms and approaches', because they will 'clarify why, when and how something works'. Researchers turn to qualitative methods, according

Table 4.2 Comparing the traditional research approaches

Quantitative research	Qualitative research
Underpins rationale with theoretical perspectives/scientific method	Inductive (observations and/or findings to theory); evident in grounded theory OR Deductive (theory to observations and/or findings)
Objectivist paradigm	Interpretivist/Constructivist paradigm
Positivist view of social reality	Post-/anti-positivist view of social reality
The 'standard view'	Evidence imperfect and fallible
Realism	Idealism
Derivation of a hypothesis and sometimes a null hypothesis as well	Inductive: observations; analysis + assessment; conjecture + hypothesis; generalization of the theory
	Deductive: starts with an idea or theory; hypothesis; evidence; conclusion; feedback into the research
Generalizable as data are reliable and unbiased so findings can be extrapolated to the rest of the population	Validity because the new knowledge draws on understandings of research subjects
	Not generalizable as analysis relies on the interpretation of researcher
Validity, reliability and objectivity of the research	Credibility, dependability, confirmability of the research
Deterministic as phenomena can be predicted by acknowledging scientific laws	Naturalistic as data are collected in the setting of everyday life
	Subjectivity because research practice and knowledge production are neither neutral nor objective, but partial
	Complexity as analysis explores depth as opposed to inferences
What is the relationship between x and y?	How does x relate to y?
	Enables deeper exploration of the situation and subsequent
	Requires reflection on the data in relation to the situation
RCT (randomized controlled trials) commonly recognized method	Interviews, observation, focus groups, secondary discourse analysis, questionnaires
Social surveys' epidemiology, structured interviews, systematic meta-analysis reviews, secondary document analysis (e.g. content analysis)	

to Gergen and Gergen, 'in the hope of generating richer and more finely nuanced accounts of human interaction'.[7] The authors continue by saying that supporters of the qualitative approach highlight the absence of 'the critical ingredient of human understanding' when empirical research is selected over a qualitative one. It remains difficult to convince purist empirical quantitative researchers of the intrinsic value of qualitative and mixed methods research findings. The inclusion of a critical and action-orientated research approach in mixed methods offers a conduit for adding academic rigour to the adoption of a mixed-methods research approach.

Figure 4.2 illustrates how this third methodological movement blends different research approaches.

The logic of the design affects the credibility of the research and its findings, again adding weight to the value of this 'third methodological movement'[15] in ensuring that the design is appropriate to the situation under investigation. The elephant in the room remains the fact that RCT is seen in medical spheres as the best and most powerful form for gathering research evidence. Tritter's proposed resolution is through reflection: 'The credibility afforded different kinds of data is a reflection of different kinds of disciplinary cultures'.[17] This reflection can be on practice (by the researcher and the research subjects) and in practice (the research subjects), thus affording the evidence some triangulation (Oversby, p. 241)[14] as depicted in Figure 4.2. This figure does not position the role of reflection in the process. Figure 4.3 presents the characteristics which the researcher needs to be aware of when using a mixed-methods research approach.

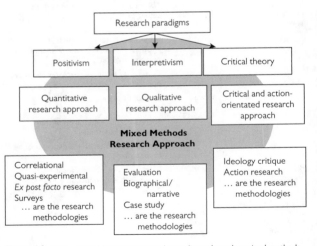

Figure 4.2. A blending of the three research paradigms through a mixed-methods approach.

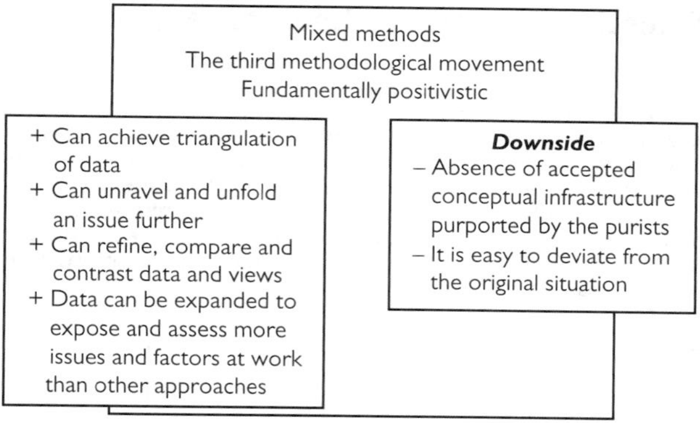

Figure 4.3 A summary of the mixed-methods research approach and its characteristics. From Haynes, based on Newby.[15]

Robson[16] highlighted the fact that the scientific attitude incorporates scepticism, while Tritter's[17] comment pertaining to the need for careful and detailed planning underpins this view that the qualitative researcher must be able to address in defence of his chosen methodological approach. The criteria underpinning the value of qualitative evidence are, according to Tritter, 'antithetical to qualitative methods and interpretative data analysis'.[17] It is worth noting that in healthcare many of the decisions are made by managerial or polite elite who may not be clinically trained and thus fail to comprehend fully and appreciate the findings from a qualitative or mixed-methods research project.

The use of a mixed-methods approach helps research into attitudes, values, beliefs and performance that are not criterion-referenced. This field of research can be intriguing but more difficult to design for the collection of appropriate data. Miller and Brewer[13] outline the historical perspective of this complicated genre of social research, dating back to Thurstone in 1928 with his attitude-measurement scale and Likert's five-point scale of measuring any qualitative commodity. Fishbein and Ajzen[6] explored belief, attitude, intention, and behaviour in their seminal study. A number of healthcare topics, such as depression and ME, would benefit from an exploration of these frames of reference (attitude, belief, values, self-esteem) by examining the evidence in order to expose their root causes.

Selecting the methodological approach

The social researcher should embark on designing the research with an open mind. Newby's approach might be the most logical for any novice education researcher to take as it provides a platform from which to structure the project.[15] He looks at 'dissecting the research question', something that is not done enough, and whose absence often results in the adoption of a flawed research and strategic approach (see Figure 4.4).

Once the situation has been clearly identified and a research question posed, then the research questioning can lead the researcher to selecting the research method and its concomitant methodological data-gathering tools and analytical strategies.

Research issue
The situation

Research question
Why is the situation happening?

Research questioning
What factors are influencing the situation?
for example…What is happening?
Why is this happening?
What happened initially?
What will happen?
What will the effect be?
What should we do?
Is this (approach) working?

Figure 4.4 Newby's steps in dissecting the research question.[15]

Research methods

The *methods* are the tools that will be used in collecting the data. It is important to be aware of the *kind* of data needed to answer the research question(s), and collect accordingly. Table 4.3 outlines some opposing approaches to consider when choosing a method.

Essentially, it is the sampling procedure selected to gather the data that will vary depending on the research perspective of the project. Quantitative sampling needs to consider the types of probability sampling *and* non-probability sampling methods that will yield data to address the research issue that the sample size will affect greatly. Table 4.4 provides a summary of these sampling procedures.

Table 4.3 Opposing approaches to gathering data

Quantitative	Qualitative
Numbering	Wording
Predetermined or controlled	Open-ended or responsive
Measuring	Capturing uniqueness
Short-term	Long-term
Comparing	Capturing particularity
Describing	Interpreting
Description	Explanation
Objective	Subjective
Regularities	Uniqueness
Looking in from the outside	Looking from the inside

(Adapted from Cohen et al. 2011, p. 414)[4].

It has been fairly well established in this chapter that the recommended research approach would blend quantitative and qualitative methodologies with critical theory in order to harvest data to get to 'those root causes of the situation' in healthcare and medical education research. Mixed-methods methodological approaches to sampling are presented in Table 4.4 with data from Newby[15] and Johnson.[9]

Table 4.4 A summary of research methodologies to gathering data for quantitative–qualitative–critical theory and mixed-methods sampling

Methodology	Focus	Information assembly
Case studies	Can learn from the particular situation	Interview to explain, explore and describe
Evaluation	Question focus	Any in order to understand, test compliance, improve and inform
Ethnography	Researcher focus	Observation and conversation (unstructured interviews) to understand and explain
Action research	Change focus	Reflection to change, build, improve, and develop
Ideology critique	Explore the 'too self-evident'	Elicit 'critical' or 'emancipatory' knowledge
Biography/ narrative	Discourse analysis	Interpretive + ethnographic account of participant's perspective to understand the symbolism of an issue/the situation

The reality of using these methodologies

What do these methodologies look like and comprise in terms of research? A brief overview of each tool is presented. The cited references will provide in-depth protocols once the research approach and methodology that best complements researching the situation has been selected.

Case studies

The case study is both a research method and methodology. As a data collection tool, the case study provides a rich platform for obtaining qualitative data because it is 'the study of an instance in action'.[1] A key feature of the case study is that it approaches a research situation 'holistically' (Verschuren)[18]. Yin[20] describes five key components of case study research design:

- Study question
- The study propositions (if any)
- The unit(s) of analysis
- The logic linking the data to the propositions
- The criteria for interpreting the findings

Ethnographic and qualitative research

Ethnographic research lies within qualitative research and is the study of cultures and people within cultures. Every group or society has a culture in which they function. It is from that culture that meaning is given to everyday actions and objects. The researcher must acknowledge that the questions that are asked will be influenced by the individual's experiences and values. For example, tacit and implicit knowledge about a social group cannot be ignored and may be invaluable when interpreting a situation.

Interviews are a way to gather this implicit knowledge and opinions, providing valuable narrative data from human subjects. Kvale[12] suggests that human subjects are treated as knowledge generators instead of factors or variables, with the interviewer being the research tool. If the researcher can gain trust and establish a rapport with the interviewee(s), he or she can potentially elicit good information unavailable through other forms of research.

There are several types of interview formats. Adopting a suitable style depends on the type of questions the investigation seeks to answer. Cohen and colleagues[4] offer four different interview formats:

- Informal/unstructured conversational interview
- Interview guide approach loosely adhered to scripted questions
- Standardized, open-ended interview based on scripted questions
- Closed, quantitative interview with preset questions and answers from which the respondents have to choose. This format is good for quantifying the data, but it forces the interviewee to fit his or her experiences with the selection of answers and this may distort reality.

Observations are another fundamental tool in qualitative and critical-theory research, such as ethnography and action research. Observations can help to identify and establish the conditions of a given situation or topic. They can provide evidence of quantitative *facts* and/or *behaviours*. Interpretations by the researcher should be noted immediately or soon after an observation if any are to be made. It is important that interpretations are not confused with *fact* in the noting process. Self-awareness and reflection are important throughout the data collection process.

Observations allow for greater flexibility, interest, and creativity than other tools of data collection, such as tests or questionnaires. Anything can happen in a real-world context. For example, one may witness an event only once and yet it should still be included in the analysis. Unlike in physical sciences research, where one is looking for reproducibility, social research allows for a more dynamic approach to understanding the world.

There are four types of observer as described by Gold[8] and cited by Cohen and colleagues:[4] the complete participant; the participant as observer; the observer as participant; complete observer. Observing should not be a random process but instead one undertaken with predetermined foci and direction.

Role play by the researcher requires insight, behavioural change, and to some extent, empathy. As a data collection tool it is not as well-known but it is a useful technique for gaining insight into how people react to certain social environments, for example, useful in an ethnographic study. It can also be used to encourage individuals to change their behaviour, values, perceptions, and attitudes in a certain way[21].

Evaluation

Evaluation, according to Johnson,[9] focuses on the appraisal of the programme or process, and reflection on practice and in practice are central in the analytical stage. The focus of an evaluation (Table 4.4) can be elicited through direct talk, interviews, and questionnaires. The latter are one of the most important tools in a researcher's toolkit, and not only for this methodology. A questionnaire allows the researcher to collect information without being present and can be distributed widely to generate large quantities of data. A good questionnaire format can be tricky to develop and will take time to construct.

It is critical that a questionnaire is piloted before being administered. A simple mistake in a question's wording, such as omitting to state 'select the *best* answer' when there is more than one correct answer. This oversight can result in respondents ticking more than one box in a check-box answer format, resulting in difficult data interpretation and poor reliability in data analysis.

Cohen and colleagues[4] have adapted Sellitz and colleagues' 19-point guide list when constructing a research questionnaire:
- Question content
- Question wording
- Responding to the question
- Question order and sequence
- Action research

Action research

Action research is a good methodology for individuals directly involved with their environment of study. It is a practical tool that can be used to improve local conditions and situations. Action research is a collaborative effort and requires an understanding of both the researcher's own practice as well as the practice of others. Continuous, constructive self-reflection is critical.

Case studies are another method often employed within action research. Some methods of data collection within a case study include documentation, interview, observation, and analysis of artefacts. Figure 4.5 represents the relationship between a situation or problem and using reflection to seek and apply solutions.

Ideology critique

Johnson[9] depicts this methodology as asking 'questions that may be considered too self-evident to be put into question, encouraging critical engagement with ideological claims. It attempts to look beneath the obvious and self-evident in order to examine contradictions and counter arguments and claims.' Handled effectively, this methodology could underpin such research with the academic rigour necessary to substantiate the research findings.

Biographical narrative

Personal accounts, current or past, provide the researcher with insight into the situation and may reveal some root causes of a problem because this anecdotal but nonetheless qualitative evidence documents the participant's perspective. Narrative is a flexible methodology that can provide evidence missed by any other data-harvesting approach. Discourse analysis should be undertaken bearing in mind the effect of the participant bias of the data.

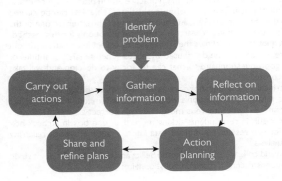

Figure 4.5 The cyclic actions of action research.[11]

Reproduced from Jordan J, Perry E, Bevins S. Is anyone listening? Action Research and Science Teacher Voice. *Education in Science* April 2011, pp. 12–13, with kind permission of Julie Jordan.

What to do with the data gathered

As this stage of the research process is as yet some way in the future, only a brief overview of a few strategies and tools to interrogate and interpret the data gathered is offered. Knowing what can be done with and to the data while selecting the methodologies to be used helps to focus the preparation of tools such as interview and questionnaire questions so that they will be compatible with the analytical tools.

Quantitative data can be 'crunched' and subjected to numerous statistical tests mentioned earlier in the chapter with which a healthcare worker from a traditional science background will be both familiar and comfortable. These test outcomes will be used to provide the evidence to reject the null hypothesis and present the hypothesis as a fact underpinned by the research itself.

Qualitative data comprises a range of evidence, much of which is subjective and anecdotal. These data can be quantified using NVIVO and SPSS software. Both these programmes use a system of coding, which can again lead to further subjectivity, depending on the nature of the methodology utilized. The programmes present the data in tabulated, graphic, and nodal formats that will facilitate interrogation and interpretation. These graphic representations of the findings will be more accessible to the novice social researcher and the audience to whom these will be presented.

Other forms of data representation include concept (mind) mapping and Ishikawa or fish-bone diagrams to identify cause and effect[10] as presented in Figure 4.6. Ishikawa diagrams can be used to represent data and help the researcher drill down into data to identify root causes of the situation (taken from ✒ www.project-management-skills.com/fishbone-diagram.html).

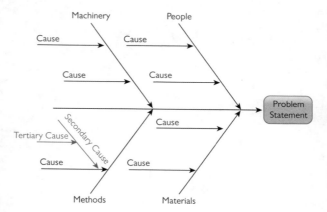

Figure 4.6 An outline of an Ishikawa diagram (taken from
✒ www.project-management-skills.com/fishbone-diagram.html).

Regardless of the original answers the researcher derived for the ontological, epistemological, and methodological questions, or the research paradigm followed, the data will present the researcher with a conclusion. Whether that conclusion is what was hoped for, expected or an antithesis thereof, the researcher needs to present these data to the audience to explain what has been ascertained.

This penultimate stage of the research process requires that all decisions pertaining to the methodological approach and criteria (reliability, replicability, and validity of the method and data) need to be succinctly presented and justified in a systematic review. The rigour of the written work is crucial, particularly if the findings will be presented as a grounded theory in induction mode, true to the interpretivist research paradigm. Wallace and Poulson[19] provide an insightful introduction to writing in the genre of social and educational research

The paper written and/or presented will need to defend every stage of the process succinctly and rigorously to convince sceptics of the validity of the research findings and their value as a socially constructed instrument to address and/or understand the situation/problem.

Ultimately, the social researcher, novice or experienced, exists within a socially constructed world wherein he or she is continually confronted by situations that can best be addressed by social research, usually most effectively through a mixed-methods approach.

References

1. Adelman C, Kemmis S, Jenkins D. Rethinking case study: notes from the Second Cambridge Conference, in H Simons (ed.), *Towards a Science of the Singular*. Centre for Applied Research in Education, University of East Anglia, Norwich, 45–61, in Cohen L, Manion L, and Morrison K *Research Methods in Education* 7th edn. London: Routledge, 2011.
2. Broom A, Willis E. Competing paradigms and health care research, in M Saks and J Allsop (eds) *Researching Health: Qualitative, Quantitative and Mixed Methods*. London: Sage, 2007, 16–31.
3. Bryman A. *Social Research Methods*, 4th edn. Oxford: Oxford University Press, 2012.
4. Cohen L, Manion L, Morrison K. *Research Methods in Education*, 7th edn. London: Routledge, 2011.
5. Cook DA. Randomised controlled trials and meta-analysis in medical education: What role do they play? *Medical Teacher*. Early Online 2012;1-6 doi: 10.3109/0142159X.2012.671978.
6. Fishbein M, Ajzen I. Belief, attitude, intention and behaviour: an introduction to theory and research. Reading, MA: Addison-Welsey, 1975.
7. Gergen K, Gergen M. Social Construction and Research Methodology, in W Outhwaite and SP Turner (eds), *The SAGE Handbook of Social Science Methodology*. London: Sage Publications, 461–78.
8. Gold RL. Roles in sociological field observations. *Social Forces* 1958; 36(3):217–23.
9. Johnson J. Deciding paradigms and methodologies, in J Oversby (ed.). *ASE Guide to Research in Science Education*. Hatfield: Association for Science Education, 2012a, 189–99.
10. Johnson J. Analysing data, in J Oversby (ed.), *ASE Guide to Research in Science Education* Hatfield: Association for Science Education, 2012b,189–99.
11. Jordan J, Perry E, Bevins S. Is anyone listening? Action Research and Science Teacher Voice. *Education in Science* April 2011, pp.12–13.
12. Kvale S. *Interviews*. London: Sage Publications, 1996.
13. Miller RL, Brewer JD (eds). *The A–Z of Social Research*. London: Sage Publications, 2003.
14. Oversby J (ed.). *ASE Guide to Research in Science Education*. Hatfield: Association for Science Education, 2012.
15. Newby P. *Research Methods for Education*. London: Pearson-Longman, 2010.
16. Robson C. *Real World Research: A Resource for Users of Social Research Methods in Applied Settings*, 3rd edn. Chichester: John Wiley & Sons, 2011.

17. Tritter J. Mixed methods and multidisciplinary research in health care in M Saks, J Allsop (eds). *Researching Health: Qualitative, Quantitative and Mixed Methods*. London: Sage Publications, 2007, 301–18.

18. Verschuren PJM. Case study as a research strategy: Some ambiguities and opportunities. *International Journal of Research Methodology* 2003; 6 (2):121–39.

19. Wallace M, Poulson L. Critical reading for self-critical writing, in M Wallace and L Poulson (eds). *Learning to read critically in Educational Leadership and Management*. London: Sage Publications, 2003.

20. Yin RK. *Case Study Research: Design and Methods*, 3rd edn. Applied Social Research Methods Series, Volume 5. London: Sage Publications, 2003.

21. Bolton GM, Heathcote D. *So You Want to Use Role-Play? A New Approach in How to Plan*. Stoke on Trent, UK: Trentham Books, 1999.

Further reading

Cooper HM. *Research Synthesis and Meta-evaluation: A Step-by-Step Approach*. Thousand Oaks, CA: Sage, 2010.

Mackie JL. Causes and conditions. In E Sosa and M Tooley (eds), *Causation*. Oxford: Oxford University Press, 1993, 33–55.

Marshall C, Rossman GB. *Designing Qualitative Research*. Newbury Park, CA: Sage, 1995.

Chapter 5

Navigating research methods: evidence-based medicine (EBM)

What is EBM and how is it relevant?

Evidence-based medicine arose from what can be considered a cognitive itch and has evolved into an entire cause or movement. The basis for this is the gradual realization that doctors are not demigods and they can make mistakes. Decisions can have high stakes and a single *faux pas* could be fatal. It is interesting that this change in perception by the medical fraternity is somewhat behind that of public opinion. Ask the average person on the street what he or she thinks about evidence-based practice and you're likely to elicit a puzzled response: 'well, what on earth were previous clinical decisions based on?' Good question indeed, and one that we are still trying to answer. What does all of this mean in practice? Well, it translates to applying best research evidence to populations or individual patients.

- From cognitive hunch to movement
  - Humans are not perfect
  - Scientific knowledge increases but medical decisions can have very high stakes
  - Mistakes are costly and can be fatal
  - Moral obligation to first do no harm
- Changing perceptions of the physician vs public
  - What were previous decisions based on?
  - Where was the evidence?
- Defining practices
  - Conscientious and judicious use of current best evidence from research in managing patients

Evolution, EBM, and seven honest men

Turning the time machine back some centuries, illness was looked upon by some as a curse, and treatments such as trephination or drilling holes in the skull were used to let out evil spirits. The code of Hammurabi, the sixth Amorite king of Babylon, for instance, meant that surgeons who made mistakes would lose their hands. However, even from those historic times doctors practised advanced surgery and they had developed pharmacopoeia, whilst Hippocrates laid down the principles of medical ethics. Despite their distance from us in terms of both historical time and geographical location, our medical predecessors all had one thing in common: the employment of seven honest men to further their quest: what? where? when? who? why? how? and how much? These were the earliest seeds of evidence-based medicine. However, the intellectual and moral conception of EBM occurred over two centuries ago when Thomas Beddoes implored Sir Joseph Banks to encourage data sharing, archiving, analysis, and publication in the interest of patients. This was complemented decades later when Pierre Louis performed the first recorded outcomes research and introduced numerical methods and clinical evaluation to give rise to the systematic approach of EBM. The Galashiels-born epidemiologist, Cochrane, began a movement encouraging evidence-based practice. Cochrane's work continues to expand through the eponymous centres and collaborations still extant. Interestingly, however, the term EBM itself was first coined by Eddy and published by the McMaster group two and a half decades ago.

Professor Archie Cochrane (1909–88)
- 1972 published *Effectiveness and Efficiency*
- Advocacy of evidence-based practice
- Cochrane centres and collaboration

David Sackett, Gordon Guyatt, and David Eddy
- Sackett and Guyatt developed explicit methodologies to determine best evidence
- EBM as a term first used by Eddy in 1990 and published by Guyatt and colleagues in 1992

In a discussion between White and Cochraine, the two giants of epidemiology, less than 10% of healthcare was grounded in hard evidence just three decades ago. We are not much better off today, able to justify only perhaps one-quarter of our practices, but research plays an important role in continuing to strengthen the evidence base upon which rests current clinical and healthcare practices.

From time to time we all tend to plea ignorance. However, it is individual ignorance where the liability is highest, whilst collective ignorance may be a shortcoming of the EBM process.

Patients and the public still have an unbending faith in expert opinion. However, the ex-cathedra statements of experts have been debated by Noyes as long as a century and a half ago and EBM approaches this area with caution.

> 'In every subject of scientific study the progress of investigation and the accumulation of knowledge must reach a point where it becomes a serious task to master all its facts or to be acquainted with all that has been written about it. When a great number of zealous observers are bending their energies in a common pursuit, it happens after a time that not the oldest and most eminent among them can possibly attain to a perfect acquaintance with all that is known about it.'

Dr Noyes (1856)

EBM today utilizes a mixed box of tools taken from science, engineering, and statistics aiming to treat through valid guidelines or facilitate individual decisions based on evidence. The business of evaluating studies ranges from the very human journal club to highly sophisticated IT-driven data mining.
- Uses science, engineering, and statistical techniques
  - Meta-analysis
  - Risk-benefit analysis
  - Randomized controlled trials (RCTs)
  - Other well-designed studies
- Treats patients using most valid scientific literature
  - EBG (evidence-based guidelines)—guidelines, policy, and regulations
  - EBID (evidence-based individual decisions)—individual decisions (concerns about EBID are greater than for EBG)
- Evaluates the best studies on specific topics
  - Journal clubs—human-centric
  - Data mining—automated

The logic behind taking an evidence-based approach is quite simple. The approach seeks to convert problems into answerable questions, looking at the population, intervention, comparisons, and outcomes. The ultimate product of information analysis ought to eventually make itself known and the best example of this is the published paper.

However, just as some of George Orwell's animals are more equal than others, evidence too is differential in value and the Oxford Centre for EBM defines this continuum ranging from RCTs and other large studies, to unchallenged expert opinion, as presented in the hierarchy of evidence in Chapter 1.

Critical appraisal of studies is a good starting point, focusing particularly on results and their application potential. Clinical effectiveness is another key area underpinned by evidence and guidelines at one end, and change and its evaluation at the other.

For the clinical researcher it is imperative to appraise any meta-analytic data critically, keeping in mind that only one-quarter of all data are available online, individual studies in meta-analyses can sometimes be small and lack comparability (perhaps cleverly woven together using an I statistic), negative studies may be unpublished, and similar RCTs cannot just be 'averaged out' in terms of treatment effect. In addition, evidence-based measurements can help prioritize tests, evaluate their diagnostic capacity, and make them clinically meaningful.

Meta-analysis
- Research findings may be contradictory
- Pooling can increase weight of evidence
- Critically appraise meta-analyses
  - Breadth of search strategy (comparability of the results across the studies included, i.e. inclusion of positive and negative results)
  - Direction of results (10 positive and 5 negative RCTs)
  - Size of individual studies (small = caution)

Measurements
- Likelihood ratios to prioritize tests
- Area under curve, receiver operating curve (AUC-ROC) = sensitivity–specificity ratio of tests
- Number needed to treat (NNT) to make tests clinically meaningful

EBM is not without its fair share of dilemmas and criticism. It can be difficult to navigate over 2 million papers per annum. Whilst EBM is considered a gold standard, many practices lack literature and RCTs may not always be ethical or even reflect reality. Ethnic minorities and the elderly remain under-researched and there can be considerable skews in funding priorities. The introduction of EBM into medical insurance claims further obscures the picture and often we are left asking whether it is scientific rigour, truth, or patient benefit that is most important.

Why use EBM? Any opportunity for patient benefit or empowerment can be useful. EBM produces open-minded sceptics who will hopefully make good use of public funds. If nothing else, EBM has greatly improved our reading habits!

Further reading

Davidoff F, Haynes B, Sackett D, et al. Evidence based medicine. *BMJ* 1995;310:1085–6.
Griffiths M. Evidence based medicine. Must be applied critically. *BMJ* 1995;311:257.
Oxman AD, Sackett DL, Guyatt GH. Users' guides to the medical literature. I. How to get started. The Evidence-Based Medicine Working Group. *JAMA* 1993;270:2093–5.
Rosenberg W, Donald A. Evidence based medicine: an approach to clinical problem-solving. *BMJ* 1995;310:1122–6.

Chapter 6

Navigating research methods: critical appraisal

Introduction

Definition

Critical appraisal is the process of systematically evaluating research to judge its usefulness and validity in a given context. Critical appraisal provides a systematic framework to appraising evidence and assessing its quality, taking into consideration the relevance of research, its internal validity, applicability, and the results and main conclusions drawn from it. It forms an integral part of evidence-based practice and is essential in assisting clinical decision making and guiding clinical practice in view of the vast scientific literature available.

Checklists

To date, there is no gold-standard tool for conducting critical appraisal. Nevertheless, a number of checklists have been developed which provide a useful framework for appraising research. These checklists are specific to the type of research examined (qualitative or quantitative) and the study design, and include guidelines for evaluating:
- randomized controlled trials
- systematic review
- cohort studies
- case-control studies
- surveys

Checklists generally begin with a set of standard questions that can be used to appraise evidence regardless of study methodology. These standard questions are often organized around the four main sections found in research papers: introduction, methods, results, and discussion (Table 6.1). Using these questions can help extract important information and can provide the basis for evaluating the quality of research.

Table 6.1 Standard checklist

Question	Relevant section of paper
Is the study relevant to a key question?	Title, abstract
Why was the study done?	Introduction
How was the study done? Internal validity	Methods
What are the main findings?	Results
What are the implications of the findings?	Abstract, discussion
External validity	Introduction, discussion
What else is of interest?	

Screening questions

A further two sets of questions can then be used to evaluate the quality of the evidence (Table 6.2). These sets of questions are specific to study design and methodology and are generally divided into two question types: screening questions and detailed questions. Screening questions are used to identify papers that are relevant to one's research topic. This is achieved by asking the following questions:

- Does the research address a clearly focused research question?
  Research should be focused in terms of the population studied, the intervention given, and the assessed outcomes.
- Was the type of study used appropriate? Consider the study design and whether it is appropriate to the research question.

Screening questions are important since a paper can be of little value if it does not address an important topic and if it does not add to current knowledge.

Table 6.2 Checklist for controlled trials

Section 1: Screening questions	
The study addresses a clearly focused question.	Yes No Not clear
The study is a randomized controlled trial.	Yes No Not clear

IF the answer to both of the above questions is YES, then complete Section 2 of the checklist. Otherwise state reason for rejection:
1. Paper not relevant to key question ☐
2. Other reason ☐ (please specify):

Section 2a: Detailed questions (internal validity)		
1.	Subjects were randomized to treatment groups.	Yes No Not clear
2.	Subjects and investigators are kept 'blind' about treatment allocation.	Yes No Not clear
3.	The study had an appropriate sample size and power calculations are provided.	Yes No Not clear
4.	The treatment and control groups are similar at the start of the trial.	Yes No Not clear

Table 6.2 (*Contd.*)

5.	The treatment and control groups are followed up and data collected in a similar way.	Yes No Not clear
6.	All relevant outcomes are measured in a standard, valid and reliable way.	Yes No Not clear
7.	What percentage of the individuals or clusters recruited into each treatment arm of the study dropped out before the study was completed?	Yes No Not clear
8.	All the subjects are analysed in the groups to which they were randomly allocated (often referred to as intention to treat analysis).	Yes No Not clear
9.	Where the study is carried out at more than one site, results are comparable for all sites.	Yes No Not clear

Section 2b: Detailed questions (external validity)

1.	What are the overall findings of the review?
2.	Could these results be due to chance?
3.	What are the implications of this study for practice?
4.	Are the conclusions justified?
5.	Are the results of this study directly applicable to the patient group targeted by this guideline?

Detailed questions

Studies that fulfil the requirement of the screening section can undergo more in-depth assessment using the detailed questions. These address two important aspects of a study: internal and external validity.

- Is the research internally valid? Questions are often centred around how well the research has been conducted and what measures were undertaken to reduce bias. Assessing internal validity helps establish the extent to which results from the research reflect the true results taking into account study design and methodology.
- Is the research externally valid? This helps clarify the extent to which the results from the study can be generalized or are applicable to the targeted population group.

Based on the internal and external validity of research, it is possible to identify high-quality studies that can potentially guide clinical practice and influence decision making (Tables 6.3, 6.4, 6.5, 6.6).

Table 6.3 Checklist for systematic reviews and meta-analyses controlled trials

Section 1: Screening questions	
The study addresses a clearly focused question.	Yes No Not clear
The study is a systematic review or meta-analysis.	Yes No Not clear
The review includes studies that address the review's question and that have an appropriate study design.	Yes No Not clear

IF the answer to the above questions is YES, then complete Section 2 of the checklist. Otherwise state reason for rejection:
1. Paper not a systematic review/meta-analysis ☐
2. Paper not relevant to key question ☐
3. Other reason ☐ (please specify):

Section 2a: Detailed questions (internal validity)	
1. A description of the methodology used is included.	Yes No Not clear
2. The literature search is sufficiently rigorous to identify all the relevant studies.	Yes No Not clear
3. Study quality is assessed and taken into account.	Yes No Not clear
4. There are enough similarities between the studies selected to make combining them reasonable.	Yes No Not clear

Section 2b: External validity and applicability
1. What are the overall findings of the review?
2. Could these results be due to chance?
3. What are the implications of this review for practice?
4. Were all important outcomes considered?
5. Are the conclusions justified?

Table 6.4 Checklist for cohort studies

Section 1: Screening questions	
The study addresses a clearly focused question.	Yes No Not clear
The study is a cohort study.	Yes No Not clear

IF the answer to the above questions is YES, then complete Section 2 of the checklist. Otherwise state reason for rejection:
1. Paper not a cohort study ☐
2. Paper not relevant to key question ☐
3. Other reason ☐ (please specify):

Section 2a: Detailed questions (internal validity)	
Sample selection	
1. The cohort is representative of a defined population (selection bias).	Yes No Not clear
2. Sample size is justified.	Yes No Not clear
3. Response rates are provided.	Yes No Not clear
4. Differences between respondents and non-respondents are considered.	Yes No Not clear
Assessment	
5. The outcome is accurately measured to minimize measurement or classification bias.	Yes No Not clear
6. The exposure is accurately measured to minimize measurement or classification bias.	Yes No Not clear
7. Adequate follow-up.	Yes No Not clear
8. Comparison is made between subjects who completed the study and those who were lost to follow-up.	Yes No Not clear

Table 6.4 (*Contd.*)

Confounding		
9. All important confounding factors are identified.	Yes	
	No	
	Not clear	
10. Potential confounders are considered in the design and/or analysis.	Yes	
	No	
	Not clear	

Statistical analysis		
11. A description of the statistical methods is provided.	Yes	
	No	
	Not clear	
12. The estimates of risk are precise and confidence intervals are provided.	Yes	
	No	
	Not clear	
13. Bradford Hills criteria are considered.	Yes	
	No	
	Not clear	

Section 2b: External validity and applicability
1. What are the overall findings of the study?
2. Could these results be due to confounding?
3. What are the implications of this study for practice?
4. Are the conclusions justified?

Table 6.5 Checklist for case-control studies

Section 1: Screening questions	
The study addresses a clearly focused question.	Yes No Not clear
The study is a case-control study.	Yes No Not clear

IF the answer to the above questions is YES, then complete Section 2 of the checklist. Otherwise state reason for rejection:
1. Paper not a case-control study ☐
2. Paper not relevant to key question ☐
3. Other reason ☐ (please specify):

Section 2a: Detailed questions (internal validity)	
Sample selection	
1. The cases/controls are representative of a defined population (selection bias).	Yes No Not clear
2. The cases/controls are defined precisely using an appropriate inclusion and exclusion criteria.	Yes No Not clear
3. Sample size is justified.	Yes No Not clear
4. Response rates are provided.	Yes No Not clear
5. Differences between respondents and non-respondents are considered.	Yes No Not clear
6. Cases are either matched, population-based, or randomly selected.	Yes No Not clear
7. There is a sufficient number of cases and controls.	Yes No Not clear
Assessment	
8. The exposure was accurately measured to minimize measurement or classification bias.	Yes No Not clear

Table 6.5 (*Contd.*)

Confounding	
9. All important confounding factors are identified.	Yes No Not clear
10. Potential confounders are considered in the design and/or analysis.	Yes No Not clear

Statistical analysis	
11. A description of the statistical methods is provided.	Yes No Not clear
12. Estimates or risk are precise. Consider p-values and potential confounders.	Yes No Not clear

Section 2b: External validity and applicability
1. What are the overall findings of the review?
2. Could these results be due to confounding?
3. What are the implications of this study for practice?
4. Are the conclusions justified?

Table 6.6 Checklist for cross-sectional studies

Section 1: Screening questions	
The study addresses a clearly focused question.	Yes No Not clear
The study is a cross-sectional study.	Yes No Not clear

IF the answer to the above questions is YES, then complete Section 2 of the checklist. Otherwise state reason for rejection:
1. Paper not a cross-sectional study ☐
2. Paper not relevant to key question ☐
3. Other reason ☐ (please specify):

(*continued*)

Table 6.6 (Contd.)

Section 2a: Detailed questions (internal validity)	
Sample selection	
1. The study sample is representative of a defined population (selection bias).	Yes No Not clear
Assessment	
2. The outcome is accurately measured to minimize measurement or classification bias.	Yes No Not clear
3. The exposure was accurately measured to minimize measurement or classification bias.	Yes No Not clear
Confounding	
4. All important confounding factors are identified,	Yes No Not clear
5. Potential confounders are considered in the design and/or analysis,	Yes No Not clear
Statistical analysis	
6. A description of the statistical methods is provided,	Yes No Not clear
7. The estimates of risk are precise and confidence intervals are provided,	Yes No Not clear
Section 2b: External validity and applicability	
1. What are the overall findings of the review?	
2. Could these results be due to confounding?	
3. What are the implications of this study for practice?	
4. Are the conclusions justified?	

Tables 6.2–6.6 have been adapted from the CASP and SIGN critical appraisal check-lists.

Further reading

Hill A, Spittlehouse C. *What is critical appraisal?* Cambridge: Hayward Group Ltd, 2009.
Crombie IK. *The pocket guide to critical appraisal.* London: BMJ Publishing Group, 2003.

Navigating research methods: clinical audit

Why audit?

Audits are implemented to ensure that quality standards are met in the provision of patient care. This could include assessing the structure, process, and outcome of therapeutic intervention(s) and other aspects that contribute to patient care. Audits should be transparent and focus on improving patient care and safety.

Purpose of an audit:
- To review and improve the standards of patient care and the outcomes by identifying deficiencies so they can be addressed.
- To contribute to the professional and educational development of those concerned with patient safety and care.
- To initiate the development of evidence- and research-based practice.
- To contribute to risk and resource management.

Audits can cover a wide variety of areas and are not limited solely to actual medical interventions. Some examples include:
- Accuracy of diagnosis
- Appropriateness of treatment regimes
- Quality of referral letters
- Timeliness of interventions
- Type and quality of information given to participants

An excellent resource for conducting an audit is the NICE Principles for Best Practice in Clinical Audit, released in 2002.

Does it make a difference?

There is some debate regarding the effectiveness of conducting an audit, since this measure is not itself supported by an evidence base. However, when done effectively, a well-defined audit can contribute to improvements in clinical practice. Evaluation is essential to measuring practices. When the correct procedures of an audit cycle are implemented, the results have the potential to affect the hospital setting positively and improve patient care and safety.

The audit cycle

Although there are many different resources that can be used when completing the audit cycle, all generally rely on the same methodology and general process. Before beginning an audit it is important to consult the audit team in your facility to ensure you are following the steps as specifically outlined by the team. The steps listed are a general overview and will prompt some of the questions you need to consider throughout the process. Your local audit team is usually an excellent resource and is best consulted in the early stages of audit planning.

Step 1: Identify the problem
- What is the purpose of the audit?
- What problem do you aim to address? Why?
- What measure are you considering to address this problem?
- Has an audit been conducted in this area before? In your hospital?
- Who are the main people to consult for this problem?
- Is this problem a priority in your organization?

Step 2: Define the standard
- Where can you find clinical guidelines relating to your problem?
- What are the standards for your chosen measure?
- What standards have been used if this audit was previously conducted? Have these standards changed/been updated?

Step 3: Collecting data
- Can you use an existing audit questionnaire? If yes:
- Was it conducted in your hospital?
- Is it relevant to your hospital?
- Is it up to date?
- Will you be able to compare your results to the results from the previous audit?

If you need to develop a questionnaire:
- Is more than one question needed to obtain the required information?
- Can the respondents understand the questions?
- Are the questions unambiguous?
- Is the format easy to follow?
- Is the response you want clear (i.e. yes/no)?
- Is the question open to interpretation?
- Do you have any leading questions (these should be avoided)?
- Have you used negative terms which may be confusing?
- Have you piloted the questionnaire? On whom?
- Has this been reviewed by the audit team?
- How will you analyse this data?
- Have you ensured that the analysis plan is in place before the questionnaire is delivered?
- Have you streamlined the data? For example, including several open-ended questions will increase the time required for analysis, potentially without necessarily gaining new information.

Step 4: Analysing data

- Have you followed your analysis plan? Did it work?
- How do your results compare to the standards?
- Can you compare this to any other audits? If so, how does it compare?
- When conducting statistical analysis, achieving statistical significance from a research perspective may not always be possible. Although the results may not have statistical significance, they may still be clinically significant.

Step 5: Improving practice

- What are your key findings?
- What limitations did you find in the data which can be used to improve the re-audit?
- Who should you discuss these key findings with before wider dissemination? (Generally this includes anyone who was involved in the audit process, or will be affected by the changes.)
- After these discussions, how will you disseminate the findings? Possibilities include:
  - Posters
  - Dedicated seminars to present results
  - Adding into existing seminars
- Remember, this is not a name, blame, or shame game! All involved should work together towards improving patient care and safety.

Step 6: Sustainability and re-audit

- How will you continue the dissemination?
- Have you followed up on discussions with key people to see if changes have been implemented/had an impact? How often?
- The audit cycle can be seen as a spiral as it is a continuous process which builds upon its results for a sustained impact. The spiral process drives the audit to a higher level of quality.

What if there are no standards?

- Use the best-practice model to follow the safest clinical methods.
- For subjects that do not have a best-practice model, aim to follow the safest clinical standards

Points to consider

Feasibility

- Do you have the capacity to complete an effective audit?
- Have you gained approvals from the relevant groups in your hospital?
- Will you pilot the audit and then expand based on impact?
- Based on quantity of data, will you have time to analyse the data, or should you limit the size of the audit? It is better to do a small audit well rather than collecting too much data which is too difficult to analyse.
- Will this audit have a direct impact on your patient care and safety in the hospital? If not, why are you conducting the audit?

Validity
- Do you know exactly what you want to measure?
- Does your audit measure what it is supposed to measure?
- Based on reading your questionnaire, what do others think your audit is measuring? Does this match what you think it is measuring?
- Have the tools used in the audit been calibrated correctly?

Reliability
- Are you consistently measuring what you plan to measure?
- How will you add consistency in data collection? This is particularly important when more than one person is involved in data collection.

Sensitivity
- Is your measure sensitive enough?
- How do you know that you have chosen the correct and most sensitive measure to address your problem?

Writing the report
Introduction
- This will mainly be based on step 1 of the audit cycle.
- What is the problem? Why does it need to be addressed?
- Why is an audit the best approach?
- What measure are you using? Why?
- What standards will you use?

Methodology
- This will mainly incorporate steps 2 and 3 of the audit cycle.
- Where was the audit conducted? (hospital, ward, etc.)
- How many people, wards, etc. were audited?
- Who was involved in the audit process?
- How was the questionnaire developed? Provide a copy of the questionnaire as a table or appendix.
- How was the data collected?
- Who collected the data? (One or more people?)
- What was the time frame for data collection?
- What methods did you use to analyse the data? (Step 4)
- How have you ensured that the audit is reproducible?

Audit findings
- How many people/wards were audited?
- What did you find?
- Be sure to make use of graphs, tables as appropriate (visual representations of data are important for dissemination, but should not be misleading) (Step 5).

Recommendations and re-audit
- How do your results compare with the standards?
- Have you identified any good practice?
- Have you identified any room for group improvement? Be specific and realistic.
- Have you identified any room for individual improvement? Be specific and realistic.

- Have you identified some potential barriers to change?
- How will you use these audit results?
- Have you created an action plan for implementation of change with a realistic timeline?
- How will you follow up to ensure your actions have had an impact?
- When should the re-audit be conducted?
- Should any changes be made to the audit before the re-audit?

References and the Appendix should include all applicable references and any documents which are necessary to reproduce the audit.

Acknowledgements: acknowledge the contributions of all relevant hospital departments and individuals involved in the audit.

Clinical audit vs clinical research

Clinical research aims to identify an unknown factor which may have an impact on patient safety and care. Clinical audits are conducted when the treatment is known and we want to compare a specific location (hospital, ward, etc.) to the standards/guidelines (Table 7.1). Clinical research asks 'what is the right thing to do?' while a clinical audit asks 'are we doing the right thing the right way?' Table 7.2 and Figures 7.1 and 7.2 represent the sources of useful information for various aspects of clinical audit.

Table 7.1 Differences between clinical audit and clinical research

	Clinical audit	Clinical research
Ethical approval	No (only approval from the audit team)	Yes
Null hypothesis	No	Yes
Power calculation	No	Yes
Statistical analysis	Yes	Yes
Results apply beyond the patients used	No	Yes
Duration	Ongoing and continuous	May be one-off
Collection of new data	No (usually via patient records and follow-up)	Yes

Table 7.2 Sources of useful information

Question	Likely source
Where can I go to find clinical guidelines?	NICE, National Electronic Library, Health Guidelines Database, National Guideline Clearinghouse (USA) SIGN
Where can I go to find criteria for clinical audit?	Clinical guidelines, performance indicators
Where can I go to find service standards?	National Service Frameworks National Centre for Health Outcomes Development Specialist Health Services Commission for Wales (SHSCW)
Which organizations have information about clinical audit?	Royal Colleges and other professional bodies
Where can I find examples of clinical audits?	Bibliographic databases
Where else can I go to get advice?	Newsgroups and other quality improvement networks

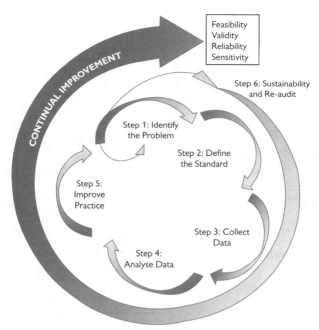

Feasibility
Validity
Reliability
Sensitivity

CONTINUAL IMPROVEMENT

Step 6: Sustainability
and Re-audit

Step 1: Identify
the Problem

Step 2: Define
the Standard

Step 5:
Improve
Practice

Step 3: Collect
Data

Step 4:
Analyse Data

Figure 7.1 Spiral diagram of the clinical audit process.

Setting standards and finding the evidence

Clinical guidelines
- *NICE*
- SIGN

Systematic reviews
- Cochrane Library
- Clinical Evidence
- Centre for Reviews and Dissemination
- Health Evidence Bulletins

Service standards
- National Service Framework
- National Centres for Health Outcome Development

Organizations offering support
- Medical Royal College and other professional bodies
- Clinical Audit Associations

Discussion groups
- CHAIN
- Clinical audits
- Clinical governance group

Sharing the know-how

Quality improvement initiatives
- Beacons programme
- Innovation in Care programme
- Service delivery practice database
- Impact and Bandolier
- National Primary Care Collaborative
- CLIP database

Clinical governance
- Clinical Governance Research and Development unit
- NHS Clinical Governance Support Team
- National Assembly for Wales Clinical Governance Support and Development Unit (CGSDU)
- Commission for Health Improvement
- WISDOM

Assessing the impact

Clinical audit assessment
- Health Service Management Centre, University of Birmingham

Finding further resources

Specialist gateways
- OMNI
- NMAP
- NeLH and its virtual Branch Libraries

Figure 7.2 Useful resources for clinical audits.

Further reading

Benjamin A. Audit: how to do it in practice. *BMJ* 2008;336(7655):1241–5.

NICE. *Nutrition support in adults: oral nutrition support, enteral tube feeding and parenteral nutrition*. Clinical Guideline 32. NICE, 2006.

Grimshaw JM, Shirran L, Thomas R, et al. Changing provider behavior: an overview of systematic reviews of interventions. *Med Care* 2001;39(8 Suppl 2):II2–45.

University of Dundee. *Clinical Audit & Research for Healthcare Professionals*. 2002. Unit 7 – Implementing Clinical Audit.

Setting the scene and ICH GCP in clinical and healthcare research

What is the purpose of good clinical practice (GCP)?

GCP is an international quality standard that should be followed when conducting clinical research to ensure that the rights and well-being of patients are protected and the resulting data are valid.

GCP has been coordinated across Japan, the USA, and Europe, setting out best practice and core principles.

Why do we need GCP?

There have been several disasters in the history of clinical research that have created the need for a standard in good clinical practice. Some of these include:

- Events resulting in the Nuremburg Code 1946
- Tuskegee Syphilis Study 1932–72
- Guatemala 1945
- Elixir of sulfanilamide 1937
- Thalidomide 1950s

History of research ethics and GCP

Nuremberg Code

A well-known chapter in the history of research with human subjects opened on 9 December 1946 when a US military tribunal took criminal proceedings against 23 leading German physicians and administrators for their willing participation in war crimes and crimes against humanity. Among the charges were that German physicians conducted medical experiments on thousands of concentration camp prisoners without their consent. Most of the subjects of these experiments died or were permanently disabled as a result. As a direct result of the trial, the Nuremberg Code was established in 1948 and stated that 'the voluntary consent of the human subject is absolutely essential', making it clear that subjects should give consent and that the benefits of research must outweigh the risks. Although it did not carry the force of law, the Nuremberg Code was the first international document which advocated voluntary participation and informed consent.

Tuskegee Syphilis Study (1932–72)

An equally well-known chapter in history occurred during a research project conducted in the US. Six hundred low-income African–American males in the Department of Corrections, 400 of whom were infected with syphilis, were monitored for 40 years. Free medical examinations were given, however subjects were not told they had syphyilis; instead they were told they had bad blood. The study looked at the course of the disease over time and did not treat the subjects for the disease even though a proven cure (penicillin) became available in the 1950s. The study continued until 1972 with participants being denied treatment. Many subjects died of syphilis during the study, which was stopped in 1973 when the details were published. In 1997, under mounting pressure, President Clinton apologized to the study subjects and their families.

Guatemala (1945)

In 2011, it was reported that further experiments were conducted by the US government in the 1940s in Guatemala. Fifteen hundred Guatemalans, including men, women, and children, were deliberately infected with syphilis and other sexually transmitted diseases to test the early antibiotic penicillin. Again, subjects were not informed of the study and did not give their consent.

Elixir of sulfanilamide (1937)

Sulfanilamide was an antimicrobial drug. In 1937, it was decided to make the formulation into a liquid preparation. The elixir required a dilutent and they found that diethylene glycol dissolved sulfanilamide. Diethylene glycol (or antifreeze) was a toxin and resulted in a large number of patient deaths from its therapeutic use. This disaster led to the Food and Drug Act being implemented in America in 1938 which required proof of safety before the release of a new drug.

Thalidomide (1950s)

In the late 1950s thalidomide was approved as a sedative in Europe. It was not approved in the US by the Food and Drug Administration (FDA). The drug was prescribed to control sleep and nausea throughout pregnancy but it was soon found that taking this drug during pregnancy caused severe deformities including phocomaelia (seal-like limbs) in the foetus. US Senate hearings followed and in 1962 the Kefauver Amendment to the Food, Drug and Cosmetic Act were passed into law to ensure drug efficacy and greater drug safety. For the first time, drug manufacturers were required to prove to the FDA and other authorities the effectiveness of their products before marketing them.

The ethical cornerstone of research

The Nuremberg Code led to the Declaration of Helsinki which forms the ethical cornerstone of medical research.

In 1964, the World Medical Association established recommendations guiding medical doctors in biomedical research involving human subjects. The Declaration governs international research ethics and defines rules for 'research combined with clinical care' and 'non-therapeutic research.' The Declaration of Helsinki was revised in 1975, 1983, 1989, 1996, 2000, 2008, and 2013, and is the basis for good clinical practice standards used today. There is debate about which version of the Declaration should be used. The European Directives refer to the 1996 version, the Clinical Trial Regulation refers to the 2008 version, while the US no longer refers to the Declaration at all. The problem centres around two paragraphs in the 2000 version concerning the use of placebo and providing continued treatment at the end of a clinical trial.

Further information regarding the Declaration of Helsinki can be found in Chapter 10.

International harmonization in good clinical practice

Disasters have shaped the history of GCP and led to its current identity and created worldwide changes to legislation. Between 1962 and the present, many changes were made in legislation, yet there is one standard that is truly seen as the global standard: ICH GCP (International Conference on Harmonisation of Good Clinical Practice).

The ICH process

ICH is a joint initiative involving both regulators and industry as equal partners in the scientific and technical discussions of the testing procedures that are required to ensure and assess the safety, quality, and efficacy of medicines. The focus of ICH is on new drugs, the majority of which are developed and marketed in Europe, Japan, and the US. Therefore, it was agreed that the scope would be confined to these three regions where more than 80% of all medicines are consumed.

During the 1960s, the pharmaceutical industry was becoming more international and seeking global markets but the registration of medicines remained a national responsibility. Although different regulatory systems were based on the same fundamental obligations to evaluate the quality, safety, and efficacy, the detailed technical requirements had diverged over time to such an extent that industry found it necessary to duplicate many time-consuming and expensive test procedures in order to market new products internationally. The urgent need to rationalize and harmonize regulation was impelled by concerns over rising costs of healthcare, escalation of the cost of research and development, and the need to meet the public expectation that there should be a minimum of delay in making safe and efficacious new treatments available to patients in need.

The three regions involved in the ICH process set up a steering committee consisting of two representatives from the regulatory authorities and the manufacturers of each regions. This committee then set up three expert working groups to look at quality, safety, and efficacy issues of research (Figure 8.1).

The steering group and expert working groups identified topics to be harmonized and a five-step process was put in place (Table 8.1).

Although there are only three expert working groups, the ICH topics are divided into four major categories and ICH topic codes are assigned according to these categories.

Q. Quality topics

- Product quality—stability, validation, pharmacopoeias, etc.
- Quality of the raw product

Examples:
Q1 Stability testing
Q9 Risk management

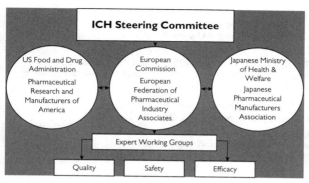

Figure 8.1 The ICH process.

Table 8.1 Five steps of the ICH guideline development	
Step 1	The committees set up working groups to write the drafts
Step 2	Drafts are reviewed by the Steering Committee and Committee for Proprietary Medicinal Products (CPMP)
Step 3	Drafts put out for consultation
Step 4	Final draft endorsed by CPMP and time frame for implementation established (please note that there can be several draft stages)
Step 5	The ICH guideline accepted into national framework (not laws)

S. Safety topics

- Toxicology, carcinogenicity, reproductive toxicology, etc.
- Safety of the raw product

Examples:
S1 Carcinogenicity testing
S2 Genotoxicity testing

E. Efficacy topics

- Details on how to conduct clinical research

Examples:
E2 Clinical safety data management
E4 Dose-response studies

It is the efficacy guidelines that affect clinical research.
- E2 Guideline for Expedited Reporting of AEs
- E3 Clinical Study Reports: Structure and Content
- E5 Ethic Factors in the Acceptability of Foreign Data
- E7 Clinical Trials in Special Populations—Geriatrics

- E8 General Considerations for Clinical Trials
- E9 Statistical Considerations
- E10 Choice of Control Groups
- E11 Clinical Trials in Children

ICH has existed for more than 20 years and the process it adopted continues. There are new guidelines being added; the latest E guidelines E15 and E16 relate to pharmagenomics.

M. Multidisciplinary

- Some topics did not fit into S, Q, or E

Examples:
M4 on the Common Technical Document
M5 to address the identified terminology differences

Box 8.1 (*Contd.*)

2.8

Each individual involved in conducting a trial should be qualified by education, training, and experience to perform his or her respective task(s).

2.9

Freely given informed consent should be obtained from every subject prior to clinical trial participation.

2.10

All clinical trial information should be recorded, handled, and stored in a way that allows its accurate reporting, interpretation, and verification.

2.11

The confidentiality of records that could identify subjects should be protected, respecting the privacy and confidentiality rules in accordance with the applicable regulatory requirement(s).

2.12

Investigational products should be manufactured, handled, and stored in accordance with applicable good manufacturing practice (GMP). They should be used in accordance with the approved protocol.

2.13

Systems with procedures that assure the quality of every aspect of the trial should be implemented.

The responsibilities

The main responsibilities are indicated in Box 8.2 and the guidelines assign each task to a single person. This clear line of responsibility also gives clear accountability within research roles. More detailed information regarding roles may be found in subsequent chapters of this book.

Box 8.2 The responsibilities of all involved in clinical research

Ethics committee
- Safeguarding rights, safety, and well-being of trial subjects
- Review of documentation provided by applicants
- Establish composition and function
- Establish clear procedures

Principal investigator (see Chapter 11 for details)
- Adequate medical care of trial subjects
- Overall responsibility for conduct of trial and compliance with protocol
- Informed consent
- Adequate resources producing reports

Chief investigator
- Overall responsibility for the design, conduct, and reporting of the study
- Responsible for his or her employees and through them to the sponsor
- Directly accountable to the care organization(s) where the research takes place

Sponsor (see Chapter 12 for details)
- Quality assurance and quality control systems
- Trial management and data handling
- Monitoring and audit
- Investigator selection
- Financing
- Safety information and reporting
- Investigational products
- Initiate and manage the study
- The sponsor is normally the chief investigator's employer alone or in collaboration with the care organization/university

---

Essential documentation

The last three chapters of ICH GCP E6 cover documentation (Box 8.3). Chapter 6 defines the requirement for a protocol. Chapter 7 defines the investigator brochure (IB). Chapter 8 discusses the essential documentation.

> **Box 8.3 Documentation**
> (see Chapter 22)
>
> **The protocol**
> The most essential document in a study is the protocol (detailed information is contained in Chapter 15). The protocol is a document that describes:
> - Objectives
> - Design
> - Methodology
> - Statistical considerations, and
> - Organization
> - Usually also gives the background and rationale of a study
>
> The content of the protocol should conform to:
>   ICH GCP Guideline, Chapter 6, 'Clinical Trial Protocol and Protocol Amendments'.
>   Most companies and institutions will have their own protocol templates in place.
>   The protocol must be clear, concise, and before use must receive ethics committee approval and regulatory authority approval where indicated.
>   Further considerations when writing a protocol can be found in Chapter 15 of this book.
>
> **Investigator brochure**
> Chapter 7 of ICH GCP E6 outlines the requirements of the investigator brochure (IB).
>   An investigator brochure is a compilation of the clinical and non-clinical data on the investigational medicinal product or products which are relevant to the study of the product or products in human subjects. This document is for investigators to aid their decision to undertake a trial or not.
>   The IB contains a description of possible risks and side effects, and must be updated regularly. It is essential that the most recent version is held at investigator site.

Box 8.3 (*Contd.*)

Essential documents

ICH GCP definition states: 'Essential Documents are those documents which individually and collectively permit evaluation of the conduct of the trial and the quality of the data produced. These documents serve to demonstrate the compliance of the Investigator, sponsor, and monitor with GCP and all applicable regulatory requirements'.

Chapter 8 of ICH GCP outlines the essential documentation and the purpose of the documents. It lists the documents needed before, during, and after a study and identifies the location where documents are needed: with the sponsor/investigator. Most documents have to be filed in **both** locations. There are some exceptions.

The following only appear in the *sponsor files.*

Pre-study

8.2.13	Sample of IP labels
8.2.16	Certificate of analysis of IP
8.2.18	Master randomization list
8.2.19	Pre-trial monitoring report

During study

8.3.9	Certificate of Analysis

After study

8.4.4	Audit certificate
8.4.5	Close-out monitoring report
8.4.6	Treatment allocation decode

The following only in the *investigator files.*

Pre-study

During study

8.3.12	Signed informed consents
8.3.13	Source documents
8.3.21	Subject ID list
8.3.22	Subject enrolment log

After study

8.4.3	Completed subject ID log
8.4.7	Report to EC/Regulatory authority

Any information with patient-identifiable information will remain in the investigator file only.

For how long should essential documents be kept?

ICH GCP states that documents should be kept for two years after the last marketing application in an ICH region. This was an undefined term. Some countries have legislative requirements for retention of essential documentation (e.g. EU GCP Directive for clinical trials in investigational medicinal products 2005/28/EC states that documents should be kept for five years after study completion). The Clinical Trials Regulation 536/2014 mandates 25 years after study completion. The protocol should define the timeline for documentation retention and should reflect the legislative requirements.

Archiving

Sponsors and investigators must archive essential documents. The archives must be secure and there should be restrictive access to named individuals. The sponsor files and the investigator files must be stored separately and the sponsor should not have access to the investigator's copy. The investigator's copy is the tamper-proof version of the data and may be inspected by the regulatory authorities to ensure that the data have not been manipulated or changed in any way by the sponsor.

Sponsors may utilize commercial archives to store data but they have to ensure that facilities meet requirements and have to audit the archives regularly to ensure conditions continue to be met.

Many investigators are also unable to archive on site due to shortage of space. Some also store data in commercial archives.

Investigator commercial archives

The investigator files must be stored securely in tamper-proof boxes. There must be a record of who is allowed access to the material. The sponsor should not have access to the data.

Whether or not documents are stored on or off site, the following must be considered:

- The facilities must be safe, secure, and acceptable conditions of temperature, humidity, and fire risk must be met

The off-site storage of investigator files may be arranged by the sponsor and the following procedures should be in place:

- Boxes should be sealed and over-signed by the investigator to witness the sealing
- Sealed boxes are not to be opened again unless in the presence of the investigator
- Boxes must be kept in a separate (third-party) location, not at the sponsor's location

Archived data must be kept for the appropriate time and must be made available for inspection even after the trial is completed.

ICH GCP and level of detail

ICH GCP is *not* detailed enough to explain how someone should do his or her job or how to comply with the requirements. It does not offer a solution to every problem. The guidelines had to harmonize practices in the US, Japan, and Europe, and are therefore written in an interpretative way.

How do institutions and companies implement ICH GCP? Where are the interpretations documented? Each institution or company has standard operating procedures (SOP) that document that institution or company's interpretation of the guideline.

Example question: 'In what time frame should the investigator report a serious adverse event (SAE) to the sponsor?' Many would answer: 'within 24 hours.'

The guideline is not that specific as it does not give a specified time interval. The guideline states 'immediately' which is interpreted to mean 'within 24 hours' by many institutions and companies. Some may have different criteria; for example, one working day. With the full implementation of the CT Regulation 536/2014 it will be a legal requirement to report within 24 hours.

It is the SOPs that define how a company operates within the ICH GCP guideline but these also incorporate legislative and local requirements.

ICH GCP resulted in the ability to conduct globalized studies through standardization. There is less duplication of research as regulatory authorities accept data from other countries. There is one standard for GCP, documentation, and the conduct of studies.

Worldwide legislation

Although ICH GCP is regarded as the worldwide standard, it operates alongside national legislation.

In the US, the Food and Drug Administration (FDA) has published the Code of Federal Registers (CFR). In Europe, the European Directives (2001/20/EC and 2005/28/EC) and the Clinical Trial Regulation (536/2014) give the legislative requirements for clinical trials in investigational medicinal products. In China, there is the SFDA, in India Schedule Y.

All have firm footing in ICH GCP which is to be followed no matter what research is being conducted.

Relevance of GCP principles in non-pharmaceutical/non interventional healthcare research

In the UK, pharmaceutical research or CTIMPs (clinical trials in investigational medicinal products) must always be conducted according to the principles of GCP and in compliance with EU legislation.

The principles and origins of GCP have been set out earlier in this chapter. As previously mentioned, these standards have been rolled out internationally so that there is harmonization across Japan, Europe, and the US in order to ensure that all research is conducted to GCP standard.

Non-pharmaceutical/non-interventional healthcare research has no legal requirements to adhere to ICH GCP and is carried out under different research governance frameworks. All, however, have their principles based on ICH GCP.

Although governance for non-pharmaceutical/non-interventional healthcare research is not legislative and may vary slightly between institutions, the research must still comply with some good research standards in order to be accepted for publication or to receive funding from stakeholders. The Research Governance Framework for Health and Social Care (RGF) governs all research in the NHS. This framework must be followed for any research involving human participants. The Health Research Authority in the UK is now charged with the formulation of the policies that will define the future framework for research governance.

Overall, the quality requirements for research that is non-pharmaceutical/non-interventional are less prescriptive but no less rigorous. The management of a study will be different for CTIMPs and non-pharmaceutical/non-interventional research so it is important to have confirmation before research starts as to whether the experiment is classed as a CTIMP trial or not.

CTIMP or non-pharmaceutical/non-interventional

Clinical trials involve the use of drugs/procedures called investigational medicinal products (IMPs). If the research study involves IMPs and is interventional, then it is classified as a CTIMP and the study will be regulated according to European legislation and GCP.

An IMP may be:
- An established drug (with or without marketing authorization)
- A compound that is presented (in pharmaceutical form) as potentially effective in prevention, treatment, or diagnosis of a disease
- An advanced therapy, e.g. gene therapy with a proposed pharmaceutical function
- Not a device or a surgical intervention

For some studies, deciding if the study is a CTIMP can sometimes be unclear. The definitions of what constitutes an IMP may not quite describe the compound under investigation.

The distinction between an IMP and non-IMP lies in the claim of the product being investigated. A food supplement will count as an IMP if there is a health claim about it; that is, it has benefits in the treatment of a disease and the study is investigating this. However, if there is no health claim but the study is merely looking at its physiological effect on the body then it would be classified as a foodstuff, and so a similar experiment can be performed without registering the compound as a drug and consequently adhering to European regulation.

For example, if a study is performed on a food supplement such as fish oil that it is hypothesized will have an effect on reducing blood pressure in hypertensive subjects, then the experiment will probably involve administering the drug to participants in a controlled way and looking directly at its effects on the disease. This would be a CTIMP and researchers will need to adhere to EU Regulation.

However, if it is intended to give fish oil to participants to see what it does physiologically, and it is intended to measure blood pressure amongst other outcomes to see if it is affected, then the distinction is less clear. Is this a drug or a food?

The Medicines and Healthcare Regulatory Agency (MHRA) in the UK has oversight regarding research involving IMPs with responsibility for standards of safety, quality, and performance. It can help in the decision as to the type of study.

The MHRA website (search CTIMP) has up-to-date information regarding what studies would be classed as CTIMPs with an algorithm entitled 'Is it a clinical trial of a medicinal product?'.

There is also a section called 'Borderline Products' which explains how the MHRA will work out the classification of certain products which do not obviously fit into the CTIMP or non-CTIMP categories.

It is worth remembering that although there will not be the same legal requirements and intensive auditing controls for every part of the research process as there is with the EU Regulation, there will still be the usual need to comply with GCP and the law regarding informed consent and data protection and the Human Tissue Act.

Summary of non-pharmaceutical/non-interventional research regulations

• Law: UK-wide, devolved administrations, statute and common law
• Ethics
• Policy
• Best practice guidance

Non-pharmaceutical/non-interventional healthcare research

In the UK, once it has been confirmed that the research is non-pharmaceutical/non-interventional, the study can proceed adhering to the RGF, which has its principles taken from ICH GCP. The RGF sets standards, defines responsibilities, and allocates responsibilities to individuals and organizations involved in the research project in a similar way to GCP. In summary, the RGF framework guides the conduct of the study in accordance with ethical principles that have their origin in the Declaration of Helsinki and that are consistent with ICH GCP and other applicable regulatory requirements.

As with CTIMPs, the research begins with a protocol (this is described in Chapter 15). After peer review, the protocol is submitted to the local NHS research ethics committee (see the National Research Ethics Service, NRES) via the Integrated Research Application System (IRAS). Central to any application will be your documentation of informed consent (Chapter 9).

As with ICH GCP, the RGF guidance sets out definitions of stakeholders in research, the chief investigator (CI) is the person with overall responsibility for the design, conduct and reporting of a study. The CI and investigators must have the expertise to undertake the role as defined by RGF; this may include training in GCP, and specifically consent training. The guidelines state that there should be certificated evidence of GCP training; they do not specify how often such training is required, but many institutions stipulate that GCP training must take place every two years. This training may either be via personal contact or by e-learning. In the UK, the National Institute for Health Research (NIHR) and other institutions provide such training.

If a study involves NHS sites, then appropriate NHS contracts will have to be in place such as honorary contract, honorary research contract, and letter of access. Disclosures are also important and the NHS has a Research Passport Scheme, which deals with this for external investigators.

The RGF definition of a sponsor is similar to that for ICH GCP and will usually be the CI's employer either alone or in collaboration with a care organization, university, etc. The basic difference between CTIMP and non-pharmaceutical/non-interventional research lies in the degree of documentation for CTIMP that must adhere to European legislation, but the underlying principles of ICH GCP must be applied to both.

Conclusion

The application of ICH GCP in all clinical trials has increased the confidence with which everyone, including the regulatory agencies, can view the results of a clinical trial. ICH GCP has improved the standards of research. It allows the regulatory authorities to ensure that products are safe and effective for their intended use. Simultaneously, the increasing globalization of research has been paralleled by the development of corresponding global medicinal regulations, but all have their roots firmly based on ICH GCP. Unless non-pharmaceutical/non interventional research is seen to have been conducted to GCP standards, the data is unlikely to be accepted for publication.

Further reading

ICH GCP E6 Guidelines ℘ www.ich.org

EU Clinical Directive 2001/20/EC ℘ http://ec.europa.eu/health/human-use/clinical-trials/regulation/index_en.htm

EU GCP Directive 2008/28/EC ℘ http://ec.europa.eu/health/human-use/clinical-trials/regulation/index_en.htm

EU Clinical Trial Regulation 536/2014 ℘ http://ec.europa.eu/health/human-use/clinical-trials/regulation/index_en.htm

Informed consent in a research setting

Introduction

Informed consent is a legal requirement for all studies involving human participants, whether or not they are studies investigating medicinal products or research which are not clinical trials.

This chapter summarizes the process for obtaining consent correctly for non-trialists and describes the more highly regulated consent process for clinical trials investigating medicinal products (CTIMPs).

Consent for research not investigating medicinal products

Definition
Formally, consent may be defined as agreement to an action based on knowledge of what the action involves and its likely consequences.

In practice, this means that any participants in a study must be fully informed about the study, must agree to take part freely without coercion, and are aware that they can withdraw their consent at any stage. How you plan to take consent will be central to the process of gaining ethical approval for a study. Consent can only be taken once you have gained ethical approval for your study.

Obtaining consent correctly is not simply a case of the participant signing a form; it comprises a formal process of informing the participant about the study clearly and in language that is understandable to him or her.

The participant must also be aware of his or her right to withdraw consent at any time, without the need to provide an explanation.

Capable adults
The consent process summary described here only applies to capable adults; additional legal procedures are required for children or adults who lack the capacity to provide informed consent.

A capable adult is someone who is not a child (i.e. an individual over the age of 16 in the UK) and who is not mentally incapacitated in such a way that he or she would be unable to understand fully the research study in which he or she is participating.

Process of informing the participant
Once ethical approval is gained for a study, the process of gaining consent from the participants can begin. Central to this will be informing them about the study.

The ethical application will have included copies of documents that are to be used to inform participants—advertising material, information sheets, consent forms, and template of approach letters to participants. Only documents that have had ethical approval may be used.

Participants have to know what they will be expected to do and what the risks and burdens to them will be.

Approaching the participant
It is not permitted to simply 'cold call' people and ask them directly to participate. Invitation to participate in a study is usually made via a letter or a poster, or in person.

The approach can only be made in a way previously approved by the research ethics committee. Approach letters or posters should be brief and give a general idea of what the study involves and what the participants are expected to do.

If potential participants are interested in the study then the next step in gaining consent would be to give them the study information sheet and invite them to meet and talk with a study representative and have the study explained in more detail.

Once fully informed, the participant should be given at least 24 hours to decide whether to take part or not.

Participant information sheet

The participant information sheet is an important part of the process of informing the participant. It is an important study document and must be written in non-technical English that is easy to understand. It should be version controlled and dated.

The potential participant must be given a copy of the study information sheet to read privately and then allowed time to decide whether to participate or not.

The information sheet must include:
- A simple study summary
- The purpose of the study and why the participant is invited
- What will happen to the participant during the study
- Clarity that consent may be withdrawn at any stage
- Advantages/disadvantages to the participant
- Honoraria details
- Details of confidentiality, data protection (i.e. what will happen to samples and any data collected)
- Who has reviewed the study and who is organizing the study
- Who can the participant complain to if he or she is unhappy with any aspect of the study

Consent form

The consent form will be the legal document that participants sign to indicate that they have been taken through the informed consent process described.

Completed consent forms are part of the official study documentation and they should be kept in the site file. Two forms should be signed by each participant so that both you and your participant can keep an original. The participants should also initial a copy of the information sheet that must be kept

The design of forms will be different for individual studies, but should all include basic details such as:
- name
- title of study (this may be a simplified version of the full title)
- ethics number

The rest of the form usually comprises a series of statements/questions that the participant must read and agree to before participating. These should be clearly and simply written, and best practice is to have a box beside each statement for the participant to initial to confirm they have read and understood each one. Typical statements are:
- I confirm that I have read and understand the information sheet dated ... (version) for the above study and have had the opportunity to ask questions.

- I understand that my participation is voluntary and that I am free to withdraw at any time, without giving any reason, and without my medical care or legal rights being affected.
- I consent to my general practitioner being notified of my participation in this research and to being informed of my results.

Summary of consent process for capable adults

- Information about your study that is given to the participant must be unambiguous and straightforward. Information sheets should be easy to understand.
- Participants must understand why you are conducting the research and exactly what their participation will entail.
- They should be given time to decide whether or not they wish to take part.
- They must know what the goals of your study are and what the benefits and risks might be to them or to others.
- Most importantly they must understand that their participation is voluntary and that they must not feel coerced in any way.
- Participants should understand that they can withdraw from the study at any time without explanation or any recrimination.
- Participants must have signed a consent form which will be kept as part of the formal study documentation. They will have an original to keep.

Consent for research focusing on clinical trials investigating medicinal products

To ensure the rights, safety, and well-being of trial subjects and be legally valid, consent for research must be provided voluntarily by a person who has been fully informed and who has the capacity at the time it is requested to make the decision. This chapter describes the process of consent for research focusing on clinical trials, referring to the relevant international standards or European legislation.

Specific standards and laws are enforceable when consenting to clinical trials investigating medicinal products (CTIMP); however, the principles may be applied to other research. In 2001, the European Communities Clinical Trial Directive 2001/20/EC (CT Directive) was introduced and extended in 2005/28/EC. This lays down certain end results for trials that each Member State must achieve, and each country adapts its national law to meet the goals. As each country is free to decide how to achieve the goals set out in the Directive, there is some variation to each nation's law on consent. In the UK, the Medicines for Human Use Clinical Trials Regulations were introduced in 2004 to implement the goals of the CT Directive. The CT Directive requires adherence to International Conference on Harmonisation (ICH) of Good Clinical Practice (GCP) standards for research that were introduced in 1996. This is an international ethical and scientific quality standard including specific guidance on consent. The standards are consistent with the ethical principles for medical doctors contained in the Declaration of Helsinki 1996. Although GCP standards are a legal requirement for CTIMPs, they were introduced as an international research governance standard, therefore the principles apply to all other research. In some circumstances, specific issues regarding consent are not specified in the Directives, Regulation or ICH GCP when the nation's common law or guidance of professional bodies may be applied; for example, the guidance on consent for medical treatment.

To protect the patient and minimize the risk of legal or disciplinary action, the research team must ensure consent procedures adhere to:
• CT regulations and common law
• research protocol
• clinical trial agreement
• standard operating procedures
• policies (hospital/university/pharmaceutical industry)
• research governance standards
• professional body/employer/union agreements

Health professionals who are part of the research team should follow guidance of their professional body, union, and employer to ensure they adhere to the requirements and therefore have their support in the event of legal action.

The information in the next section of this chapter offers a brief outline of the key points relevant to the continuous consent process, including information given to the participant, how to assess capacity, and the withdrawal of consent. Wider issues regarding the role of the research team and protection of vulnerable groups are included.

Information

The subject must be adequately informed about the aims, methods, anticipated benefits and risks or discomfort associated with the study, and it must be made clear that they are free to abstain or withdraw. To ensure structure, ICH GCP defines elements of consent that must be included in both the written information sheet and consent discussion (Box 9.1).

Information provided to potential participants in research requires approval by the research ethics committee (including posters, brochures, or information sheets). This is to ensure lay terminology is used and that the information is not coercive. Study information provided to the clinical or research teams does not require ethics approval. Researchers are actively encouraged to gain feedback from the public (patient–public involvement, PPI) regarding their study and this is increasingly a requirement of funding applications. This is a system funded by the NIHR as part of its commissioning and management processes. There are guides on PPI on how to include members of the community and the public in research. The PPI solutions website is helpful but many hospitals have salaried positions to

---

Box 9.1 ICH GCP 4.8.10 Elements of consent

- Trial involves research
- Purpose of the trial
- Trial treatments and probability of random assignment
- Trial procedures to be followed
- Subject's responsibilities
- Experimental aspects of the trial
- Foreseeable risks or inconveniences (to subject, embryo, foetus, or nursing infant)
- Reasonably expected benefits to the subject
- Alternative procedures or course of treatment, their benefits and risks
- Compensation available in the event of trial-related injury
- Pro-rated payment if any (not for minors or incapacitated adults)
- Expenses to participate
- Participation is voluntary, they may decline or withdraw at any time
- The trial monitor/auditor/ethics or regulatory authority may have access to participants' medical records to verify trial procedures and data without violating confidentiality
- Records will be kept confidential and identification of subjects remains confidential
- The subject/legal representative will be informed of information relevant to his or her willingness to continue to participate
- A contact person will be available to obtain further information and regarding any trial-related injury (provide direct contact details rather than a hospital switchboard)
- Expected duration of the subject's participation in the trial
- The approximate number of subjects in the trial

help researchers include the public in their studies. ℘ www.patientpub-licinvolvement.com

Feedback from those with similar conditions or experiences allows the investigator to make changes prior to formal submissions to information sheets or study design that may otherwise have deterred subjects. The lay interpretation of wording used in information sheets can be valuable. For example, describing 'randomized' as being similar to 'tossing a coin' may appear to show a lack of consideration for what may be a significant decision on their treatment.

The level of information must be presented according to the participant's level of comprehension. Expert patients such as those with chronic conditions may require a higher level of clinical information. Incapacitated adults or children should be offered an assent form that allows them to contribute to the consent decision. Different levels of information may be provided to reflect a child's level of understanding rather than noting his or her age but the levels ought to represent these age ranges:

• Children and young people 11–15 years
• Children 6–10 years
• Children less than 5 years
• Legal representative/parent/guardian

The information sheet should be concise. Lengthy information sheets of more than four sides may deter participants from taking part, especially in stressful acute situations. However, in other situations it may be essential to provide more detail. The information sheet must have the hospital/other logo and a version number consistent with the consent form.

Information sheets may be prepared in different languages. However, some interventions may require communication between the clinical team and the participant at any time of the day or night to discuss his or her response to the treatment or to report adverse events. In such cases, it is necessary to ensure that interpreters can be available whenever required prior to recruiting the participant. Also, funding should include financial provision for this service.

Participants must be allowed 'ample time' to read the information and ask questions. The regulations do not specify a set time period and unless it is stated in the protocol, this is determined by the time available before intervention must start. This may be as little as an hour to consent for a blood sample, whereas interventions with possible long-term effects may be longer to allow the participant time to seek further information, discuss with family or health professionals, etc. In practice it is useful to provide an information sheet, explain the study, then ask the person consenting how much time he or she would like before you return to discuss the study with him or her.

Capacity

The researcher must assess the capacity of the person requested to provide consent. A person's capacity may change, even during the consent process. Following the initial consent discussion and having provided the study information sheet, the researcher may ask open questions such as 'can you tell me what you thought of the study?' The response made or the questions

Box 9.2 Framework for assessing capacity

To determine if a person has capacity, the person must demonstrate that he or she:

- understands and can retain information material to the decision, its purpose, principles, benefits, risks, and alternatives available
- understands the consequences of having or not having the intervention
- retains information for long enough to be able to make a reasoned judgement as to whether or not to participate
- can communicate the decision by any means, verbal or non-verbal

participants ask will demonstrate whether they have retained the information and balanced the risks and benefits. There is no formal tool for determining capacity for clinical trials, but the information in Box 9.2 provides a useful framework to assess capacity (Box 9.2).

Capacity can change depending on the situation due to other stresses or the person's state of mind, including elements such as confusion, panic, trauma, shock, pain, or medication. The ability to retain information during stressful situations may be improved by providing a continuous consent process by reinforcing information at different stages. Participants may be asked to consent in advance in case they become eligible at a later stage; this allows more time for them to consider their decision. It is also helpful if a stressful period is envisaged at some stage in the future, allowing the participant to avoid making a decision on new information at a more stressful time. Patients given information pre-operatively if they become eligible following surgery (e.g. pain management interventions) may not have the capacity to finalize consent when they become eligible post-operatively. To overcome this problem, they can be asked to consent ahead of time and then asked to reconfirm their consent when appropriate.

Capacity and vulnerable groups: children and incapacitated adults

The Directive and Regulation provide specific guidance for the protection of vulnerable groups including children and adults who are incapacitated at the time consent is required. Those classed as vulnerable subjects also include those who may be unduly influenced by the expectations of their role or hierarchical structure such as healthcare employees, those serving in the armed forces, and persons in detention, refugees, or the unemployed.

Specific conditions are in place to protect vulnerable groups. The intention is that they are only included in CTIMP trials when the same results cannot be obtained from others with capacity to consent and a direct benefit to the individual from the intervention is expected or for the group they represent (Box 9.3).

The EU Paediatric Regulations 2006, the CT Directive, and the EU Clinical Trial Regulation aim to ensure medicines for children are subject to high-quality research under conditions that afford the best possible protection. There is increasing awareness that conducting trials should be balanced

Box 9.3 Principles for protection of minors or incapacitated adults: Clinical Trials Directive 2001/20/EC, summary points of Articles 4 and 5

- Informed consent of a parent or legal representative is obtained that represents the participant's presumed will
- Information—the minor or incapacitated adult has received information to his or her capacity of understanding from staff experienced with such individuals regarding the trial, and the anticipated risks and benefits
- The explicit wish (child or incapacitated adult) to refuse participation or to withdraw from the clinical trial is considered by the investigator
- No incentives or financial inducements are given except compensation
- Some direct benefit for the 'group of patients' is obtained; such research should relate to a clinical condition from which the minor/incapacitated adult suffers, or be of such a nature that it can only be carried out on this group
- Scientific guidelines have been followed
- Clinical trials are designed to minimize pain, discomfort, fear, and any foreseeable risk
- Ethics committee with expertise in paediatrics/disease of incapacitated patient population approval is required
- The interests of the patient always prevail over those of science and society

against the ethical concerns about giving medicinal products to a population in which they have not been appropriately tested. EU guidance on ethical considerations recognizes that parents may need more detailed and explicit information because they bear the responsibility for the child, unlike in adult trials where they are responsible for themselves.

Legally acceptable representative

The Directive allows 'an individual or juridical or other body authorised under applicable law to consent, on behalf of a prospective subject to the subject's participation in a trial'. A legal representative may also make a decision to participate or withdraw consent. In the UK, this must not be a person connected with the conduct of the trial. A parent may consent for a child. In an emergency for both children and incapacitated adults, the Regulation sets out a hierarchy of consent:

- Personal legal representative
- Professional legal representative (doctor primarily responsible for the medical treatment, or person nominated by the healthcare provider)

The Regulation has been amended to allow protocols to be designed to allow deferred consent for studies that require action urgently.

As the CT Directive makes specific provision for assessing capacity and which individuals comprise vulnerable groups, common law on capacity does not apply to CTIMP. However, assessing capacity for other research may be covered by national law; for example, in the UK the Mental Capacity Act 2005 covers treatment and other non-trial research.

Emergency consent for trials that require urgent action

In emergency situations, approval may be given to allocate the treatment and requesting consent as soon as possible afterwards. Research studies often evaluate interventions already used in clinical practice. In emergency situations, the proposed intervention may be less effective if delayed due to consent. The participant may not have capacity to make an informed decision. ICH GCP states that measures to participants in emergency situations must be defined in the protocol and approved by the ethics committee. The UK and the US makes provision for deferred consent. The EU Member States have differing views and approaches so local requirements must be checked and met. In the UK this is subject to ethics approval, and the items in Box 9.4 will be considered.

Box 9.4 Emergency consent for trials requiring urgent action: UK statutory instruments

An unconscious person or child can enter a clinical trial without prior consent from a legal representative, subject to the following:

• The treatment is required urgently
• Urgent action is required
• It is not practical to obtain consent from the participant or a legal representative
• Prior approval has been granted by the Research Ethics Committee

---

This law aims to minimize any delay to commencing the intervention that may unduly affect the efficacy. The participant or his or her legal representative will be asked to consent at a later stage, and if the participant declines, he or she may withdraw information already collected. Asking participants to consent in emergency situations may add to their stress levels. Ethics committees take this into consideration when considering emergency deferred consent. It may be more appropriate to discuss consent to use data at a later stage, especially for interventions that may otherwise have been provided as part of standard care.

Parental responsibility—the law regarding parental responsibility varies in different Member States. Box 9.5 illustrates the definition of parental responsibility in the UK.

In most cases a child will only be included in a study when consent is available from a parent with parental responsibility. In some countries, the law only requires one parent to sign the consent form, however, it is preferred that both parents are included in the consent discussion and share the decision. If there is disagreement it is usually advisable not to include the child in the study. In exceptional situations when the study is deemed to be in the child's best interest (e.g. oncology protocols) this would be discussed further with the clinical team.

> **Box 9.5 Parental responsibility: UK definition as found in the Children's Act 1989 Part 1 amended by the Adoption and Children's Act 2002**
> - Married parents
> - Unmarried mother
> - Unmarried father only if acquired by a legal parental responsibility order or a legal agreement order
> - Unmarried father if registered on the birth certificate for children born after 1 December 2003
> - Step-parent if natural parents agree to a legal parental responsibility order
> - Child's legally appointed guardian (not foster parent unless residence order exists)
> - Residence order if acquired by the father or another person
> - Local Authority order if the child is in care (part 1 sections 31 and 33)

Age of a child 'minor' to consent

In many Member States, the age for a minor to consent is 18 years. In the UK, the legislation states that a child may consent to a clinical trial when he or she is aged over 16 years and if he or she is able to demonstrate capacity. Alternatively, parents may consent for a child up to the age of 18 years (age of majority). An information sheet and assent form should be provided for children to allow them to contribute to the decision. A child may decline to participate in a clinical trial and the investigator is expected to take the child's decision into consideration. In the UK, children may provide consent for medical treatment as the intervention is intended to be in their best interest. It is difficult to argue that the intervention in a clinical trial can be in their best interest, particularly in a randomized controlled trial based on 'equipoise' or uncertainty in the expert medical community as to whether a treatment will be beneficial.

Voluntary participation and withdrawing consent

The investigator's team is required to ensure participation is voluntary and that participants are free to withdraw at any time. There must be no incentives or financial inducements made to vulnerable groups or patients; these are only permitted for healthy volunteers. Patients may feel obliged to take part when approached by the clinician responsible for their care, thus it is important that the clinicians approach consent without coercion or unduly influencing a subject to participate. To protect the participant's confidentiality regarding their eligibility, it is preferable that the clinical team approach the potential participant to ask if they may introduce the researcher to the individual. Also, participants may be reassured that clinical team members are informed about the study and that they are being approached to participate. Researchers do not routinely have access to a patient's medical notes and when using patient databases to contact possible participants, the contact should initially be made by the clinical team.

Participants must also feel free to withdraw at any time unless there is a risk associated with not completing the procedure. If a participant chooses to withdraw consent, he or she may be asked to consider two options:
- Allow use of data already collected but withdraw further participation
- Withdraw use of the data and further participation

Screening

Screening data can be used to explore the consent process, recruitment rates, and compliance by routinely recording the number 1) eligible, 2) consented, 3) declined, 4) withdrawn. Factors that influence recruitment may lead to changes in the study design or those associated with:
- competing studies—patients approached for multiple studies
- complex information sheets
- risks or discomfort associated with the intervention
- high involvement of patient's time
- stress of the situation

When decline rates are high, the protocol and information sheets can be reviewed and participants' reasons for declining examined to ascertain what deters participants. When a small proportion of participants decline this may be a positive indicator that the consent process has been delivered without pressure/coercion. Lower recruitment rates at a particular site can be investigated to determine whether this is due to lack of eligible patients, the researchers' approach, or possible impact of competing studies.

Determining eligibility

As the researcher may not be responsible for the clinical care of a patient, it is recommended that the individual's clinician assesses the eligibility criterion prior to the intervention and records that he or she has 'determined eligibility' in the medical notes. This ensures that a decision on eligibility takes into account the current clinical condition. It also provides the clinician with an opportunity to inform the researcher when his or her patient's participation may be contraindicated.

Formal recording of the consent process

The consent form must be signed and dated by the participant or legal representative and researcher who conducted the informed consent discussion. In exceptional cases when a person is unable to sign the form, oral consent in the presence of a witness may be given. There should be no need for the investigator to countersign the form when they have formally delegated the role. Countersigning consent forms may be inappropriate unless the investigator is present to assess the participant's capacity when signing the consent form. Participants may need to be re-consented if changes are made to the study that are relevant to their participation. Also, in long-term studies, a child should be re-consented when he or she reaches the age of majority.

The consent form may have separate signature boxes for any optional aspects of the study and to confirm those consenting have read the information sheet and have had an opportunity to ask questions. This may protect the researcher, as in stressful situations participants may not recall being given the information.

Research team role in consent

The chief or principal investigator is responsible for delegating the research roles, having assessed the health professional is registered, appropriately trained, and competent. The Declaration of Helsinki and ICH GCP emphasize the importance of the participant being informed by an appropriately qualified and experienced research team. The investigator may delegate the consent process to registered health professionals (including nurses and pharmacists), or they may delegate elements of the role such as screening and providing the initial information sheet. This will depend on the specific requirements of the Member State's law, the clinical trial agreement, protocol, the employer, professional bodies, and union. The decision may depend on the possible risk to those participating in the study and the level of expertise required to provide informed consent; for example, phase I studies may limit consent to the investigator. It is advisable to state which professionals will be involved in the consent process in the protocol as this will then be subject to approval of the ethics committee and the competent authority.

Each team member must demonstrate that he or she is 'competent, confident and formally delegated', and he or she may be required to provide evidence that his or her training includes relevant aspects of the law on consent, the trial protocol, ICH GCP, relevant clinical experience, and knowledge of the study. The risk of invalid consent may lead to legal action by a participant or disciplinary action by the employer or professional body against the health professional. In the UK, any physical contact with research subjects without consent is unlawful and constitutes assault or battery. In the event of legal or disciplinary action, the researcher may be required to provide an audit trail of their training, and demonstrate that he or she has adhered to the requirements stated earlier.

The investigator is advised to describe the process of consent and should include in this description which registered health professionals will undertake the process. In some situations, a medically qualified person will be required to:

- determine the participant's eligibility prior to the intervention (with clinical knowledge of the participant's care)
- discuss the study if/when requested by the participant
- assess capacity if there is any doubt

Developing a research culture

A participant's decision to consent for research may be influenced by the research 'culture' in the country or the healthcare setting. Research that is openly advertised provides reassurance to participants that the study is transparent and known to the public and other health professionals. In a hospital situation this may be achieved by displaying general research and study posters, and providing trial training to clinical teams. Newsletters are a valuable way of updating and motivating clinical teams. It is important to provide awareness training to the clinical team as patients will often ask for their views. Providing information continuously to participants throughout the study will reassure them and help reaffirm their willingness to continue. Participants may influence other patients to take part. A positive experience in a trial may lead them to take part in other trials or advising others to participate.

Further reading

Directive 2001/20/EC of the European Parliament and of the Council of 4 April 2001 on the approximation of the laws, regulations and administrative provisions of the Member States relating to the implementation of good clinical practice in the conduct of clinical trials on medicinal products. Official Journal of the European Communities, 2001.

Directive 2005/28/EC of 8 April 2005 laying down principles and detailed guidance for good clinical practice as regards investigational medicinal products for human use as well as the requirements for authorisation for the manufacturing or importation of such products. Official Journal of the European Union 2005.

The Medicines for Human Use (Clinical Trials) Regulations 1031 (2004), UK Government ℘ www.legislation.gov.uk/uksi/2004/1031/contents/made

E6 Guideline for Good Clinical Practice (R1). International Conference on Harmonisation of Technical Requirements for Registration of Pharmaceuticals for Human Use, 1996. ICH Harmonised Tripartite Guideline.

Declaration of Helsinki. Recommendations Guiding Medical Doctors in Biomedical Research Involving Human Subjects, 1996. World Medical Association.

EU Ad hoc group for the development of implementing Directive 2001/20/EC, Ethical Considerations for Clinical Trials on Medicinal Products Conducted with the Paediatric Population 2008. ℘ www.ec.europa.eu/enterprise/pharmaceuticals/eudralex.vol-10/ethical-considerations.pdf

Mental Capacity Act, 2005: UK Government.

Allmark P, Mason S. Improving the quality of consent to randomised controlled trials by using continuous consent and clinician training in the consent process. J Med Ethics 2006;32(8): 439–43.

Regulation (EC) No 1901/2006 of the European Parliament and of the council of 12 December 2006 on medicinal products for paediatric use and amending Regulation (EEC) No 1768/92. Directive 2001/20/EC Directive 2001/83/EC and Regulation (EC) No 726/2004. Official Journal of the European Union.

Medicines for Human Use (Clinical Trial) Regulations Amendment Statutory Instrument No 1928 2006: UK Government.

Medicines for Human Use (Clinical Trials) Regulations Blood Safety and Quality Amendment Statutory Instrument No 941 2008: UK Government.

Food and Drug Administration, Exception from Informed Consent for Studies Conducted in Emergency Settings FDA regulation (21 CFR 50.24). ℘ www.fda.gov/RegulatoryInformation/Guidances/ucm126482.htm

Children Act 1989. ℘ www.legislation.gov.uk

Adoption and Children Act 2002. ℘ www.legislation.gov.uk/ukpga/2002/38/contents

Ethics of clinical and healthcare research: general considerations, Mental Capacity Act, Human Tissue Act

The responsibilities of the ethics committee and its role in the protection of vulnerable subjects

Responsibilities of an ethics committee

Ethical considerations touch many aspects of life but here we are restricting our considerations to the responsibilities of an independent ethics committee (IEC) in healthcare and clinical research. One major difference between ethical considerations in general and ethical considerations as applied to clinical research is that the latter now operate within a legal framework in most countries. Definitions, standards, and responsibilities have been agreed by the International Conference on Harmonisation (ICH), published in its guidelines, and incorporated into national guidelines and even some laws. The legal status, composition, function, operations, and regulatory requirements pertaining to an IEC differ between countries but they should allow the IEC to act in agreement with the international standards defined in ICH GCP.

Under ICH GCP, an ethics committee (EC) is defined as an independent body (a review board or a committee, institutional, regional, national, or supranational), constituted of medical professionals and non-medical members, whose responsibility it is to ensure the protection of the rights, safety, and well-being of human subjects involved in a trial, and to provide public assurance of that protection, by, among other things, reviewing and approving/providing favourable opinion on the trial protocol, the suitability of the investigator(s), facilities, and the methods and material to be used in obtaining and documenting informed consent of the trial subjects.

In some countries (e.g. the US) the responsibilities of an EC are carried out by an institutional review board (IRB). The ICH definition of an IRB is an independent body constituted of medical, scientific, and non-scientific members, whose responsibility is to ensure the protection of the rights, safety, and well-being of human subjects involved in a trial by, among other things, reviewing, approving, and providing continuing review of trial protocol and amendments and of the methods and material to be used in obtaining and documenting informed consent of the trial subjects. In practice, the responsibilities of an independent EC and an IRB can be considered synonymous and this chapter refers to ECs only.

Although ICH GCP should be considered as a whole, it defines 13 principles that have their origin in the Declaration of Helsinki. The sixth principle of ICH GCP is that a trial should be conducted in compliance with the protocol that has received prior EC approval/favourable opinion. The use of the alternative wording 'favourable opinion' is to allow for the fact that ECs do not take on the responsibilities of a sponsor with respect to any research proposals that they review and approve. By approving or giving a favourable opinion they are really indicating that they have no objection to the proposed research being conducted.

In order to carry out its responsibilities, an EC reviews a comprehensive list of documents describing the proposed research and, depending on its working practices, it may also interview persons proposing the research in order to understand the proposal more clearly. Face-to-face discussions between researchers and an EC ensures both parties take their responsibilities seriously and can lead to improved science for the project as well as better protection for the subjects. The committee can review any additional document it feels necessary to fulfil its responsibilities. The EC should give its decision in writing within a reasonable time and review any amendments to the approved protocol before they are implemented. It is required that the EC conducts ongoing review of the research—for example, at yearly intervals—and it may request additional written information for the trial subjects if appropriate to protect their rights, safety, or well-being.

These duties summarized here for ethics committees may appear reasonable but it has to be acknowledged that ethics committees were not represented as part of the ICH process when GCP guidelines relating to ECs were being drawn up. Some committees consider ethics to be beyond the reach of the law and any interference from outsiders was initially resented. Indeed, in some countries such as the UK, ECs functioned entirely outside the legal framework prior to 2004 and some committees resented losing their autonomy. Education of the members has been successful in reducing the opposition to bringing the clinical research ethics review system within a defined framework. In the UK, ECs work to extensive and detailed standard operating procedures (SOPs) to ensure all aspects of GCP are achieved and subjects are protected, even if the results of the research are not intended to be used as part of a marketing authorization application.

Protection of subjects

The third principle of GCP is that the rights, safety, and well-being of the trial subjects are the most important considerations and should prevail over interests of science and society. A subject is an individual who participates in a clinical trial, either as a recipient of the investigational product(s) or as a control. In the world of clinical research all subjects are vulnerable to some degree.

In order to protect subjects, it is now a principle of GCP that freely given informed consent should be obtained from every subject prior to his or her clinical trial participation. Informed consent is a process by which a subject voluntarily confirms his or her willingness to participate in a particular trial, after having been informed of all aspects of the trial that are relevant to the subject's decision to participate. Informed consent is documented by means of a written, signed, and dated informed consent form.

In obtaining and documenting informed consent, the investigator should comply with the applicable regulatory requirement(s), and should adhere to GCP and to the ethical principles that have their origin in the Declaration of Helsinki. Prior to the beginning of the trial the investigator should have the EC's written approval/favourable opinion of the written informed consent form and any other written information to be provided to subjects. This should be revised whenever important new information becomes available that may be relevant to the subject's consent. Any revised written informed consent form and written information should receive the EC's approval/favourable opinion in advance of use. The subject or the subject's legally acceptable representative should be informed in a timely manner if new information becomes available that may be relevant to the subject's willingness to continue participation in the trial, and the communication of this information should be documented.

Neither the investigator nor the trial staff should coerce or unduly influence a subject to participate or to continue to participate in a trial.

None of the oral and written information concerning the trial, including the written informed consent form, should contain any language that causes the subject or the subject's legally acceptable representative to waive or to appear to waive any legal rights, or that releases or appears to release the investigator, the institution, the sponsor, or their agents from liability for negligence.

The investigator, or a person designated by the investigator, should fully inform the subject or, if the subject is unable to provide informed consent, the subject's legally acceptable representative, of all pertinent aspects of the trial including the written information and the approval/favourable opinion by the EC. The language used in the oral and written information about the trial, including the written informed consent form, should be as non-technical as practicable and should be understandable to the subject or the subject's legally acceptable representative and the impartial witness, where applicable.

Before informed consent may be obtained, the investigator, or a person designated by the investigator, should provide the subject or the subject's legally acceptable representative ample time and opportunity to inquire about details of the trial and to decide whether or not to participate in the trial. All questions about the trial should be answered to the satisfaction of the subject or the subject's legally acceptable representative. Prior to a subject's participation in the trial, the written informed consent form should be signed and personally dated by the subject or by the subject's legally acceptable representative, and by the person who conducted the informed consent discussion.

If a subject is unable to read, or if a legally acceptable representative is unable to read, an impartial witness should be present during the entire informed consent discussion. After the written informed consent form and any other written information to be provided to subjects, is read and explained to the subject or the subject's legally acceptable representative, and after the subject or the subject's legally acceptable representative has orally consented to the subject's participation in the trial and, if capable of doing so, has signed and personally dated the informed consent form, the witness should sign and personally date the consent form. By signing the consent form, the witness attests that the information in the consent form and any other written information was accurately explained to, and apparently understood by, the subject or the subject's legally acceptable representative, and that informed consent was freely given by the subject or the subject's legally acceptable representative.

Requirements for informed consent

Both the informed consent discussion and the written informed consent form and any other written information to be provided to subjects should include explanations of the following:

- That the trial involves research.
- The purpose of the trial.

- The trial treatment(s) and the probability for random assignment to each treatment.
- The trial procedures to be followed, including all invasive procedures.
- The subject's responsibilities.
- Those aspects of the trial that are experimental.
- The reasonably foreseeable risks or inconveniences to the subject and, when applicable, to an embryo, foetus, or nursing infant.
- The reasonably expected benefits. When there is no intended clinical benefit to the subject, the subject should be made aware of this.
- The alternative procedure(s) or course(s) of treatment that may be available to the subject, and their important potential benefits and risks.
- The compensation and/or treatment available to the subject in the event of trial-related injury.
- The anticipated pro-rated payment, if any, to the subject for participating in the trial.
- The anticipated expenses, if any, to the subject for participating in the trial.
- That the subject's participation in the trial is voluntary and that the subject may refuse to participate or withdraw from the trial, at any time, without penalty or loss of benefits to which the subject is otherwise entitled.
- That the monitor(s), the auditor(s), the EC, and the regulatory authority(ies) will be granted direct access to the subject's original medical records for verification of clinical trial procedures and/or data, without violating the confidentiality of the subject, to the extent permitted by the applicable laws and regulations and that, by signing a written informed consent form, the subject or the subject's legally acceptable representative is authorizing such access.
- That records identifying the subject will be kept confidential and, to the extent permitted by the applicable laws and/or regulations, will not be made publicly available. If the results of the trial are published, the subject's identity will remain confidential.
- That the subject or the subject's legally acceptable representative will be informed in a timely manner if information becomes available that may be relevant to the subject's willingness to continue participation in the trial.
- The person(s) to contact for further information regarding the trial and the rights of trial subjects, and whom to contact in the event of trial-related injury.
- The foreseeable circumstances and/or reasons under which the subject's participation in the trial may be terminated.
- The expected duration of the subject's participation in the trial.
- The approximate number of subjects involved in the trial.

Prior to participation in the trial, the subject or the subject's legally acceptable representative should receive a copy of the signed and dated written informed consent form and any other written information provided to the subjects. During a subject's participation in the trial, the subject or the subject's legally acceptable representative should receive a copy of the signed and dated consent form updates and a copy of any amendments to the written information provided to subjects.

When a clinical trial (therapeutic or non-therapeutic) includes subjects who can only be enrolled in the trial with the consent of the subject's legally acceptable representative (e.g. minors, or patients with severe dementia), the subject should be informed about the trial to the extent compatible with the subject's understanding and, if capable, the subject should sign and personally date the written informed consent.

A non-therapeutic trial (i.e. a trial in which there is no anticipated direct clinical benefit to the subject) should be conducted with subjects who personally give consent and who sign and date the written informed consent form. Non-therapeutic trials may be conducted with subjects with the consent of a legally acceptable representative provided the following conditions are fulfilled:

• The objectives of the trial cannot be met by means of a trial in subjects who can give informed consent personally.
• The foreseeable risks to the subjects are low.
• The negative impact on the subject's well-being is minimized and low.
• The trial is not prohibited by law.
• The approval/favourable opinion of the EC is expressly sought on the inclusion of such subjects, and the written approval/favourable opinion covers this aspect.

Such trials, unless an exception is justified, should be conducted with patients having a disease or condition for which the investigational product is intended. Subjects in these trials should be particularly closely monitored and should be withdrawn if they appear to be unduly distressed.

In emergency situations, when prior consent of the subject is not possible, the consent of the subject's legally acceptable representative, if present, should be requested. When prior consent of the subject is not possible, and the subject's legally acceptable representative is not available, enrolment of the subject should require measures described in the protocol and/or elsewhere, with documented approval/favourable opinion by the EC, to protect the rights, safety, and well-being of the subject and to ensure compliance with applicable regulatory requirements. The subject or the subject's legally acceptable representative should be informed about the trial as soon as possible and consent to continue and other consent as appropriate should be requested.

Vulnerable subjects

Some subjects are especially vulnerable, such as individuals whose willingness to volunteer in a clinical trial may be unduly influenced by the expectation, whether justified or not, of benefits associated with participation, or of a retaliatory response from senior members of a hierarchy in case of refusal to participate. Examples are members of a group with a hierarchical structure, such as medical, pharmacy, dental and nursing students, subordinate hospital and laboratory personnel, employees of the pharmaceutical industry, members of the armed forces, and persons kept in detention. Other vulnerable subjects include patients with incurable diseases, persons in nursing homes, unemployed or impoverished persons, and patients in emergency situations, ethnic minority groups, homeless persons, nomads, refugees, minors, as well as those incapable of giving consent.

Mental Capacity Act

The Mental Capacity Act (MCA) (2005) applies in England and Wales and states that research with individuals (adults) who lack the capacity to consent must have the ethics of the research scrutinized and approved by an 'appropriate body' as defined in law. In England and Wales, the 'appropriate body' must be a recognized research ethics committee. Scotland follows the Adults with Incapacity (Scotland) Act.

Key points

- MCA applies to 16–17-year-olds and adults (18 years and over) who lack capacity **to make a particular decision or take a particular action for themselves at the time** the decision or action needs to be taken.
- Guidance on the Act notes that lack of capacity may be permanent or temporary. It could be state-related (e.g. due to drug or alcohol use) or the person concerned could gain capacity for decision-making or action (within the legal definition) with appropriate support/training. The key point relates to capacity *at the time* of consent.

Key questions

- Is the research related to the 'condition' that causes the lack of capacity, or to the treatment of those with that condition?
- If 'no', then the study should proceed without involving the participant who lacks mental capacity. If 'yes', the additional question below applies:
- Could the research be undertaken effectively with people who have capacity to consent?
- If 'yes', the study should exclude those without mental capacity. If 'no', then inclusion of people without capacity can be justified.

Exceptions to the MCA

Guidance on the Act states that it does not *generally* apply to:

- research with **children and young people** under the age of 16 years.
- **clinical trials** that are covered under the Medicines for Human Use (Clinical Trials) Regulations 2004.
- research that only involves **data that has been anonymized** (it cannot be traced back to individuals). Confidentiality and data protection laws do not apply in this case.
- some research involving **human tissue**:
  - under the Human Tissue Act 2004 (please see the last section of this chapter), research that deals only with human tissue that has been anonymized does not require consent. This applies to both those who have capacity and those who do not. But the research must have ethical approval, and the tissue must come from a living person.
  - if researchers collected human tissue samples before 31 August 2006, they do not need a person's consent to work on them, but they will normally have to get ethical approval.
- some research using **confidential patient information**, under regulations made under section 251 of the NHS Act 2006 (formerly known as section 60 of the Health and Social Care Act 2001), for which you would need to apply to the Patient Information Advisory Group for approval on behalf of the Secretary of State.

The role of the consultee

A potential participant has the right to disagree with the decisions that others (such as relatives or carers) might make. If it is established that an adult does not have the capacity to decide whether to participate, the Act requires use of a specified consultee.

- If possible, this should be a personal consultee who should be someone whom the person who lacks capacity would trust with important decisions about their welfare, for example, a family member or close friend of the person, but not a paid carer or other professional such as a social worker.
- If no personal consultee can be identified, a nominated consultee should be proposed; that is, someone who is prepared to be consulted by the researcher but who has no connection with the research study—for example, someone from a relevant organization such as a local church or the person's GP, providing they have no connection with the study.

Summary points

- Refer to the Code Of Practice for the Act, and Guidance on Nominating a Consultee
- The requirements that a research project must meet in order to be approved by an ethics committee include:
  - potential for benefit vs burden and risk
  - extent to which the research really needs to involve people who lack capacity
  - when people should be allowed to withdraw from research as well as the specific responsibilities of researchers
- There are ambiguities in the guidance, and in the wording of the Act itself, particularly for studies that don't meet the narrow definition of research.

What are an ethics committee's key responsibilities?

An EC must be satisfied that there is a need to involve potentially vulnerable adults (e.g. those with severe learning disabilities) and their participation must be justified to the committee. You should ensure that you have familiarized yourself with the relevant legal position, where it is intended to conduct research with adults who may not be able to give a legally valid consent to take part in research.

Where the proposed research subject is in a dependent relationship to the researcher (e.g. where the research subject is a student), the researcher must make it clear that a decision to take part or not in the project will in no way affect the individual's relationship with the researcher and the researcher must ensure that this is the case.

The implementation of the EU Directive on Clinical Trials since 2004 and subsequent amendments to allow the inclusion of incapacitated adults in an emergency situation (e.g. UK SI 2006/2984), and minors in emergency (e.g. UK SI 2008/941). These and the Clinical Trial Regulation have helped to harmonize this requirement within the EU and an acceptable way forward has been found to conduct research in those unable to consent for themselves in most EU Member States. GCP allows for research in the emergency situation where consent may not be possible, and if such research is to continue the role of the EC is pivotal in ensuring that an acceptable form of 'consent' is included. Under GCP, subjects may receive payment, particularly when they are not expected to derive any benefit from the treatment under investigation, such as in phase I studies; however, payments must be pro-rated and approved by the EC beforehand. The EC has a pivotal role to play in the protection of vulnerable subjects.

The requirements for consideration by an ethics committee for review of a clinical trial

Ethics review

Under GCP, the EC is responsible for safeguarding the rights, safety, and well-being of all trial subjects. This usually involves the EC reviewing the research proposal and the sites at which it is proposed to conduct the research.

It is now a legal requirement in most countries of the world that each protocol must be reviewed and approved by an independent ethics review committee before a trial can commence. When ICH GCP was drafted, ECs were not consulted, and industry-sponsored researchers suddenly began making additional demands of them in terms of documentation. These requests were along the lines of: was the EC compliant with GCP, did it have a written constitution, or who were the members present when a particular trial was reviewed? Many ECs resented this interference with their function (as they saw it), but today, through improved education and training of its members, most committees discharge their duties in a very professional and responsible way.

When ICH GCP was introduced, EC members were not the only group of people to be affected. There has also been some resistance from the academic community to comply fully with GCP when not performing medical research intended for a licence submission. They feel that in some clinical trials, the increased resource required to achieve ICH GCP standards is disproportionate to the identifiable risks to which research participants are exposed. On the other hand, it does not seem justifiable that research participants should have any lower standards of protection when involved in academic research. The GCP Directive does allow Member States in Europe to introduce special arrangements for non-commercial studies conducted in authorized indications—for example, the provision of an Investigator's Brochure may be achieved by providing a Summary of Product Characteristics (SmPC)—but GCP will still apply.

Another aspect of GCP that is resource-intensive and difficult for the academic community to provide in multicentre studies is monitoring. Even regulatory authorities and ECs are now adopting a risk-based approach to monitoring where the type of healthcare intervention being tested and the risk to research participants is taken into consideration when determining the type and frequency of monitoring visits to the investigator's site.

To review a research proposal it is suggested in ICH GCP that a comprehensive list of documents are reviewed by the EC. The protocol and investigator's brochure are obvious candidates, but the list also includes subject recruitment procedures, including any advertisements, written patient information, and the informed consent signature form.

The protocol is a document that describes the objective(s), design, methodology, statistical considerations, and organization of a trial. The protocol usually also gives the background and rationale for the trial, but these could be provided in other protocol-referenced documents. Because protocols are large documents, and their structure and content varies considerably between research proposals, it is difficult for EC members to find the relevant information contained within quickly. Therefore, in some countries (e.g. the UK), applicants are asked to complete an application form. This presents to the EC the information it wishes to review in a standardized format and is intended to make the review comprehensive and easier for EC members to undertake. Due to the wide variety of research proposals which need EC review, the application form is a formidable document and can run to 100 pages. It can be a useful exercise to complete a draft EC application form before the protocol is finalized. Although most information in the application form should also be present in the protocol, this has not always been the case in this author's experience. Completing an EC application can improve the content of a protocol.

Ethics committees are responsible for the protection of subjects so in addition to reviewing details of the research proposal, they review in detail the recruitment and consent process. This includes not only the written subject information to be given to prospective subjects and the informed consent form to be signed, but also exactly how potential subjects will be identified. Research is increasingly being conducted into lifestyle diseases, and potential subjects will not all be routinely attending a hospital or general practice clinic. Advertising to the general public for research subjects is now permitted in many countries, but the proposed advertisements must be reviewed by the EC as part of its role. An EC may request additional written information for the trial subjects if appropriate to protect their rights, safety, or well-being. The committee can review any additional document it feels necessary to fulfil its responsibilities.

When research is proposed involving those below the age of consent, the process for identification of parents/guardians, all the written and other information (e.g. videos) provided, and documentation of consent, and assent if appropriate must all be carefully scrutinized by the EC.

If a trial is proposed which may include adults unable to consent for themselves, consent should be sought from a legally acceptable representative. The implementation of the EU Directive on clinical trials since May 2004 and subsequently the Clinical Trials Regulation has helped to harmonize this requirement within the EU and an acceptable way forward has been found to conduct research in those unable to consent for themselves in most EU Member States. GCP allows for research in the emergency situation where consent may not be possible and if such research is to continue, the role of the EC is pivotal in ensuring that an acceptable form of 'consent' is included. The requirements for consideration by an EC for review of such a clinical trial must comply with the legislation of the country concerned, whilst being practical and achievable for the researchers.

Under GCP, subjects may receive payment for their time and travel expenses, particularly when they are not expected to derive any benefit from the treatment under investigation, such as in phase I studies. Any compensation payable to the subjects has to be declared; payments must be pro-rated and approved by the EC beforehand.

ECs should check that in the event that the research participant suffers harm through his or her participation, adequate insurance is in place or the sponsor has adequate resources available to pay compensation to any subjects harmed.

Another aspect of the requirements for consideration by an EC for review of a clinical trial is whether the investigator and research site(s) are appropriate to carry out the proposed research. In order to assess the investigator it is usual for the investigator's curriculum vitae to be submitted to the EC. This should include details of research experience and GCP training. Details of the site may be known to members of an EC or the EC can ask for a written description of the site and its facilities to assess its suitability.

Having received the research proposal, the committee should give its decision within a reasonable time. In Europe, a time limit of 60 days is imposed for standard products, with one round of questions permitted. Research involving novel therapies can take longer.

After approval it is becoming increasingly common for the sponsor or investigator to wish to amend the research proposal. An EC must review and 'approve' any amendments to the approved protocol before they are implemented. Even if the protocol is not amended, it is a requirement that the EC conducts ongoing review of the research, for example, at yearly intervals.

Thus it can be seen that the requirements for consideration by an EC for review of a clinical trial are detailed and numerous. For a trial within a development programme to be considered ethical, it is usually necessary to provide not only details of the trial itself but also some high-level information regarding the programme so it can be determined where a particular study fits. Only by evaluating the overview in addition to looking into the detail of a research proposal can the EC take on its full responsibility to protect the safety and well-being of all trial subjects.

Ethics committee composition, functions, operation, and procedures

Interesting historical facts

Following the well-publicized medical research horrors that were described at the Nuremberg trials, during which it was revealed that Nazi physicians had undertaken experiments on prisoners without their consent and without regard for the individual's well-being, the Nuremburg Code was published in 1949. It described the principles of informed consent and this became the basis for the Declaration of Helsinki made by the World Medical Association at its annual meeting in Helsinki in 1964. Just prior to this, in 1962 the Drug Amendment Act had been approved in the US. This became the Food and Drug Administration (FDA) Regulations governing clinical research which obliged investigators to inform the FDA of any proposed clinical trials, required the submission of pre-clinical data to support the proposed trials, and required informed consent of the trial subjects to be obtained and that the trial results would be reported. The FDA Regulations of 1962 were subsequently expanded to include Good Manufacturing Practice in 1963, Institutional Review Boards in 1971, and Good Clinical Practice in 1977. This was the start of a framework of legislation and guidelines that are now in place covering the majority of clinical research in almost every country in the world.

However, when the first ECs were established in relation to healthcare and clinical research during the mid- to late twentieth century, there were no rules specifically for them. As the need for medical research to undergo independent ethics review became clear, committees of the 'great and the good' were formed to provide this service on a local basis, usually covering just a single hospital. These early committees grew up without the benefit of experience.

Countries gradually developed their own guidelines for good clinical practice (GCP), and ethics review was part of these; for example, the guidelines from the Royal College of Physicians, London, 1971 concerning ethical review of research. Israel introduced ethical research guidelines in 1980, the Nordic countries and Austria in 1983, Greece in 1984, and the Association of the British Pharmaceutical Industry (ABPI) guidelines covering research in general practice were first issued in 1986. Finland, France, Germany, and Ireland also had their first GCP guidelines issued in 1987; Canada and Japan in 1989, and the European Committee for Proprietary Medicinal Products (CPMP) GCP guidelines were issued in 1990. The World Health Organization (WHO) issued its set of GCP guidelines in 1993, by which time it was becoming increasingly obvious that a global standard for GCP was required. The International Conference on Harmonisation of Technical Requirements for Registration of Pharmaceuticals for Human Use (ICH) recognized this need in 1991 and set up an Expert Working Group to draft a guideline on GCP. This was issued as a finalized guideline (ICH E6 GCP Consolidated Guideline) in May 1996 and adopted by the three main ICH regions: CPMP in Europe, published in the Federal Register in the US and adopted by the Ministry of Health and Welfare in Japan, in the following year. This GCP guideline also attracted considerable interest from those countries and organizations outside the three main ICH regions such as Canada, South Africa, Australia, and the World Health Organization. Thus the ICH GCP Guideline, which includes detailed guidance on ethical review, quickly became the most widely accepted and followed GCP guideline globally.

In 2001, the EU introduced Directive 2001/20/EC that required Member States to implement GCP in the conduct of clinical trials on medicinal products for human use from 1 May 2004. All 28 Member States now have legislation in place to achieve this.

Current situation

It is important to realize that the ICH GCP guideline, EU Directives, and subsequent EU Regulation cover all phases of clinical research, including phase IV studies.

Much of the drive for one standard of GCP is due to the multinational nature of clinical research and the consequent need to have common standards of ethics, behaviour, and process so that the data are equally acceptable to regulatory authorities worldwide. The guideline should be followed when gathering clinical trial data that are intended to be submitted to regulatory authorities, and the principles can be applied to all clinical investigations that may impact on the safety and well-being of human subjects. The composition, functions, and operations as described are taken from ICH E6 GCP guideline and may vary locally, but the general principles described here should be implemented to give at least the minimum standard of protection for human subjects involved in healthcare or clinical research.

Composition, functions, and operations

ICH GCP states that the EC should consist of a reasonable number of members, who collectively have the qualifications and experience to review and evaluate the science, medical aspects, and ethics of the proposed trial. The basic recommendations are that the EC should include:
- at least five members.
- at least one member whose primary area of interest is in a non-scientific area.
- at least one member who is independent of the institution/trial site.

Only those EC members who are independent of the investigator and the sponsor of the trial should vote or provide an opinion on a trial-related matter. So that this can be verified, a list of EC members and their qualifications should be maintained. The EC should perform its functions according to written operating procedures, should maintain written records of its activities and minutes of its meetings, and should comply with GCP and with any applicable regulatory requirement(s).

Regarding decisions, it states that an EC should make its decisions at announced meetings at which at least a quorum, as stipulated in its written operating procedures, is present. Only members who participate in the EC review and discussion should vote/provide their opinion and/or advice. The investigator may provide information to the committee on any aspect of the trial, but should not participate in the deliberations of the EC or in the vote/opinion of the EC. An EC may also invite non-members with expertise in special areas for assistance. In the UK it has become normal practice to invite the investigator and representatives of the sponsor to attend the EC meeting to answer any questions the committee members may have on the research proposal before the committee goes into a closed session to deliberate and reach a decision.

Reading the guidelines and legislation concerning ethics review, one might easily conclude that following review of a research proposal, an EC issues its opinion as favourable/approved or not favourable/not approved. However, this is rarely the case. Straightforward approvals and outright rejections are relatively rare. Very often the initial response from an EC is a conditional approval in which the EC makes requests or suggestions for changes to, for example, the written patient information. Final approval or favourable opinion is then issued by the EC following submission of the requested amendments to the original research proposal.

Procedures

ICH GCP states that an EC should establish, document in writing, and follow its procedures; in other words it should have standard operating procedures (SOPs). These SOPs should describe its composition (names and qualifications of the members) and the authority under which it is established. Most ECs are established under the administrative framework of a hospital or university covering a town, city, or administrative region. However, in Europe a local EC may take on a national role in order to provide a single opinion per Member State, and how this is achieved will be laid down in national laws, guidelines, or SOPs.

Meetings must be scheduled, and members notified, in order for the EC to conduct its meetings. At the meetings both an initial review of new research proposals and continuing review of approved trials should be undertaken. The frequency of continuing review should be determined, as appropriate, but is often annual on receipt of a progress report. Another aspect of the ongoing review is to provide, according to the applicable regulatory requirements, expedited review and approval/favourable opinion of minor change(s) in ongoing trials that already have the approval/favourable opinion of the EC. It should be included in EC SOPs and investigators reminded that no subject should be admitted to a trial before the EC issues its written approval/favourable opinion of the trial.

Investigators should also be reminded that no deviations from, or changes to, the protocol should be initiated without prior written EC approval/favourable opinion of an appropriate amendment, except when necessary to eliminate immediate hazards to the subjects or when the change(s) involves only logistical or administrative aspects of the trial (e.g. change of monitor(s), telephone number(s)). Also, investigators should promptly report to the EC deviations from, or changes to, the protocol to eliminate immediate hazards to the trial subjects, or any changes increasing the risk to subjects and/or affecting significantly the conduct of the trial.

What happens in the case of protocol amendments?

Investigator should also inform the EC of all substantial amendments by completing a notice of substantial amendment. Substantial amendments include:

- change to the design or methodology the study, or to background information affecting its scientific value
- changes to the procedure undertaken by the participant: any changes relating to the safety or physical or mental integrity of participant, or to the risk/benefit assessment for the study
- significant changes to the study documentation such as participant information sheet, consent forms, questionnaires, letters of invitation, letters to GP or other clinicians, information sheet for relatives or carers
- change of sponsor(s) or sponsor's legal representative
- appointment of new chief investigator or key collaborative
- a change to the insurance or indemnity arrangement for the study
- temporary halt of a study to protect participant from harm, and the planned restart of a study following a temporary halt
- a change to the definition of the end of the study
- any other significant changes to the protocol or the terms of the EC application

Some changes, however, will have no significant implication for participants or for the conduct, management, or scientific value of the study and can be regarded as 'non-substantial' or 'minor amendments'. Non-substantial amendments do not need to be notified. These include:

- minor changes to the protocol or other study documentations, e.g. correcting errors, updating contact points, minor clarification
- update of the investigator brochure (unless there is a change to the risk/benefit assessment for the trial)
- changes to the chief investigator's research team (other than appointment of key collaborators)
- changes in funding arrangements
- changes in documentation used by the research team for recording study data
- changes in the logistics arrangement for storing or transporting samples
- extension of the study beyond the period specified in the application form

Please note, changes to the contact details for the sponsor (or the sponsor representative), chief investigator, or other study staff are minor amendments but should be notified to the EC for information. In the UK, the chief investigator and/or sponsor's representative should notify both the main research ethics committee (REC) and the relevant local REC if a principal investigator's contact details have changed.

Investigators are also to report to the EC all adverse drug reactions that are both serious and unexpected. Also to be reported is any new information that may affect adversely the safety of the subjects or the conduct of the trial. In return, the EC is required to notify promptly and in writing the investigator/institution concerning its trial-related decisions/opinions, the reasons for its decisions/opinions, and procedures for appeal of its decisions/opinions.

The importance of communication with as well as records retained by the ethics committee

Communication between sponsors, investigators, and ECs has improved a lot in recent years, and with the prospect of ECs and regulatory authorities to be able to work together and access the same application information, the potential for further improvement is good. Guidelines have not really kept pace with the advances in electronic document management and the communication that is now possible, but it is to be hoped that bureaucracy will not stifle the introduction of new technology whose purpose is to improve patient safety and protection.

Communication with the EC

Since ECs have had a role to play in clinical research, communication between the investigator and the EC has never been more important. Communication has to happen before, during, and after a trial, and a trial cannot be conducted legally without it. ICH requires that before initiating a trial, the investigator/institution should have written and dated approval/favourable opinion from the EC for the trial protocol, the written informed consent form, any consent form updates, subject recruitment procedures (e.g. advertisements), and any other written information to be provided to subjects. As part of the investigator's/institution's written application to the EC, the investigator/institution should provide the EC with a current copy of the investigator's brochure. If the investigator's brochure is updated during the trial, the investigator/institution should supply a copy to the EC. During the trial, the investigator/institution should provide to the EC all documents subject to review. If the investigator is performing a trial on behalf of a commercial sponsor, most ECs will accept communication directly from the sponsor, with a copy to the investigator, as many documents originate from the sponsor.

An example of such a document is a progress report. The investigator should submit written summaries of the trial status to the EC annually, or more frequently, if requested by the EC. However, in a multicentre, possibly multinational study, it is the sponsor who has the overview of the trial and is able to provide progress reports. Also, it is the investigator who should promptly provide written reports to the sponsor, the EC and, where applicable, the institution, of any changes significantly affecting the conduct of the trial, and/or increasing the risk to subjects. However, in a multicentre study such changes are often driven by events at other investigational sites and communication is initially with the sponsor and then with all the other affected parties.

Once a study is approved by an EC, the investigator and the sponsor should comply with the applicable regulatory requirement(s) concerning the reporting of suspected unexpected serious adverse drug reactions (SUSAR) to the regulatory authority(ies) and the EC. In general, this means that the sponsor should expedite the reporting to all concerned investigator(s)/institution(s), to the EC(s), where required, and to the regulatory authority(ies) of all SUSARs. The EC's role to maintain the ongoing safety of enrolled subjects means that it should be promptly made aware of any such adverse events, including those events occurring at investigator sites outside the area for which they are responsible. In some studies, adverse events will be centrally monitored by an independent data monitoring committee on an ongoing basis and this committee may also communicate with ECs approving the study.

For reported deaths, the investigator should supply the sponsor, the independent data monitoring committee (if relevant) and the EC with any additional requested information (e.g. autopsy reports and terminal medical reports) so that safety can be kept under review at all times.

Although it does not happen very often, if the investigator terminates or suspends a trial without prior agreement of the sponsor, the investigator should inform the institution where applicable, and the investigator/institution should promptly inform the sponsor and the EC and should provide the sponsor and the EC a detailed written explanation of the termination or suspension. More often it is the sponsor that suspends or terminates a study prematurely and therefore initiates the communication with the investigator and EC. The investigator should promptly inform the institution where applicable and provide the EC with a detailed written explanation of the termination or suspension.

It is also possible that the EC terminates or suspends its approval/favourable opinion of a trial, so the investigator should inform the institution where applicable and the investigator/institution should promptly communicate with the sponsor and provide the sponsor with a detailed written explanation of the termination or suspension.

Upon completion of the trial the investigator, where applicable, should inform the institution; the investigator/institution should provide the EC with a summary of the trial's outcome, and the regulatory authority(ies) with any reports required. Again, the final report often originates from the sponsor in commercially sponsored multicentre trials.

In order to demonstrate appropriate ethics review, the sponsor should obtain from the investigator/institution the name and address of the investigator's/institution's EC, a statement obtained from the EC that it is organized and operates according to GCP and the applicable laws and regulations and documented EC approval/favourable opinion and, if requested by the sponsor, a current copy of protocol, written informed consent form(s) and any other written information to be provided to subjects, subject recruiting procedures, and documents related to payments and compensation available to the subjects, and any other documents that the EC may have requested.

ICH GCP states that if the EC conditions its approval/favourable opinion upon change(s) in any aspect of the trial, such as modification(s) of the protocol, written informed consent form, and any other written information to be provided to subjects, and/or other procedures, the sponsor should obtain from the investigator/institution a copy of the modification(s) made and the date approval/favourable opinion was given by the EC. If the study is industry sponsored, it is often the sponsor that makes the amendments to submitted trial documents and resubmits the amended documents to the EC for approval.

Although ICH GCP states that the sponsor should obtain from the investigator/institution documentation and dates of any EC re-approvals/re-evaluations with favourable opinion, and of any withdrawals or suspensions of approval/favourable opinion, in practice ECs often copy correspondence with the investigator directly to the sponsor so that communication takes place as quickly and efficiently as possible.

Records to be retained by an EC

The EC may be asked by investigators, sponsors, or regulatory authorities to provide its written procedures and membership lists, therefore ECs need to keep appropriate records. But what are appropriate records to be retained? The answer has two parts; what documents should be kept by the EC, and for how long? ICH GCP helpfully says the EC should retain all relevant records (e.g. written procedures, membership lists, lists of occupations/affiliations of members, submitted documents, minutes of meetings, and correspondence) for a period of at least three years after completion of the trial, and make them available upon request from the regulatory authority(ies).

So it would appear that ICH provides an adequate answer to this question. However, in the real world life is never that simple; healthcare administrative structures change, new ECs may be formed whilst old ones are disbanded. Even where the administrative framework is stable, is three years long enough? What about the situation where a subject who suffered harm as a result of his or her participation in a clinical trial decides to sue the EC who approved the research? The subject's harm may only become apparent several years after trial participation. It is also possible to imagine the situation where following the licensing of a medicine, more widespread clinical use reveals it to have harmful effects. Can the EC demonstrate that it carried out its duties and responsibilities adequately at the time, especially with respect to the protection of subjects? Similarly, detection of investigator fraud can take time and involve the inspection of records going back many years. Therefore, retention of documents for just three years may be inadequate to protect the EC from investigations that may happen in the future, and a period of five to ten years is probably more appropriate. The Clinical Trial Regulation requires the sponsor keep essential documentation for 25 years upon completion of the study.

ICH GCP is clear about what documents should be submitted to an EC for review: the EC should obtain trial protocol(s)/amendment(s), written informed consent form(s) and consent form updates that the investigator proposes for use in the trial, subject recruitment procedures (e.g. advertisements), written information to be provided to subjects, investigator's brochure (IB), available safety information, information about payments and compensation available to subjects, the investigator's current curriculum vitae and/or other documentation evidencing qualifications, and any other documents that the EC may need to fulfil its responsibilities—quite a long list!

The EC should review a proposed clinical trial within a reasonable time (a maximum of 60 days for standard products within Europe), and document its views in writing, clearly identifying the trial, the documents reviewed and the dates for approval/favourable opinion, or any modifications required prior to its approval/favourable opinion. If the application is unsuccessful, disapproval/negative opinion, or termination/suspension of any prior approval/favourable opinion should be notified within the same time frame. Therefore, an EC should keep all of this documentation for whatever period is defined in its SOPs, which should be for at least three years.

If research is being carried out in the UK, the following legislation, policies, and common-practice guidance apply to the retention of records relating to research carried out in the NHS.

- Data Protection Act 1998 (DPA)—Schedule 1, Part 1, Principle 5 states that personal data processed for any purpose or purposes shall not be kept for longer than is necessary for that purpose or those purposes. However, the Medicines for Human Use (Clinical Trials) Amendment Regulations 2006—sections 18 and 28 states that the sponsor and the chief investigator shall ensure that the documents contained, or which have been contained, in the trial master file are retained for five years after the conclusion of the trial. The sponsor and the chief investigator shall ensure that the medical files of trial subjects are retained for at least five years after the conclusion of the trial. The Clinical Trial Regulation stipulates records should be kept for 25 years upon completion of the trial.

When UK law refers to EC documents, it states that an EC shall retain all the documents relating to a clinical trial on which it gives an opinion for (a) where the trial proceeds, at least three years from the conclusion of the trial, or (b) where the trial does not proceed, at least three years from the date of the opinion (The Medicines for Human Use (Clinical Trials) Amendment Regulations 2006). UK law is therefore in agreement with ICH GCP and the EU Directive.

Various organizations (e.g. sponsors, funders, regulatory bodies, ECs, trusts, universities) may stipulate for how long records should be kept. However, meeting any of these requirements in relation to research involving the National Health Service must be consistent with UK law and Department of Health guidance.

Human Tissue Act 2004

Introduction
In the UK, research with human tissue takes place either under ethical approval by an independent EC or under the aegis of a Human Tissue Licence. The former allows use of samples under the specified terms of the EC approval and any planned use outside of this requires a substantial ethical amendment. A Human Tissue Licence under the terms of the Human Tissue Act, is overseen by the Human Tissue Authority (HTA). Biorepositories require explicit ethical approval and in addition, a Human Tissue Licence may also be required.

Background: what it is and how it came about
The Human Tissue Act 2004 (HT Act) came into force on 1 April 2006, consolidating and replacing the Human Tissue Act (1961), Anatomy Act (1984), and the Human Organ Transplants Act (1989). It sets out a legal framework for regulating the storage and use of human organs and tissue from the living and removal, storage, and use of tissue and organs from the deceased.

Fully implemented on 1 September 2006, the HT Act was introduced following public enquiries into 'scandals' involving the removal, use, and retention of human tissue without proper consent. Although the initial enquiries centred on activities at the Royal Infirmary and the Royal Liverpool Children's Hospital, Alder Hey, it became clear that post-mortem organ removal, examination, and retention without consent was commonplace throughout NHS institutions and widely regarded by the medical profession as 'normal practice'. The resulting changes in legislation were designed to clarify the law and restore public confidence. Overseeing the current legislation is the Human Tissue Authority (HTA) by licensing and inspecting organizations that store and use human tissue for research, organ donation and transplant, post-mortem examination, and public exhibitions.

The HT Act mainly covers England, Wales, and Northern Ireland, with the exception of the UK-wide offence of DNA 'theft' or having human tissue with the intent to analyse its DNA without qualifying consent. Its counterpart in Scotland is the Human Tissue (Scotland) Act 2006.

What does the HT Act cover?
The HT Act focuses on two fundamental issues: licensing and consent. Licensing allows specific activities to be carried out at specified premises under the supervision of a named designated individual (DI), whilst appropriate consent allows the lawful storage and use of 'relevant material' for certain 'scheduled purposes'.

Licensing
The activities licensed by the HTA under the HT Act are:
- carrying out of an anatomical examination
- conducting a post-mortem examination
- removal of relevant material from a deceased person
- storage of relevant material from a deceased person (other than for a specific ethically approved project)

- storage of anatomical specimens
- storage of relevant material from a living person for research (other than for a specific ethically approved project) or for human application
- public display of a body or material from a deceased person

The HTA is also responsible for carrying out inspections to ensure that the licence conditions are being upheld.

Key licensing requirements

The licensing requirements outlined by the HTA broadly follow four themes; consent, governance and quality systems, premises, facilities and equipment, and disposal. Compliance with these is evaluated by the HTA on application and at subsequent inspections.

- Consent—under the HT Act, there should be provision for informed consent and this must be obtained in accordance with the HTA Code of Practice on Consent.
- Governance and quality systems—to ensure the quality and integrity of material, management systems should include relevant documented policies and procedures, training and competency records, traceability of material, adverse event reporting, audits and record management.
- Premises, facilities and equipment—premises need to be fit for purpose, with environmental conditions that avoid potential contamination, and facilities and equipment which are suitable for storage, transport, and delivery, thereby maintaining material integrity.
- Disposal—there should be a clear and sensitive policy for disposing of human organs and tissue which is written in accordance with the HTA Code of Practice for disposal of human organs and tissues and complies with health and safety requirements. The reasons for disposal and the methods used should be clearly documented, along with any consent or authorization. These requirements also include disposal of surplus material from medical treatments, diagnostic purposes, research, or material which is no longer to be used or stored for a scheduled purpose.

Key roles

There are a number of key roles associated with an HTA licence, with defined responsibilities. Everyone working with human tissue, however, has a responsibility of knowing what the HT Act is and how it affects their activities.

- Designated individual (DI)—this is a named individual who has a legal duty to ensure that the requirements of the licence are met. The DI does not have to be medically qualified but should hold a suitable position to allow him or her to carry out his or her duty.
- Licence holder (LH)—this can be an individual and the same person as the DI but is preferably and usually the corporate body, e.g. NHS Trust.
- Persons designated (PD)—these individuals are designated by the DI and may be named in the licence. They do not have a legal duty but must have an adequate understanding of the HT Act in order to direct others in relation to the requirements.

Licensing exemptions

There are some specific activities which are exempt from licensing under the HT Act. These exemptions include but are not limited to the following:

- Storage of material for less than a week while being conveyed from one place to another.
- Storage of relevant material for transplantation, where the material is an organ or part of an organ or the storage is for less than 48 hours.
- Tissue held prior to processing with the intention to extract DNA, RNA or other subcellular components that are not 'relevant material' (i.e. rendering the tissue acellular), providing the processing takes hours or days and less than a week.
- Storage of tissue and cells for a research project that has appropriate ethics approval. If storage is continued after the project has ended, a licence will be required. In addition, consent is not required to store and use tissue from the living for an ethically approved research project if it has been anonymized.
- Material from deceased persons more than 100 years old.
- Storage of material from a person who died before the HT Act came into force.
- Storage of relevant material from the body of a deceased person for the purpose of research which has been ethically approved by an EC or for a specific research project for which such ethical approval is pending.
- Storage of relevant material which has come from the body of a living person where the intended use is for determining cause of death, obtaining information which may be relevant to another person, education or training related to human health or qualifying research.

For more details on specific licensing exemptions, please see the HTA website.

Appropriate consent

Once an establishment is licensed under the HT Act for the appropriate activities, consent is the next crucial element underpinning the legislation. Consent relates to the 'scheduled purposes' for which material might be removed, stored, or used. Having established that consent is necessary, the Act requires 'appropriate consent', which is defined in terms of the person who may give consent. This is either the consent of the person concerned, his or her nominated representative or, in the absence of either of these, the consent of a person in a qualifying relationship with him or her immediately before he or she died. The standards expected with respect to the HT Act are laid out by HTA in the Code of Practice on Consent, including a requirement for those seeking consent to be adequately trained and competent to do so, and provisions for taking tissue from the living, the deceased, adults who lack capacity, and children.

What are 'scheduled purposes'?

General purposes requiring appropriate consent include:
- anatomical examination
- determining cause of death
- establishing after a person's death the efficacy of any drug or other treatment administered to him or her

- obtaining scientific or medical information about a living or deceased person which may be relevant to any other person (including a future person)
- public display
- research in connection with disorders or the functioning of the human body
- transplantation

Consent to use material from deceased persons is also required for clinical audit purposes, education or training relating to human health, performance assessment, public health monitoring, and quality assurance.

What is 'relevant material'?

'Relevant material' under the HT Act includes material from a human body, other than gametes, which consists of or includes human cells. In essence, this includes body parts and organs such as bone, skin, and brain, biopsies, blood, tissue blocks, microscope slides, and any human bodily fluid or waste product that might contain cells such as saliva, breast milk, faeces, and urine. Relevant material does not include embryos outside the human body, or hair and nail from the body of a living person.

Tips and advice

- Check if the organization is licensed with the HTA for the relevant scheduled purposes, and who the DI is.
- Know what the HT Act is and what it covers.
- Fully understand the requirements and standards to be met under the HTA's regulatory framework and any individual responsibilities.
- Establish whether material collected requires consent, is classed as 'relevant material', and is intended for use under the licensed 'scheduled purposes'.
- Know what tissues are held within the establishment, what is 'relevant material' and what is not, when the material was collected, and whether consent was given.
- Have processes in place for tracking tissue from consent to disposal, including sample inventories, consignment/delivery notes, audit trails, and document retention.
- Ensure those seeking consent are suitably trained and competent.
- Best practice is to obtain consent wherever practicably possible, even if not legally required under the HT Act. Consent can be project-specific consent for storage and use or, where applicable, generic for storage and future use.
- Go to the HTA website for more advice, or contact them directly at enquiries@hta.gov.uk

Further reading

Declaration of Helsinki ℔ www.wma.net/en/30publications/10policies/b3/

Clinical Trials Regulation ℔ www.mhra.gov.uk/Howweregulate/Medicines/index.htm

International Conference on Harmonisation of Technical Requirements for Registration of Pharmaceuticals for Human Use ℔ http://www.ich.org/

Dixon-Woods M, Angell EL. Research involving adults who lack capacity: how have research ethics committees interpreted the requirements? *Journal of Medical Ethics* 2009;35: 377–81.

Human Tissue Act 2004 ℔ http://www.legislation.gov.uk/ukpga/2004/30/contents

Human Tissue Authority website ℔ www.hta.gov.uk/

Human Tissue (Scotland) Act 2006 ℔ www.legislation.gov.uk/asp/2006/4/contents

HTA Code of Practice for Consent ℔ www.hta.gov.uk/legislationpoliciesandcodesofpractice/codesofpractice/code1consent.cfm

HTA Code of Practice for Disposal ℔ www.hta.gov.uk/legislationpoliciesandcodesofpractice/codesofpractice/code5disposal.cfm

Role and responsibilities: investigator and research team

Introduction

The good clinical practice (GCP) guidelines (ICH E6) have as their clear primary objective the need to safeguard and protect the rights, safety, and well-being of clinical trial subjects, and as their clear secondary objective ensuring the collection of high quality and verifiable data.

Responsibility for achieving these objectives is divided among three identified parties, the IEC/IRB, the investigator, and the sponsor. Each party has a chapter of the ICH E6 guidelines outlining its responsibilities. The ICH E6 devotes one chapter per each party. The independent ethics committee (IEC) or institutional review board (IRB, in the US) is responsible for the safeguarding and protection of the rights, safety, and well-being of subjects, and therefore appears first in Chapter 3 of the guideline. Immediately following in Chapter 4 is coverage of the responsibilities of the investigator who actually treats the trial subjects and thus directly affects the trial subject. The third party, the sponsor, is covered in Chapter 5. The main tasks of the sponsor with regards to the trial subjects lie in the provision of support and guidance to the research teams and in ensuring consistency in the generation of data. The sponsor sets up the parameters of the trial, based upon expected event rates and the best risk/benefit assessment the research team can make. The sponsor's other main task is to ensure the quality of data by applying quality control (QC) and quality assurance (QA) procedures as the trial is underway.

The investigative site staff is in a unique position as they have direct contact with the trial subjects. Any action taken to safeguard the rights, safety, and well-being of the trial subject has a direct impact on the subjects.

The role of the investigator

The role of the investigator is crucial as he or she is both qualified and responsible for leading the research team conducting a clinical trial as well as bringing together the following key elements of the clinical research process. These include:
- Ideas and collaborations
- Support
  - Clinical
  - Scientific
  - Financial
  - Sponsorship (may be responsible if uncoupled from financial support)
- Ethical approval
- Site resources
- Standard operating procedures
- Commitment from appropriately appointed site personnel
- Approval by other relevant bodies and/or stakeholders

In investigator-initiated studies, any intellectual property rights related to the clinical trial rest with the investigator and/or the institution he or she is representing.

There are different types of investigators in a clinical trial, and these include:

- Principal or chief investigator (PI or CI). The PI has overall responsibility for the study at the site. The CI may well fulfil the duties of the PI but also holds overall responsibility, often for multiple sites
- Deputy PI or CI can deputize for the principal/chief investigator and may hold an equivalent level of responsibility, particularly in multiple site trials over a large geographical region
- Co-investigator or sub-investigator (may be more than one per trial) has secondary responsibility, usually reporting to the principal/chief investigator

The study coordinator (often a senior research nurse or other appropriately experienced healthcare professional) works closely with the investigator and has shared responsibility in certain areas, as per a CTA (clinical trial agreement).

Responsibilities of the investigator

Who holds investigators responsible? Everyone! The investigator is accountable to the following organizations or groups of individuals:

- Independent ethics committees
- Regulatory authorities (e.g. Medicines and Healthcare Regulatory Authority, MHRA)
- Institution management (e.g. the research and development (R&D) directorate/division of an NHS trust/health board or its equivalent in a university setting)
- Sponsor (e.g. a pharmaceutical company in commercial research or the management of an institution in non-commercial research)
- Trial participants, their doctors, carers, and families

In what way are investigators held responsible? The following mechanisms all require responsibility/accountability on the part of the investigator:

- Legislative frameworks (International Conference on Harmonisation—Good Clinical Practice (ICH GCP), the European Clinical Trials Directive and its incorporation into UK law, and the Clinical Trial Regulation)
- Institutional governance frameworks (based on ICH GCP and the research governance framework)
- Professional accountability
- Moral obligation
- Scientific obligation
- Responsibility to patients

What are the actual responsibilities of the investigator? This list can be extensive and may vary according to the particular clinical trial in question. The following are important generic resources that the investigator is responsible for:

- resources
  - Appropriate resources at trial site(s) (potential participants, materials, money, and manpower)
  - Staff qualifications, skills, and knowledge (e.g. ICH GCP certification)

- At least one qualified physician as part of the research team, to make medical judgements
- participants
  - Adequate medical care of participants during the trial
  - Appropriate treatment of adverse events (AEs) and/or adverse reactions (ARs)
  - Continuity of care at start and end of trial
  - Attempt to understand reasons for participant withdrawal
- protocol and regulation compliance
  - Protocol deviations only to eliminate an immediate or definite hazard
  - Facilitating monitoring and auditing
  - Obtaining informed consent
- safety reporting (and where relevant, premature termination or suspension of a trial)
- data security and integrity
- appropriate storage, handling, and use of investigational medicinal products (IMPs)

Accountability

Accountability of IMP at the trial site lies with the principal investigator and an IMP must only be used in accordance with the trial protocol. There may be additional requirements as detailed in standard operating procedures (SOPs). Accountability of IMP may be delegated to the pharmacist but the investigator is still ultimately responsible. The investigator must ensure that those delegated to are qualified, competent, and aware of regulatory requirements. Responsibility for records includes ensuring that case report forms (CRFs) are completed and contain at least the following:

- Dates
- Signatures
- Appropriate and legible clinical notes

Communication is an important function of an effective research team and although this may be delegated to a sub-investigator or study coordinator, the investigator is responsible for ensuring the following:

- approvals to everyone
- amendments to everyone
- periodic reports
- end-of-study reports

The role and responsibilities of healthcare professionals in research

Healthcare professionals play a key role in clinical research, as the core principle of clinical research is that it includes the use of human trial subjects.

In phase I the subjects are typically healthy volunteers, with the exception of certain therapeutic areas like oncology or HIV/AIDS where patient volunteers are asked to participate. From phase II the trials will be run by including patients with the specific disease indication for which the investigational product is being developed.

Phase I trials are mostly run in specialized units with the use of clinical research professionals that are dedicated to phase I clinical trials.

From phase II onwards, clinical trials are typically run in regular clinics and hospitals, where a significant part of the trial site staff are regular healthcare professionals having additional tasks in a role as clinical trial site staff member.

Running a clinical trial is very different from everyday practice for healthcare professionals.

Here are two examples where things are significantly different in a clinical research setting.

Example 1: Informed consent

An informed consent (Chapter 9) within regular medical practice is a document that a patient signs to consent to a particular treatment. This consent for the largest part is intended to protect the healthcare professional and the treating institution, the clinic, or hospital. A patient is informed about the options and consents to a proposed intervention.

In clinical trials, informed consent is intended to protect the trial subject. The amount of information offered and collected is much more detailed. We are asking subjects to undergo an experimental treatment. It is a requirement to explain clearly the differences between normal practice and experimental practice. The differences between the expected risks and potential benefits of both treatments must be outlined and time must be given for participants to make a well-informed voluntary decision to take part. This includes making every effort to ensure their understanding, which includes a measurement of their understanding through question and answer moments. The differing consent procedures are not comparable.

The other example concerns medical practice versus clinical research practice. The two differ significantly. Medical practice is standard care, the everyday practice that exists in clinics and hospitals.

Example 2 concerns timings of drug administration

In medical practice a drug is to be administered every 12 hours. If, however, a patient attends hospital at 9 p.m. he or she is likely to get the first dose before 10 p.m. The next day the patient goes into the normal routine of drug distribution and administration, 8 a.m. and 6 p.m. This clearly is not every 12 hours but accommodates shift transitions, etc. In a clinical research setting, if that same patient becomes a trial subject upon presentation to the hospital, he or she may equally receive the first dose at around 10 p.m.

However, as the label indicates a dosing every 12 hours, this trial subject receives the next dose at 10 a.m. and then at 10 p.m. That makes two time points when the healthcare professional needs to be very alert to ensure that the trial subject receives the dose as per protocol.

Healthcare professionals, outside the realm of clinical trials, are treating their patients on an individual basis. Slight adjustments to standard treatment are quite common. The focus of the treatment is the patient's response to that treatment. Tests are conducted to determine the patient's response to a treatment. Treatments are changed, terminated, or initiated based upon the patient's individual response, when the desired outcome has been achieved.

In clinical trial practice, tests are conducted as indicated in the protocol. Treatments are administered as outlined in the protocol. Concomitant medication may be prohibited and should not be given. Any follow-up visits and tests must be completed as detailed in the protocol.

When a patient becomes a clinical trial subject, everything changes. For those patients it is more important to ensure consistency in treatment by following the protocol as closely as possible, ensuring as controlled circumstances as possible, enabling the best comparison of the outcome, rather than to provide a tailored, personal approach to medicine.

For healthcare professionals working in the clinical research setting, if an error occurs it is vital to record the incident. Proper documentation of exactly what happens is key. Documentation that as closely as possible reflects what actually happened is crucial to clinical trials and the ability to retrace steps and explain outliers when needed is critical.

When healthcare professionals become clinical research professionals, much changes with regard to their roles. Their primary responsibility remains to protect the rights, safety, and well-being of the trial subjects, closely followed by the responsibility to follow the protocol and ensure the highest possible standards of clinical research are maintained. The responsibilities are outlined in ICH GCP: to safeguard and protect the rights, safety, and well-being of clinical trial subjects, and ensure the collection of high-quality and verifiable data.

The other document that the healthcare professionals have to adhere to is the Declaration of Helsinki. This declaration, first issued in 1964, contains the 'Ethical Principles for Medical Research Involving Human Subjects'. This declaration, a guidance document, is drafted and published by the World Medical Association (WMA). Although primarily addressing physicians in clinical research, the WMA 'encourages other participants in medical research involving human subjects to adopt these principles' (Article 2, 2013 version).

There are some clear articles in the Declaration of Helsinki (2013 version) that outline the role and responsibility of the physicians in medical research, which all healthcare professionals in medical research are encouraged to adopt.

Article 4 declares that 'it is the duty of the physicians to promote and safeguard the health of patients, including those who are involved in medical research. The physician's knowledge and conscience are dedicated to the fulfilment of this duty'.

Also (in Article 9), 'it is the duty of physicians who participate in medical research to protect the life, health, dignity, integrity, right to self-determination, privacy, and confidentiality of personal information of research subjects'.

Finally, in Article 20 the Declaration of Helsinki (2008) states that physicians may not participate in a research study involving human subjects unless they are confident that the risks involved have been adequately assessed and can be satisfactorily managed. Physicians must immediately stop a study when the risks are found to outweigh the potential benefits, or when there is conclusive proof of positive and beneficial results.

Regarding the balance between medical care and clinical research, according to the Declaration of Helsinki, the physician may combine medical research with medical care only to the extent that the research is justified by its potential preventive, diagnostic or therapeutic value and if the physician has good reason to believe that participation in the research study will not adversely affect the health of the patients who serve as research subjects.

As much as the Declaration of Helsinki is a controversial document, the FDA no longer refers to the Declaration; in the EU, the Clinical Trial Directives refer to the 1996 version; with regard to the 2000 version, the 2002 and 2004 rewrites have not been generally accepted. However, the EU regulation refers to the 2008 version of the document.

The Declaration was rewritten in 2013 and is generally not referred to as yet.

Who is involved in trials?

Research teams come in many varieties when it comes to size and positions involved. The smallest possible team is a team of one: the investigator. Every team requires an investigator. ICH GCP (E6) describes the investigator as '[a] person responsible for the conduct of the clinical trial at a trial site. If a trial is conducted by a team of individuals at a trial site, the investigator is the responsible leader of the team and may be called the principal investigator'.

That team of individuals can consist of:

- principal investigator
- sub-investigator/co-investigator
- research nurse
- clinical research coordinator
- pharmacist
- laboratory responsible person
- protocol-specific personnel

Principal investigator

As stated, the principal investigator (PI) is responsible overall for the conduct of a clinical trial on site. The role of the PI has changed significantly over time.

The PI has largely been a figurehead in a trial in the past. The actual execution of the trial was undertaken by the team; the PI signed the necessary documentation but was often not directly involved in the day-to-day activities of the trial. On paper, the PI would be responsible overall; in practice, often the PI was not always aware of the current status of a trial.

Of course, this is a gross generalization and it would do great injustice to the investigators who actively run their trials. There was a great difference in the situation between a large (often academic) hospital and a smaller rural hospital or clinic. Also, there was a significant difference based upon geographical locations. In those countries where clinical trials have been underway for decades, the described situation occurred frequently. In the countries where clinical trials were just starting, the involvement of the PI was mostly direct and intense.

Over the past decade, the situation of the absent PI has been addressed significantly. The FDA (through the publication online of their warning letters) took a clear stand on the matter and cited investigators for not taking responsibilities. Other inspectors and auditors followed suit, and currently within the sponsor companies it is becoming the norm to keep track of the availability and involvement of the PI in the trial.

Although generally the case, a PI does not have to be a physician. There is no regulation that states this; moreover, ICH GCP actively mentions situations where the PI is not a physician. Many sponsor companies, however, have in their SOPs that they want their investigators to be physicians. This of course would influence their site selection procedure, leading to only physician investigators being selected.

The responsibilities of the PI can be categorized and summarized as follows.

With regards to subject safety the PI must:

- exhibit the highest ethical standards.
- prioritize subject safety and well-being over scientific interest.
- conduct his/her own risk/benefit analysis based upon available information of the product and previous trials with the product.
- ensure that the benefits and risks of participating in a trial are explained and understood by the subject.

In addition, the qualification of the PI is reviewed by the IEC/IRB prior to the site being approved to participate.
The PI should:
- be qualified by education, training, and experience to assume responsibility for the proper conduct of the trial.
- be familiar and compliant with ICH GCP and applicable ethical and regulatory requirements.
- provide evidence of qualifications through up-to-date *curriculum vitae* (CV) and/or other relevant documentation.

Often, the CV of the PI is a lengthy document listing all the publications the investigator has ever been involved in; however, it often lacks proper documentations of ICH GCP training and other clinical trial-related training and experience. The clinical research-relevant entries have to be documented in an up-to-date CV. The PI is responsible for ensuring that only appropriately trained and qualified staff work on their trials. The investigators are responsible for ensuring that all site staff members also document their education, qualification, and experience in an up-to-date CV.

During trial preparation the PI should:
- be thoroughly familiar with the appropriate use of the investigational product(s) as described in:
  - the protocol.
  - the investigator's brochure and/or product information.
  - other relevant information (e.g. a pharmacy binder or similar).
- be able to demonstrate the ability to recruit sufficient and suitable patients within the agreed recruitment period.
- have an adequate number of qualified staff for the duration of the trial to conduct the study properly and safely.
- have adequate facilities and equipment based upon the needs of the protocol.
- ensure that all members of the trial team are adequately trained and informed about the protocol and the investigational product(s) to be able to properly conduct their trial-related duties.
- ensure that the necessary approvals have been obtained from the IEC or IRB of both the trial documentation as well as the site's suitability.

As part of the trial preparation activities, investigators and other site staff may be invited to an investigator meeting to review study details. Pre-trial investigator meetings are typically intended to inform, train, and motivate site staff. They can be considered as part of the initiation process.

The site initiation process is typically concluded by an initiation visit. A monitor will visit the site on behalf of the sponsor and meet with the PI and all other key trial site staff to perform initial training, ensure the site's readiness to start the trial, and prepare the site for commencement of subject enrolment. The PI is responsible for ensuring the attendance of key personnel as well as him or herself personally attending the meeting. The PI is responsible for ensuring that any further training need, after the initiation visit, is addressed, and only trained and qualified staff work on the trials.

During the study, the investigator must:

- conduct the study in compliance with ICH GCP and applicable local law, with regards to ethical and regulatory requirements.
- conduct the study in compliance with the protocol and ensure that staff and patients follow all required procedures.
- adhere to the ethical principles as outlined in the current Declaration of Helsinki.
- ensure properly conducted informed consent procedures and obtain voluntary written informed consent from each trial subject prior to its participation in the trial.
- ensure that source data is kept according to the ALCOA method (Box 11.1).
- ensure that the data reported to the sponsor is accurate and verifiable to the source.
- observe, evaluate, manage, and document all effects of treatment.
- facilitate and be present at site visits where monitors verify study data, and review the progress and conduct of the study.
- foresee inadequate handling, preparation, and administration of the investigational product(s) and the documentation thereof.
- securely maintain the study documents and clinical supplies as agreed with the sponsor.
- ensure the enrolment of the agreed number of subjects who meet trial eligibility criteria.
- ensure all written communications going to (potential) subjects are approved by the IEC or IRB and the sponsor prior to using them.
- notify the IEC/IRB and/or sponsor of any issues that threaten the safety and well-being of the trial subjects.
- submit any changes or protocol amendments to the IEC/IRB for approval.
- provide a yearly update with information about protocol progress to the IEC/IRB.
- demonstrate due diligence to ensure patient compliance with trial procedures and assessments.

During the close-out phase of a trial, the investigator must arrange for archiving of the trial documentation. All essential documents need to be

---

Box 11.1 The ALCOA method stipulates that source data needs to be:

- Accurate
- Legible
- Complete
- Original
- Attributable

archived until the sponsor informs the investigator it can be destroyed. The Clinical Trial Regulation stipulates essential documents are kept for 25 years. That includes the site file documentation, the investigational product accountability documentation, the patient files and all other source documents, copies of the case report forms (CRFs), and contracts.

The investigator must also inform the IEC/IRB about the end of the trial as well as provide the final report for review.

Sub-investigator/Co-investigator

A sub-investigator is any individual member of the clinical trial team designated and supervised by the investigator at a trial site to perform critical trial-related procedures, and/or to make important trial-related decisions (e.g. associates, residents, research fellows) (ICH GCP 1.56).

A sub-investigator differs from an investigator in that a sub-investigator does all of the tasks but bears no responsibility. Everything is done under the supervision of and under the end-responsibility of the PI. Typically we can say that a sub-investigator is a physician member of the trial team, who is not the PI.

Research nurse

The research nurse is often the core person in a trial on site. Many of the tasks of a trial are conducted by the research nurse, as well as most of the planning. Trial subject visits, including the visits to the necessary departments (e.g. imaging), monitoring visits, initial triage of newly presenting potential trial subjects, are all coordinated by the research nurse.

The research nurse is often the primary contact point for a trial subject. Where research nurses are involved in the informed consent procedure there is a bond of trust between the trial subjects and the research nurses, specifically where the relationship with the investigators is often more distant due to the patient–physician relationship.

Clinical research coordinator

Clinical research coordinators (CRCs) fulfil the role of a research nurse. Their job content is very similar but they are not necessarily a nurse.

Pharmacist

In a lot of countries, the involvement of a pharmacist in a clinical trial is mandated by the fact that legally, drugs can only be sent to the care of a pharmacist. Legally then, and mostly the case within a hospital or clinic, the investigational product(s) (IP) will be maintained within the care of a pharmacist.

With regards to the trial responsibilities, however, the end responsibility of the investigational product on site still lies with the PI. The PI is, after all, responsible for the conduct of a clinical trial on site, and that includes IP storage and handling.

If there is a discrepancy between a legal requirement, site practice and the clinical trial on the other hand, good collaboration and good communications between the two roles, the pharmacist and the PI, is crucial to proper IP management.

Laboratory responsible person

In most trials, some lab work needs to be done. It may consist of standard assessments, be part of routine medical care, be a clinical trial-specific assessment, or it can be limited to the taking of bio-samples to be packed and shipped to a central lab.

Regardless of how involved a local lab is, as soon as there is involvement of the lab there needs to be a lab responsible person.

As with all tasks, the tasks of the lab are technically conducted under the supervision of the PI, who has end responsibility for the trial activities being conducted in accordance with the protocol.

Protocol specific

Based upon the protocol, the team of clinical research professionals of a site can be expanded with a variety of roles. For example, the medical imaging department may play a crucial role in a trial, or a paediatric trial may be conducted, which could lead to a child psychologist's involvement for the purpose of the informed consent procedure.

Various roles can be included depending on the protocol requirements. A simple, straightforward protocol may require a small team of site staff consisting only of a PI. This is not uncommon at all; think, for example, of a general practitioner (GP) trial.

As soon as a protocol becomes a bit more complicated, it likely involves a number of healthcare professionals to become a team of clinical research professionals and to execute a trial successfully.

Delegation of duties

The investigator is responsible overall for the conduct of a clinical trial on site. He or she may delegate any and almost all tasks and duties to the research team; however, he or she may choose not to delegate any responsibility. Of course, there is always an exception to the rule. If the PI is not a physician, there will have to be a member of the trial team who is a physician who will be delegated the responsibility of taking care of the medical needs of the trial subjects. In this case, and this case only, a responsibility of the PI can, and even has to be delegated.

Duties that are delegated to other members of the research team should be delegated only to appropriately trained and qualified site staff members. The tasks delegated should be clearly identified and logged in a delegation log. Each delegation needs to be signed by the PI prior to the delegation starting, to document properly the fact that the duty was indeed delegated by the PI.

Delegation of trial duties by no means relinquishes the PI of any responsibility. For any duty delegated, it is essential that the PI has a clear supervision.

Further reading

ICH E6 Guidelines for Good Clinical Practice.
The Commission Directive 2001/20/EC of the European Parliament and of the Council of 4 April 2001.
The Commission Directive 2005/28/EC of 8 April 2005.
The Commission Regulation 536/2014.
European Clinical Trials Directive ℘ http://ec.europa.eu/health/human-use/clinical-trials/directive_en.htm
The Medicines for Human Use (Clinical Trials) Regulations 2004 ℘ www.opsi.gov.uk/
ICH/GCP ℘ www.ich.org/
RGF ℘ http://www.cso.scot.nhs.uk/nrs/research-governance/
MHRA ℘ http://www.mhra.gov.uk/spc-pil/
Clinical Trials Toolkit ℘ www.ct-toolkit.ac.uk/

Role and responsibilities of the sponsor

The role of a sponsor

'The buck stops here.'

Harry S Truman

The role of the sponsor is a key one, the responsibilities are numerous, and the buck really does stop with this person. Even if there are shortcomings of others involved in a study such as an investigator or contract research organization, the onus for quality and integrity remains on the sponsor to put in place appropriate quality control mechanisms to identify such issues early and implement corrective and preventative measures.

This chapter will discuss the definition of a sponsor and the roles and responsibilities that it comprises. The role is critical (without a sponsor, a study may not proceed) and complex. ICH GCP lists more than 60 separate responsibilities of a sponsor, some of which are split into as many as 26 sub-sections. Many of these responsibilities are discussed in more detail elsewhere in this book (e.g. monitoring) and the aim of this chapter is to give an overall picture of the role and legal responsibilities and to focus on the systems required for successfully undertaking the role of sponsor.

ICH GCP defines the sponsor as an individual, company, institution, or organization which takes responsibility for the initiation, management, and/or financing of a clinical trial.[1] This definition is also used in the EU Clinical Trials Directive,[2] and a slightly simpler version is found in the UK Medicines for Human Use (Clinical Trials) Regulations 2004 (SI 1031) (UK Clinical Trials Regulations),[3] which transpose the EU Clinical Trials Directive into UK law. In relation to a clinical trial, a sponsor is the person who takes responsibility for the initiation, management, and financing (or arranging the financing) of that trial. The EU Regulation states that what is written in Directive 2004/20/EC should be upheld. The definition used by the FDA is slightly more complex. The Code of Federal Regulations Title 21, part 312.3(a)[4] defines sponsor as 'a person who takes responsibility for and initiates a clinical investigation. The sponsor may be an individual or pharmaceutical company, governmental agency, academic institution, private organization, or other organization. The sponsor does not actually conduct the investigation unless the sponsor is a sponsor-investigator. A person other than an individual that uses one or more of its own employees to conduct an investigation that it has initiated is a sponsor, not a sponsor-investigator, and the employees are investigators.'

It must also be remembered that the individual States of the US have their own laws and regulations which may affect aspects of the sponsor's role (e.g. handling of study medication).

Under the UK Clinical Trials Regulations, it is an offence to conduct a clinical trial without a sponsor, and the Medicines and Healthcare products Regulatory Agency (MHRA) requires evidence that a sponsor has accepted the role before a clinical trials authorization (i.e. UK regulatory approval) can be issued.

Who may act as the sponsor of a clinical study?

The individual or organization undertaking the role of sponsor must be agreed before a study may proceed. Deciding who should undertake the role of sponsor is straightforward in many cases, particularly where a company with intellectual property rights in a product funds a study. In this situation, the company will be the sponsor, even if aspects of managing the study are delegated to a contract research organization (CRO). For example, a pharmaceutical company is undertaking a phase 3 clinical trial of a new prostate cancer treatment at 30 hospital centres throughout the EU and has developed a protocol. The pharmaceutical product was discovered by a small biotechnology company which has licensed the rights to the pharmaceutical company. The running of the study has been delegated to a large multinational CRO which will be selecting study centres, initiating and running the study, as well as conducting audits. In this situation, the pharmaceutical company will be the sponsor of the study.

In other cases where the responsibility for initiation, management, and financing are split, discussion will be needed so that the most appropriate sponsor is determined. Examples include a study initiated and funded by a research council or charity and managed by staff it employs, working within a hospital or university. In this case, the sponsor's role would generally be undertaken by the research council/charity but might be undertaken by the hospital or university hosting the research which has a duty of care to those enrolled in the study.

In the US, trials may be sponsored by an organization such as a pharmaceutical company, a federal agency such as the National Institutes of Health or Veterans Administration, or an individual physician or healthcare provider. The Code of Federal Regulations also states that sometimes, but not always, the manufacturer of the drug being tested is the clinical trial sponsor.

Is co- or joint sponsorship possible?

Those considering taking on the role of sponsor may find the responsibilities daunting and feel that they are too much for a single entity. Certainly, very few public entities such as universities, hospitals, charities, or funding bodies have the necessary infrastructure. In particular, institutions may be unwilling to accept responsibility for work carried out by a different entity within a multicentre or even multinational study, and funding may be insufficient to pay for the administration that is necessary. Co- or joint sponsorship may therefore seem an attractive possibility.

ICH GCP does not discuss joint or co-sponsorship but regulations in individual countries may permit such arrangements; for example, the UK Clinical Trials Regulations permit groups of individuals or institutions to take on the sponsor's responsibilities. This may be as co-sponsors, where the group of individuals or institutions each have a defined subset of the overall responsibilities, or as joint sponsors, where the responsibilities are shared jointly. Joint sponsors are both jointly and severally responsible for the duties of a sponsor, so if one party does not undertake its delegated responsibilities, all are collectively responsible for the failure. An example is where a consortium of UK hospitals agrees to undertake a study and split the responsibilities among co-sponsors; one hospital will obtain regulatory approval, another will collate and interpret safety data, etc. If there is a failure within the study—for example, if safety data is not forwarded to the regulatory authorities within the applicable time frame—the responsibility will lie with the hospital that took on the responsibility for that action. If instead of a co-sponsorship agreement there had been a joint sponsorship arrangement, every centre would have been equally responsible for the failure of the one centre to forward safety data to the regulatory authority in a timely manner. This requires a high degree of mutual trust, and in general in the UK, co-sponsorship is generally the preferred option.

Co-sponsorship is not, however, permitted in other European Union countries, even though the Clinical Trials Directive[2] does not preclude it. Although there have been a couple of anecdotal cases where two sponsors have been allowed (e.g. by the French regulatory authority), the concept of co- or joint sponsorship would be exceptional. The FDA also does not recognize the concept of co-sponsorship and indeed requests details of the sponsor (singular) on the Investigational New Drug Application. Co- or joint sponsorship would therefore only be appropriate for studies conducted exclusively within the UK and/or other countries recognizing the concept of joint or co-sponsorship. It should, however, be noted that the FDA does permit sponsors to transfer responsibilities to a CRO, and this is discussed further later in the chapter.

Can an investigator be the sponsor?

The investigator may be the most appropriate sponsor for a study he or she has initiated and will be managing, even though finance may have been obtained from a grant-giving body or from a pharmaceutical company. One example is an investigator-initiated study, where an investigator from a specialist referral centre requests funding and supplies of blinded study medication from a pharmaceutical company to conduct a study looking at the effects of a new treatment on very severely ill patients. The pharmaceutical company may provide the required support on condition that the study is run to GCP standards and in accordance with local laws and regulations, for example, covering disclosure of data and confidentiality. The investigator would take the role of the sponsor and would fall within the ICH defined category of investigator sponsor.

ICH GCP defines a sponsor investigator as: '[a]n individual who both initiates and conducts, alone or with others, a clinical trial, and under whose immediate direction the investigational product is administered to, dispensed to, or used by a subject. The term does not include any person other than an individual (e.g., it does not include a corporation or an agency). The obligations of a sponsor-investigator include both those of a sponsor and those of an investigator.' Even if, as in the UK, regulations permit an individual to be the sponsor, many institutions such as universities and hospitals do not allow their employees to undertake such a role due to the responsibilities involved, such as the need for insurance and indemnity, and assurance of quality. In such a situation, a hospital may elect to become the sponsor for an investigator-initiated study.

What are the implications of taking on the role of sponsor?

The role of sponsor is crucial to the study and involves potential risks in a number of areas. It is recommended that a risk assessment is performed before a sponsor agrees to take on this role for a particular study, and risks may be mitigated by clear and comprehensive planning and documentation of responsibilities, monitoring/audit of the study, and selection of study

personnel who are appropriately qualified and trained. It is important that the sponsor considers these main areas of potential risk:
- Financial—for example, the routine expense of the study and any claims for compensation from study subjects
- Reputation of the sponsor—for example, adverse publicity resulting from safety issues
- Legal—for example, prosecution for breach of regulations such as failures in pharmacovigilance reporting

Many countries have laws governing clinical research (e.g. the US Code of Federal Regulations) and these specify that studies must be conducted to GCP standards (which specify the role of a sponsor in detail). Some specify the role of a sponsor in more detail in their legislation. Legal action may therefore be taken against sponsors who fail in their responsibilities; this could be a fine or may even involve imprisonment. The responsibilities of a sponsor should therefore not be adopted lightly.

For European studies, sponsors have the following responsibilities:
- Legal
  - To either be a legal entity in Europe, or appoint a legal representative
  - Arrange appropriate indemnity cover for study subjects
- Regulatory and ethics
  - Request the EudraCT number for a study
  - Request regulatory approval for the study from competent authorities (CA)
  - Submits amendments and requests approval for substantial amendments from the CA
  - Ensures that ethics approvals are obtained as appropriate
  - Notifies the end of the study to the CA and the IRB/IEC
  - Provides an end of study report to the CA and the IRB/IEC
- Quality
  - Ensure the quality of the study conduct
  - Ensure the quality of the study data
- Investigational medicinal product (IMP)
  - Responsible for the manufacture, packaging, labelling, and import of IMP
  - Employment of a 'qualified person' to oversee IMP
  - Provide IMP free of charge
- Safety
  - Collection of all adverse events (AE)
  - Notification of suspected unexpected serious adverse reactions (SUSARs)
  - Provides an annual safety report to the CA and IRB/IEC

The legal requirements of a UK sponsor are summarized in the following sections of the UK Clinical Trials Regulations:

Part 3: Authorization and ethics committee opinion
- Request the clinical trial authorization (CTA), amend the request if appropriate
- Produce an undertaking to allow inspection of premises in third countries if required

- Give notice of amendments to CTA, make representations about any amendments
- Give notice of amendments to the protocol
- Give notice a trial has ended

Part 4: Good clinical practice and conduct

- Put and keep in place arrangements to adhere to GCP (if no other person is specified)
- Ensure IMPs are available to subjects free of charge
- Take appropriate urgent safety measures (in conjunction with the investigator)

Part 5: Pharmacovigilance

- Keep records of all adverse events reported by investigators
- Ensure recording and prompt reporting of SUSARSs
- Ensure investigators are informed of SUSARs
- Ensure all SUSARs (including those in third countries) are entered into the European database
- Provide an annual list of suspected serious adverse reactions and a safety report

A person guilty of an offence under the UK Regulations is liable to a fine and/or imprisonment for up to two years.

When is a sponsor's legal representative required?

If the main sponsor of a clinical trial is not based in the European Economic Area (EEA) (e.g. a US or Japanese pharmaceutical company), it is a statutory requirement to appoint a legal representative based in the EEA. The legal representative may be an individual or a representative of a company and does not have to be legally qualified. The legal representative acts as the agent of the sponsor in the event of any legal proceedings within the EEA (e.g. for receipt of legal documents), and should be established and contactable at an address within the EEA.

The sponsor's legal representative does not routinely take on any of the legal liabilities of the sponsor and so won't require insurance or indemnity. However, if the representative does undertake any of the responsibilities of the sponsor (e.g. handling expedited safety reporting to regulatory authorities), the legal representative would then be regarded as a co-sponsor and hence require insurance or indemnity.

What does the sponsor do?

The NHS R&D Forum provides a comprehensive and straightforward summary of what the sponsor is responsible for:[5]

The sponsor is responsible for ensuring that specific duties are performed, properly distributed, allocated and accepted by investigators and their employing institutions and care organizations, and for the governance of the research study from conception to final completion, including design, management, and finance. The sponsor satisfies itself that appropriate checks have been undertaken to ensure that the study meets the relevant standards, and makes sure arrangements are put and kept in place for authorization, management, monitoring and reporting.

While other guidelines have different definitions and summaries, the key point in this summary is 'the governance of the research study from conception to final completion', and 'this concept of governance is crucial to the success of a study'. Clinical trials are large and complex; it is essential that there is proper oversight of the entire project and that the sponsor sets and maintains standards and systems for that oversight. The remainder of this chapter considers sponsor responsibilities in more detail.

The responsibilities of a sponsor

It is an essential principle that whilst activities may be delegated, the responsibility for quality and integrity of the study remains with the sponsor and cannot be delegated. The one and only exception to this rule is where there is a formal joint or co-sponsorship agreement in place, or, in the case of studies conducted to the FDA Code of Federal Regulations, where there has been formal delegation of sponsor responsibilities to a CRO. Almost invariably, delegation does take place within clinical trials, with the possible rare exception of small investigator initiated and sponsored studies where the principal investigator is conducting the study single handedly. Putting in place appropriate systems to check that delegation is appropriate and that delegated responsibilities are being performed to the correct standards are therefore an essential part of the sponsor's role.

Take, for example, a trial centre with a high turnover of staff, little direct involvement of the professor who is principal investigator, and a heavy routine workload in addition to clinical trial activities. If errors are made, such as missed patient assessments, lost documentation, and unreported serious adverse events, the site staff have clearly, and perhaps understandably, failed to maintain the agreed standards for running the study. Nevertheless, the responsibility remains with the sponsor: why was the study placed at this centre? Were the issues identified at initial sponsor visits or have they developed later? Was routine monitoring undertaken appropriately and if so, did it identify the issues at the site? What action was taken as a result? The sponsor's systems need to be robust enough to take appropriate preventative and corrective actions in a timely manner, to avoid such issues having a significant impact on the study.

ICH GCP specifically refers to this in relation to a CRO: 'A sponsor may transfer any or all of the sponsor's trial-related duties and functions to a CRO, but the ultimate responsibility for the quality and integrity of the trial data always resides with the sponsor. The CRO should implement quality assurance and quality control. Any trial-related duty and function that is transferred to and assumed by a CRO should be specified in writing. Any trial-related duties and functions not specifically transferred to and assumed by a CRO are retained by the sponsor.' ICH GCP also specifies: 'Prior to initiating a trial, the sponsor should define, establish, and allocate all trial-related duties and functions.'

The situation is slightly different for studies conducted under the FDA Code of Federal Regulations, where the transfer of obligations to a contract research organization is permitted. Under the Code of Federal Regulations Title 21 section 312.52, a sponsor may transfer responsibility for any or all of his or her obligations to a CRO in writing. Anything not specified in writing is assumed not to have been transferred. A CRO must comply with the same regulations and is subject to the same regulatory actions in respect of any failure. However, it is important to remember that the sponsor still retains the responsibility for this transfer of obligations and (under GCP) for 'the ultimate responsibility for the quality and integrity' of the trial data'. The sponsor would therefore be expected to be responsible for selecting a CRO to which the delegation is appropriate, and for proper oversight of the CRO throughout the study. The FDA ruling may be seen more as clarifying action that may be taken against a poorly performing CRO rather than absolving the sponsor of responsibility for the overall quality and integrity of the study.

When is the sponsor *not* responsible?

Whilst the sponsor has overarching responsibilities to delegate appropriately and put in place appropriate mechanisms to ensure the quality and integrity of the study, the investigator and site staff and the IRB/IEC also have responsibilities. Unless the principal investigator is also the sponsor, it is unlikely that the sponsor will have any direct contact with the study subjects, and only the IRB/IEC has all the information around the site facilities, subjects, and personnel that is required to make an appropriate judgement around the appropriate placement of a study.

The investigational site staff do not act as representatives or legal agents of the sponsor. Their primary responsibility is to the study subjects, including determining whether the benefits of participating in the study outweigh the risks for a specific subject, obtaining informed consent, and supervision of participants in the study. By providing information on the risks of a treatment to the investigator, the sponsor is deemed to have acted properly and it is the responsibility of the investigator to inform the study subjects of those risks.

Take the example of an investigator deciding whether to enrol an elderly patient into a trial for advanced metastatic breast cancer. Whilst the patient may be eligible for the study in terms of the protocol-specified inclusion/exclusion criteria, the investigator must make a judgement about the risks and benefits for that unique patient. What is that patient's home situation? What about the requirements to travel to additional clinic visits? Does the patient live in a rural area and rely upon public transport? Does the patient fully understand the study and the available alternative treatments, or does he or she think that 'doctor knows best', and is aggressive treatment to be preferred for this patient over palliative care? Is the patient convinced that the trial offers him or her a 'miracle cure' or are his or her expectations realistic? Only the investigator and the investigational site staff can make the appropriate judgement.

The IRB/IEC is in a position to make judgements around the suitability of the investigator, the facilities, and the local population for a particular study protocol; the sponsor generally would not have access to the kind of information upon which such a decision is based. Having made that judgement and given approval for a study, the IRB/IEC responsibility continues throughout the trial, and both ICH GCP and the FDA CFR are clear that it is the responsibility of the IRB/IEC to protect the rights and welfare of trial participants throughout the study.

Take the example of an investigator who has recently had an unsatisfactory audit that showed he had too many study patients to provide adequate oversight and care. Or a centre that is expected to soon lose access to an on-site CAT scanner due to a local reorganization, a test that is essential to the study protocol. Or a centre with a large Urdu-speaking population. The IRB/IEC must judge whether the centre has the expertise and resource required, or whether minor changes are required; for example, translation of the patient information, consent form, and diary card.

The sponsor's responsibility is to provide the investigator and the IRB/IEC with comprehensive information in a timely manner so that they may make individual decisions specific to a particular trial centre and its population. If, for example, the safety information for the study drug changes part way through the study as a link to an increased rate of pneumonia has been identified, the sponsor has the responsibility to provide the updated information, amended protocol, CRFs, and consent and re-consent forms to the site in a timely manner. The responsibility for contacting the study patients, discussing the new information with them, making individual decisions around continuation or withdrawal for each patient in light of the new information, re-consenting where appropriate, and implementing the amended protocol, remains with the investigator and site staff.

Authorizations and approvals

All authorizations and approvals should be in place before the sponsor permits the study to start. Site authorization, IRB/IEC approval, and regulatory approval are considered in more detail elsewhere in this book.

Site authorization

The sponsor must obtain the investigator's and/or the institution's agreement to conduct the study in compliance with:

- GCP
- applicable regulatory requirements (e.g. the Medicines for Human Use (Clinical Trials) Regulations 2004)
- the protocol, as agreed by the sponsor and approved by the IRB/IEC
- the procedures for data recording/reporting
- agreements to permit monitoring, auditing, and regulatory inspection
- agreements to retain trial-related essential documents until the sponsor informs the investigator/institution these documents are no longer required

The sponsor and the investigator/institution should either sign the protocol or a formal agreement to confirm this.

IRB/IEC approval

The sponsor should obtain from the investigator/institution:

- the name and address of the IRB/IEC and a statement that it is organized and operates according to GCP and applicable laws and regulations
- documented IRB/IEC approval (or favourable opinion) of the study and of the materials the sponsor has provided (e.g. a current copy of protocol, written informed consent form(s) and any other written information to be provided to subjects, subject recruiting procedures, documents related to payments and compensation available to the subjects, and any other documents that the IRB/IEC may have requested)
- if the approval is conditional upon a change or modification (e.g. a change of wording in the consent form), the sponsor should obtain a copy of the modification that has been made and the full unconditional IRB/IEC approval
- documentation and dates of any IRB/IEC re-approvals, withdrawals, or suspensions of approval

Regulatory approval

The sponsor should submit any required application to the appropriate regulatory authority for review, acceptance, and/or permission to begin the study. In the UK, the application will be to the Medicines and Healthcare products Regulatory Agency (MHRA). Regulatory approval is discussed in more detail elsewhere in this book.

Indemnity, insurance, and compensation

The sponsor is responsible for ensuring that appropriate arrangements are put in place concerning indemnity, insurance, and compensation. However, these arrangements vary between countries and it is important for sponsors to check the current legal situation in the countries they are using for a study.

The EU Regulation, EU Directive, and UK regulations make it a legal requirement for the sponsor and the principal investigator to ensure that insurance and indemnity arrangements are in place for a study. These arrangements must be reviewed by the IRB/IEC. If contract research organizations, sub-contractors, etc. are to be used then it is important that indemnity, insurance, and compensation are covered in the contracts covering such arrangements, which should also formally define legal liabilities.

It is important to remember that there are very few legal actions relating to clinical trials compared to, say, routine obstetric practice. Nevertheless, insurance and indemnity are important responsibilities of the sponsor, and under the EU Clinical Trials Directive, a clinical trial may be undertaken only if provision has been made for insurance or indemnity for liabilities of the sponsor and the investigator (although neither the Directive nor the UK Regulations specify who should make this provision). It is also important to ensure that roles and responsibilities defined for a study (e.g. within study agreements) are adequate from a legal perspective as they may potentially serve as a legal defence. In some cases, the IRB/IEC may require additional insurance or indemnity as a condition of granting approval for a specific study.

There is often confusion around insurance, indemnity, and compensation. Compensation is what a study subject will receive if they suffer injury or harm from having participated in a study. Indemnity provides protection for the study staff. Insurance is what pays for compensation and for legal costs.

Indemnity
An indemnity effectively offers no-fault compensation in the situation where harm has resulted from the clinical trial. The indemnity allows 'not at fault' claims, where on the balance of probability, participation in the study caused harm. If a study subject comes to harm, he or she may take advantage of this no-fault compensation rather than seeking legal redress. There is therefore no need for individual members of the study team or institutions such as hospitals or pharmaceutical companies to be sued for compensation and for fault to be attributed, so staff in a study are therefore protected by the indemnity.

Commercial sponsors of studies generally provide the indemnity but there is no onus on the sponsor to provide indemnity, although the sponsor must ensure that an indemnity is provided. It may be provided by the sponsor's employer (e.g. for university staff), or indemnity cover arranged with an insurer.

It must be pointed out that indemnities exclude negligence and situations where the protocol has not been followed. The indemnity will specify that malpractice and negligence are excluded and in this case, insurance will be relied upon to deal with the claim (see the next section on insurance). The indemnity will also specify that the sponsor must be notified and have control of the case. In the case of a pharmaceutical company study being run in a hospital, the hospital would not be able to handle a claim for compensation and simply rely on the pharmaceutical company to pay for any compensation; the pharmaceutical company would need to be notified (under the terms of the indemnity) and would then handle the claim and pay appropriate compensation.

There are sometimes discussions around minor protocol deviations such as a clinic visit a few days outside a visit window, and whether a pharmaceutical company might 'use' these to avoid paying compensation under an indemnity. Apart from wishing to protect its reputation, a pharmaceutical company would generally prefer to deal with what is legally a far more straightforward claim under an indemnity than a legal claim for compensation through the courts, where fault will need to be apportioned. However, where a sponsor feels that there has been significant deviation from the protocol which has resulted in or contributed to harm, then he or she may choose to void the indemnity, so that the compensation claim must be dealt with through the courts, fault established, and any compensation paid through insurance. Examples might be where an investigator has entered a patient into a study while the patient was taking proscribed medication which led to harm, or where an investigator cancelled a number of clinic visits, so leaving the patient unsupervised for a significant period.

Producers continue to have strict liability for faulty medicines, and while the indemnity would cover the situation where the investigational medicinal product was found to have caused harm, the indemnity would not generally cover harm caused by concomitant licensed medications and again, a compensation claim would have to be dealt with through the courts.

Subjects may choose to pursue a legal remedy rather than accepting a settlement under an indemnity, although if a settlement is offered under an indemnity, it generally will state that any payment will be in full settlement of the claim. In some circumstances, an interim settlement may be offered to be reviewed at a later date; for example, if it is suspected that there may be long-term implications for the subject's health that are not immediately apparent.

Insurance

As discussed earlier, indemnity (which offers no-fault compensation) cannot be used where there is fault (e.g. negligence or malpractice). In this case, insurance is used to ensure that the subject suffering harm receives appropriate compensation. In this case, the insurer must be notified of the claim and may choose to then settle the claim or allow the claim to proceed through legal channels and possibly end up in court. In some cases, the insurance on offer may be similar to an indemnity in that it is no-fault insurance; for example, universities may have insurance which offers no-fault compensation for claims arising from the design of a clinical trial. Universities, hospitals, and charitable funders normally insure against claims for harm caused by the negligence of their employees. Healthcare practitioners also hold their own personal malpractice insurance.

Many large organizations act as their own insurers (pharmaceutical companies such as Pfizer and GSK are larger than many insurers), but do offer an insurance certificate from a third party if requested. This can be useful in certain countries where the concept of self-insurance is not permitted. In the UK, the NHS and Department of Health operate within public sector policy and rather than use commercial insurance, they pool the risk of claims for negligence. NHS bodies such as hospitals agree to meet the cost of claims for negligence by NHS staff in the course of their employment, including involvement in clinical trials, and this extends to contract staff working within the NHS, although not to independent practitioners providing NHS services, where their professional liability insurance should be checked and extended if necessary. The NHS generally requires a formal agreement at the start of a study with an external sponsor, documenting the liabilities that each accepts.

UK Department of Health guidance is clear: 'NHS bodies remain liable for clinical negligence and other negligent harm to individuals covered by their duty of care. Institutions employing researchers remain liable for negligent harm caused by the design of studies they initiate. Producers continue to have strict liability for faulty medicines. The UK Regulations do not require no-fault compensation. Ethics committees will continue to consider the need for it case by case.'[6]

What about referring physicians?

It is important that the sponsor checks that anyone with even a peripheral study role has adequate insurance and indemnity. Primary care physicians may, for example, be notified of a study taking place in a local hospital and asked to refer patients who meet principal inclusion/exclusion criteria for further discussion and assessment, with a view to enrolling in the study. In the UK, the NHS R&D Forum states: 'Where an Independent Contractor such as a GP, or their practice staff, undertake research as part of their routine clinical services, their personal professional indemnity arrangements provide them with adequate cover for that activity.'[7] It quotes examples of assessing patients against defined inclusion/exclusion criteria, referring or recruiting patients to research, and screening patients and taking consent as examples of clinical activity undertaken within a research study by a clinician on his or her own patients, where the personal professional indemnity arrangements are deemed appropriate.

Compensation

The main issue in deciding whether compensation is due, either through a no-fault indemnity or through legal action, is whether the study medication or procedures actually caused, or at least on the balance of probabilities caused or contributed to, the harm to the study subject. Take the example of an elderly, overweight, hypertensive patient in a diabetes study who suffers a myocardial infarction; the patient would have been at high risk anyway, so attributing the infarction to the study medication would be complex. On the other hand, if a medication is known rarely to cause Stevens Johnson syndrome and a study subject experiences this condition, it may be relatively straightforward to determine that on balance of probability, the study medication led to harm and compensation is due.

The sponsor's policies and procedures should address the costs of treatment of trial subjects in the event of trial-related injuries. This is less of an issue in the UK, where the NHS provides free medical care at point of use, but in countries such as the US this can be a real problem as the study subject may not be able to afford to pay for immediate medical care, and claims under the indemnity or through legal action take time to process so interim decisions and payments may be appropriate.

When trial subjects receive compensation, the method and manner of compensation should comply with applicable regulatory requirements in the relevant country. In the UK, the Association of the British Pharmaceutical Industry (ABPI) has clinical trial compensation guidelines[8] which cover the indemnity and compensation in the event of injury to subjects participating in clinical trials. Whilst strictly only applicable to the UK and to ABPI member companies sponsoring studies, in practice they are more widely used and may be adopted by other commercial sponsors and may be used by sponsors with UK-based headquarters in countries with no specific guidelines available. They are generally considered to be some of the most comprehensive guidelines and include the following general principles:

• Compensation should be paid when, on the balance of probabilities, the injury was attributable to the administration of a medicinal product under trial or any clinical intervention or procedure provided for by the protocol that would not have occurred but for the inclusion of the patient in the trial.

• Compensation should only be paid for the more serious injury of an enduring and disabling character (including exacerbation of an existing condition), and not for temporary pain or discomfort or less serious or curable complaints.

• Neither the fact that the adverse reaction causing the injury was foreseeable or predictable, nor the fact that the patient has freely consented (whether in writing or otherwise) to participate in the trial should exclude a patient from consideration for compensation, although compensation may be abated or excluded; for example, in cases of negligence, including contributory negligence by the patient.

• No compensation should be paid for the failure of the medicinal product to have its intended effect or to provide any other benefit to the patients or to patients receiving placebo in consideration of its failure to provide a therapeutic benefit.

Insurance companies pool information and generally within a country, there will be guidance as to the level of compensation that it is reasonable to pay for specific injuries. It is important that compensation is appropriate to the harm suffered and to the country, although some countries permit punitive damages to be awarded. For example, if there has been negligence, an additional sum may be awarded as a 'punishment' for that negligence. ABPI guidelines recommend that if there is a difference of opinion between company and patient as to the appropriate level of compensation, the company should seek (and make available to the patient) the opinion of a mutually acceptable independent expert, and that his or her opinion should be given substantial weight by the company in reaching its decision on the appropriate payment to be made. The level of compensation should also reflect the level of risk that the subject accepted when entering the study; ABPI guidelines refer to 'the seriousness of the disease being treated, the degree of probability that adverse reactions will occur and any warnings given; [and] the risks and benefits of established treatments relative to those known or suspected of the trial medicine.'

In the case of studies conducted in developing countries where access to banking facilities may be poor, ingenuity may be required to reach a practical arrangement; for example, making payments through international money transfer services rather than a bank.

What about studies not operating to ABPI or similar compensation guidelines? Is there cover for non-negligent injury?

Commercial sponsors (e.g. pharmaceutical companies) generally operate to ABPI or similar guidelines, where the indemnity includes arrangements for no-fault, or non-negligent harm. This occurs when a study subject has suffered harm through participating in the study, but through no fault or negligence, even when the protocol and all procedures were correctly followed.

The situation may be different for non-commercial studies such as those conducted by the NHS. In this case, the indemnity may only cover the legal liability, with no-fault compensation being regarded as being a moral or ethical obligation and not a legal one. It is the role of the IRB/IEC to decide whether or not a study can go ahead in this situation and this may depend on how likely it is that no-fault harm may occur. It may be that an ex gratia payment would be possible and this should be clearly stated in the patient information.

In the UK, NHS indemnity arrangements do not cover non-negligent harm and NHS bodies cannot purchase commercial insurance cover. NHS bodies are also unable to give any undertaking to pay compensation when there is no negligence. Organizations such as universities can purchase professional indemnity cover for non-negligent harm but it is becoming increasingly expensive to do so.

Pharmaceutical companies should bear this in mind when arranging support for investigator-initiated studies or other studies where they are not the sponsor, and may choose to either stipulate that ABPI or similar guidelines are followed or arrange such cover themselves.

The responsibility for ensuring that arrangements concerning insurance, indemnity, and compensation are in the study agreements and patient information and are clear to everyone involved resides with the sponsor of a study. If a study took place without appropriate indemnity and compensation cover, the normal rules around product liability would then apply. However, it may be very difficult to determine who the subject's contract is with, for example, the sponsor, investigator, or hospital, and whether there had been any negligence or a defective product, resulting in a long, expensive, and complicated legal case.

What is different about studies in healthy volunteers?

There has been considerable public concern about healthy volunteer studies. In the UK, the ABPI has guidelines for studies in non-patient human volunteers and, as discussed in the compensation section, these may be more widely applied than by just ABPI member companies. This states that if the subject suffers any significant deterioration in health, compensation will be paid quickly and without any need to prove negligence. In general, there is not a significant difference in the ABPI guidelines for healthy volunteers and for patients enrolled in studies as both aim to make a swift and appropriate compensation payment. However, clearly no disease is being treated in a healthy volunteer and hence the risk to benefit ratios will be very different, and the risks and benefits of other available treatments will not be relevant.

How do study arrangements differ from those for marketed products?

Marketed medicinal products are covered by normal consumer protection laws that generally rely on the principle that consumers have specific expectations of safety around any product. In the EU, the manufacturer is not liable if the state of scientific and technical knowledge at the relevant time was not such that the producer might be expected to have discovered the defect with the product. However, the burden of proof is on the producer to show that it could not have been expected to know of the defect and it was not foreseeable. Simply not conducting studies or pharmacovigilance activities that might potentially show a defect such as a safety issue would not be a defence under this rule.

Some countries have specific no-fault schemes to provide compensation to those who suffer harm as a result of taking a medication or receiving a vaccine or other licensed treatment; for example, the UK vaccine compensation scheme, the New Zealand Accident Compensation Corporation which provides no-fault personal injury cover including medicine and medical treatment related injuries, and the Swedish general medicine injury compensation scheme which requires a 'preponderant probability' that an injury was caused by a medicine.

If a subject is harmed by a licensed comparator product being used in a study, then generally there would be discussions between the sponsor and the producer of the comparator. While the normal study indemnity and insurance would still apply, some producers would prefer to take responsibility for handling the case themselves and making an ex gratia payment in respect of their product, rather than permitting the sponsor of the study (who may be a competitor) to pay compensation and so potentially set a precedent.

Financing of trials

The sponsor must finance or arrange the finance for the study. The role of sponsor often is associated with the person who provides the finance for the study, but sometimes it can be the person who arranges the financing (e.g. an investigator who applies for a grant from a charity to undertake a study). The UK Clinical Trials Regulations are clear on this point: 'sponsor' means, in relation to a clinical trial, the person who takes responsibility for the initiation, management, and financing (or arranging the financing) of that trial.

In the case of a pharmaceutical company sponsoring a study, it would be expected to also provide all finance required for the study, whether direct (such as payments to investigators) or indirect (such as provision of staff to undertake monitoring). For an investigator-initiated study where the investigator is the sponsor, the investigator will need to arrange funding to cover the costs of the study from a funder (e.g. a charity or pharmaceutical company). Sponsors delegating specific responsibilities will obviously need to pay the organization that takes them on (e.g. a CRO or central laboratory).

The financial aspects of the trial should be documented in an agreement between the sponsor and the investigator/institution. This agreement should be a comprehensive, clearly worded clinical trial agreement (CTA) or contract to ensure that the sponsor and the investigator (and/or employer) know exactly what they are committed to and what payments are due during the study. In the UK, the National Institute for Health Research produces model clinical trial agreements that have been nationally agreed to cover industry-sponsored trials conducted in the NHS either directly or via a CRO, for medical technology industry-funded trials in NHS hospitals either directly or via a CRO, and a model industry collaborative research agreement to support clinical research collaborations involving the pharmaceutical and biotechnology industries, academia, and NHS organizations across the UK.[8] In the case of multinational studies, agreement must be reached on currency conversion rates, if applicable.

What costs does the sponsor take responsibility for?

The sponsor will either need to finance or arrange for finance for the following:
- The set-up, management, monitoring, audit, and reporting of the study
- Obtaining IRB/IEC and regulatory approvals
- Pharmacovigilance
- Regulatory inspections

How much should investigators be paid for commercial study work?

In some countries, it is possible to access information around private practice rates for healthcare practitioners to which clinical trial work may be aligned. However, in the UK the Office of Fair Trading now prevents the British Medical Association (BMA) from providing advice to consultants on suggested fees for private medical practice, and the BMA simply advises consultants to set their fees taking into account their time, expertise, training, and expenses.[9] Many commercial sponsors employ companies which benchmark the pharmaceutical industry and provide performance metrics, trends, and analysis in order to provide information on clinical trial costings. It is important for sponsors to pay a fair market value for work undertaken on clinical trials. Clinical trial advisory boards may also be able to provide information on likely costings. It should also be considered that there may be similar studies competing for the same subjects and payment levels may be a factor in determining in which trial the subjects are enrolled.

Although the per-patient costs may be the same, institution overheads and administration fees may vary. Hospitals and other institutions may impose charges for administration or overheads to cover items such as equipment, office support, building costs, lighting, heating, etc. In the UK, this may result in anything from 15–70% being added in addition to the per-patient investigator fee. This is an area that requires negotiation from institution to institution and it can be time-consuming. In the UK, costing templates are used to try to standardize these charges and to avoid unnecessary delays in setting up a study.[8]

The UK National Institute for Health Research provides industry costing templates for contract trials of pharmaceutical and biotechnology agents in secondary care and primary care settings and studies of medical technology. Although intended for studies involving the Clinical Research Networks in England, they may be of use to companies running trials outside the networks, but they are not intended for costing non-commercial/academic trials. The ABPI, NHS R&D Forum, Institute of Clinical Research, and industry representatives collaborated to produce the 2005 report 'Guidance to facilitate the conduct of commercially funded research in the National Health Service (secondary care)'.[9] Whilst this document is out of date in minor respects (it refers to BMA advice on private practice rates, for example), it provides valuable advice and checklists for costing a study and these may be of value to non-commercial/academic studies.

What should be included in the financial agreement with a study site?

In the UK, model agreements are available, as discussed. An agreement will generally include the following:

- The names of the parties to the agreement (e.g. the pharmaceutical company or CRO and the investigator).
- When the study is run by a CRO, the name of the sponsor on whose behalf the CRO is working.
- The protocol title, code number, and date, and numbers and dates of any amendments.
- A statement that the sponsor/CRO appoints the investigator to conduct the clinical trial, and the investigator agrees to conduct the trial according to the specified protocol, current GCP standards, and local legal requirements.
- A statement that the investigator will allow the sponsor and/or CRO staff and regulatory authority staff direct access to subjects' medical records for the purpose of source data verification, auditing, and inspection.
- A statement that the investigator will retain essential documents until notified by the sponsor (or according to local regulations).

- The estimated number of subjects to be recruited by the investigator and the specified duration. If recruitment will end once a certain total number of subjects are recruited, this should be stated.
- A schedule of payments to be made for subjects entering the study. The payment, if any, for subjects entered but not fulfilling inclusion/exclusion criteria should be specified. Any circumstances in which payments may be withheld should be stated.
- The name of the research/trust fund, or institution to which payments will be made, along with the details of their preferred method of payment (cheque or bank transfer). Payments should not be paid in the investigator's name.
- A statement that the investigator is responsible for any tax liability.
- A statement that the financial arrangements included in this Agreement do not conflict with any agreement or contract made with the investigator's employer or partner(s).
- A statement in which the investigator and other study site personnel disclose any significant equity interest in the sponsor, proprietary interest in the test product, or other significant payments from the sponsor.
- A statement that the sponsor (and CRO) will not be held responsible for the negligence of the investigator or other investigational site staff.
- Where a CRO is running the trial, a statement that the CRO has no responsibility for the manufacture of the drug or the design of the protocol and therefore will not be held liable by the site for any claim related to either the study drug or the study design.
- A statement that the investigator and site have adequate current malpractice and liability insurance.
- Indemnity or insurance arrangements, if not in a separate document.
- Details of equipment to be provided to the investigational site, for the duration of the study.
- Agreements for pharmacy, radiology, haematology, and biochemistry (unless these services are being performed by a different company).
- If the protocol is subsequently revised and makes a significant difference to the workload associated with the study, the financial agreement should also be revised.

When should study subjects receive payment?

Generally, healthy volunteers will be offered compensation for the inconvenience and discomfort that they suffer and for their time (but no payment in respect of any risk they may undertake, which would be an inducement to agree to risk and hence unethical). All study subjects, whether healthy volunteers or patients, may be offered compensation for additional costs they incur in participating in the study such as transport costs for extra clinic visits. In general, patients participating in a study would not be offered compensation for time or inconvenience as they would be expected to benefit directly from being in the study. However, if a study offers no benefit to a patient (e.g. a study comparing diagnostic techniques studying patients already known to have the condition), then a payment in respect of time and inconvenience may be considered. Another example may be a study of a minor condition requiring a high number of additional clinic visits that might be regarded as an undue burden on the patient; a payment might then be warranted.

If a payment in respect of time and inconvenience is proposed, it should be considered and approved by the IRB/IEC. Payments should not be so large as to unduly induce subjects to enrol in the study or to stay in the study when they would otherwise withdraw. Payments should accrue as the study progresses and not be contingent upon the subject completing the entire study. There may also be local laws or regulations concerning payments which should be followed.

Can study payments be adjusted for dropouts or to provide an incentive to recruitment?

This is a difficult area and will depend on circumstances. IRB/IEC reviews financial agreements for studies and some feel that reducing payments for dropouts could be an incentive to keep subjects in a trial when they should really withdraw. However, making a full payment for a subject who withdrew early means that the investigator is effectively being paid for work that was not done.

Additional payments for high levels of recruitment may be appropriate if they are directly linked to the provision of additional resources to enable the high level of recruitment to be supported or maintained. For example, an additional payment to cover the costs of an extra trial assistant to attend two clinics per week to provide support for a high number of study patients may be appropriate. However, payments linked purely to recruitment, such as a bonus payment triggered when the tenth patient is recruited, would generally be considered inappropriate as they may encourage inappropriate recruitment or pressure being put on patients to consent so that the bonus is achieved. Again, the IRB/IEC will consider the financial arrangements as part of their review of the study and incentives for recruitment, and additional payments for high recruitment will receive particular scrutiny.

In general, no or very limited payments are made in respect of subjects entering the study who do not meet inclusion/exclusion criteria. If tests are performed at entry that subsequently may mean that a patient was not actually eligible for the study, then a full payment would be made both for the work undertaken up until the point when it was realized that the patient was not actually eligible and for withdrawal procedures. For example, if it is necessary to start study treatment immediately after surgery and biopsy results subsequently show that the patient unexpectedly has a diagnosis of Crohn's disease rather than the expected ulcerative colitis, then the patient would be withdrawn and the study payment would reflect the work undertaken up to withdrawal. On the other hand, if a patient was entered into a study in clear contravention of an exclusion criterion (e.g. they exceed the upper age limit), then no payment at all may be due.

Who signs financial and other clinical trial agreements?

This will vary. It may be the investigator or a representative of the hospital or university (or in the UK an NHS Trust). In the primary care setting, the principal investigator generally signs the agreements. Signing of agreements can delay the start of a study so it is recommended that the signatory is identified early in the study planning process.

Conduct of the study to GCP standards

It is a key responsibility of the sponsor to ensure that the study is conducted to GCP standards, and specifically to implement monitoring and auditing of the study.[1] The sponsor's responsibilities are discussed in more detail in this section and additional information on monitoring may be found in Chapter 13.

GCP requirements of the sponsor

GCP specifies a large number of activities and responsibilities specifically for the sponsor, summarized as follows:

• Designate appropriately qualified medical personnel to advise on trial-related medical questions or problems
• Utilize qualified individuals throughout all stages of the trial process
• Utilize appropriately qualified individuals to supervise conduct of the trial, handle and verify data, conduct statistical analyses, and prepare trial reports
• When using electronic trial data handling and/or remote electronic trial data systems, ensure and document the fact that the system conforms to the sponsor's requirements; maintain SOPs; ensure systems maintain an audit, data, and edit trail; maintain a security system; maintain a list of the individuals authorized to make data changes; maintain adequate backup of data; safeguard the blinding; use an unambiguous subject identification code
• Retain all sponsor-specific essential documents until at least two years after the last approval of a marketing application in an ICH region and until there are no pending or contemplated marketing applications in an ICH region or at least two years have elapsed since the formal discontinuation of development of the product, or for a longer period if required by the regulatory requirement(s) or if needed by the sponsor
• If the sponsor discontinues development, notify all investigators/institutions and regulatory authorities
• Inform the investigator(s)/institution(s) in writing of the need for record retention and when trial-related records are no longer needed
• Select the investigator(s)/institution(s)
• For multicentre trials and where appropriate, organize a coordinating committee and/or select coordinating investigator(s)
• Provide the protocol and an up-to-date investigator's brochure, and allow sufficient time for review
• Ensure sufficient safety and efficacy data are available to support human exposure by the route, at the dosages, for the duration, and in the trial population to be studied
• Update the investigator's brochure as significant new information becomes available
• Specify in the protocol or other written agreement that the investigator(s)/institution(s) provide direct access to source data/documents for trial-related monitoring, audits, IRB/IEC review, and regulatory inspection

- Verify each subject has consented, in writing, to direct access to his/her original medical records for trial-related monitoring, audit, IRB/IEC review, and regulatory inspection
- If a trial is prematurely terminated or suspended, promptly inform the investigators/institutions, IRB/IEC, regulatory authority and provide the reason
- Ensure clinical trial reports are prepared and provided to the regulatory agency
- For multicentre trials, ensure all investigators conduct the trial in strict compliance with the protocol
- Design CRFs to capture the required data at all trial sites
- Document the responsibilities of coordinating investigator(s) and the other participating investigators
- Give all investigators instructions on following the protocol, complying with a uniform set of standards for the assessment of clinical and laboratory findings, and completing the CRFs.
- Facilitate communication between investigators in multicentre studies

Which GCP areas are worthy of particular attention, as they tend to be where things go wrong?

One area for a sponsor to be particularly aware of is compliance with the protocol, and in particular issues of delegation and supervision of the principal investigator. It is also relatively common for documents to be approved by regulatory agencies or IRB/IEC, or signed by the investigator, before the documents are actually finalized, and for the investigator to sign the protocol after the study is initiated.

What responsibilities does the sponsor have around monitoring?

The purposes of trial monitoring are to verify that:
- the rights and well-being of human subjects are protected.
- the reported trial data are accurate, complete, and verifiable from source documents.
- the conduct of the trial is in compliance with the currently approved protocol/amendment(s), with GCP, and with the applicable regulatory requirement(s).

Sponsors should set up systems to ensure that these purposes are fulfilled.

Monitors should be appointed by the sponsor and appropriately trained so they have the scientific and/or clinical knowledge needed to monitor the trial adequately. A monitor's qualifications should be documented. Monitors should be thoroughly familiar with the investigational product(s), the protocol, written informed consent form, and any other written information to be provided to subjects, the sponsor's SOPs, GCP, and the applicable regulatory requirement(s).

The sponsor should ensure that the trials are adequately monitored. GCP specifies that the sponsor should determine the appropriate extent and nature of monitoring, based on considerations such as the objective, purpose, design, complexity, blinding, size, and end points of the trial (Chapters 14 and 15). In general, there is a need for on-site monitoring

(Chapter 13), before, during, and after the trial as the monitor ensures that the trial is conducted and documented properly and acts as the main line of communication between the sponsor and the investigator. The monitor should follow the sponsor's established written SOPs as well as any procedures specified by the sponsor for monitoring a specific trial and he or she should submit a written report to the sponsor after each trial-site visit or trial-related communication. That monitoring report and any follow-up activities should then be reviewed by the sponsor or the sponsor's designated representative.

What do auditors and inspectors look for in the sponsor's monitoring systems?

Auditors and inspectors will review the sponsor's monitoring plan and monitoring SOPs. They will look both at the content and at the compliance with them. Of particular interest is the frequency and extent of the monitoring, which should be appropriate to the study. Monitors' qualifications will also be checked; this will include training record review. Auditors and inspectors will look at monitoring visit reports and also at the review of the reports by the sponsor and the oversight of the monitor. Last but definitely not least, auditors and inspectors will review the corrective and preventative actions taken in response to issues identified by monitoring visits in order to check that systems are in place to improve quality and are working effectively.

The provision of quality systems

Quality assurance and quality control

According to GCP, the sponsor is 'responsible for implementing and maintaining quality assurance and quality control systems with written SOPs to ensure that trials are conducted and data are generated, documented and reported in compliance with the protocol, GCP, and the applicable regulatory requirement(s)'.

Both quality assurance and quality control are important. Quality control (QC) comprises the steps taken during the generation of a product or provision of a service to ensure quality. It involves all the staff employed on a clinical study working to appropriate standards and checking their work. For example, a draft protocol would be read by several people and comments and suggestions made to improve the document; and a monitor will check data recorded at a study site and may notice a missing item and request its inclusion. These are simple everyday examples of QC. Quality assurance (QA), on the other hand, is a systematic process to determine whether the quality control system is working and effective. It involves staff with a specific QA responsibility, who check a sample of work to provide assurance that the quality standard has been met and that the QC is indeed working properly. These QA checks, or audits, are separate from routine QC and monitoring.

The sponsor is responsible for securing agreement for direct access to all study sites, source data/documents and reports, to enable monitoring and auditing by the sponsor, and inspection by regulatory authorities. These agreements will be documented in the formal clinical trial agreements and further detail is often included in the protocol.

Audits

Audits are conducted by the sponsor (whereas inspections are conducted by a regulatory authority). The purpose of an audit is to evaluate trial conduct and compliance with the protocol, SOPs, and control documents such as guidelines and checklists, GCP, and applicable regulatory requirements.

The sponsor appoints individuals independent of the study to conduct audits. The sponsor may employ staff in a QA role or may use contract auditors. Either way, the sponsor should ensure auditors are qualified by training and experience to conduct audits properly and their qualifications should be documented. The sponsor should have written procedures on what to audit, how to audit, the frequency of audits, and the form and content of audit reports and ensure these are followed. The sponsor should develop an audit plan, taking into account the importance of the study to the regulatory submission, the number of subjects, the type and complexity of the trial, the level of risk involved, and any problems that have been identified, for example, issues with a particular study assessment, or an issue with a site with relatively inexperienced staff.

After the audit, the sponsor may need to provide an audit certificate, depending on local regulations. If an audit identifies non-compliance with the protocol, SOPs/control documents, GCP, or regulatory requirements, prompt action is required by the sponsor to secure compliance. If serious and/or persistent non-compliance is identified, the sponsor should terminate the investigator's/institution's participation in the trial and promptly notify the regulatory authority.

What quality systems should a sponsor have?

The QA and QC systems established by the sponsor should provide assurance that clinical trials are conducted and data are generated, recorded, and reported in compliance with the protocol, GCP, and applicable regulatory requirements. If any duties are delegated (e.g. if a CRO conducts audits on the sponsor's behalf), then this should be documented, including details of the assessment and selection process and ongoing assessment, as well as formal delegation of duties in a contract.

QC

The sponsor should have a well-established organization for clinical research activities with a sufficient number of properly qualified and trained personnel. This may be demonstrated by organizational charts that identify the key personnel in each area and show the independence of the QA function, supplemented by the job descriptions, qualifications, and training of the staff involved in clinical trials. The sponsor should have the facilities (e.g. archiving, investigational medicinal product storage) and equipment required to undertake clinical research. Computer systems should be validated. Operating procedures should comply with GCP standards and applicable regulations and include appropriate QC activities (e.g. an SOP on monitoring should include processes for review of monitoring visit reports to check that monitoring is to an appropriate standard).

QA

The sponsor should establish an audit system and generate and implement an audit plan. It should include audits of key clinical trial processes, including monitoring, data management, safety reporting, clinical study report production, archiving, and computer system validation. Contractors and sub-contractors should also be audited. Audits should include process and system audits, as well as audits of particular studies and study centres.

Quality improvement

The sponsor should additionally have a process for communicating and addressing audit findings, including the format and distribution of audit reports, and for dealing with serious and/or persistent GCP non-compliance, so contributing to quality improvement.

What SOPs should a sponsor have?

There is no definitive list and indeed the FDA does not even specify written SOPs as a necessity for most clinical research, although most sponsors would choose to have SOPs for practical reasons.

There are indications of what SOPs would be expected to cover available in information around regulatory inspections and what inspectors will be looking for. The most comprehensive information is probably that found in EudraLex (the collection of rules and regulations governing medicinal products in the European Union). EudraLex volume 10 'The rules governing medicinal products in the European Union', Chapter IV Guidance for the conduct of GCP inspections—Sponsor and CRO, Annex IV[10] refers to reviewing sponsor/CRO operating procedures to verify their compliance with GCP and applicable regulations and covers the following areas.

Implementation and termination of the clinical trial
- Monitoring
- Investigational medicinal product
- Sample management
- Safety and adverse events reporting
- Data handling and clinical trial report
- Documentation archiving
- Sponsor audit and quality assurance system
- Delegation of duties

To take one example:

'Monitoring
The aim is to evaluate the system established for monitoring clinical trials. Determine if procedures include:
- Description of monitoring activities: planning, frequency, extent and nature of monitoring activities (visits, data review, etc.).
- Content, handling and follow up of monitoring reports.
- Agreements for direct access to source documents by the sponsor personnel (or their appointed representatives) and by regulatory authorities and confidentiality of information about subjects.'

Sponsors may wish to review Annex IV in its entirety and cross-check that their SOPs cover everything that regulatory inspectors will be scrutinizing. Conversely, they may also wish to review any SOPs that do not contain specified information, to check if the SOP is of value.

What are controlled documents?
Controlled documents is a term used to describe official documents including SOPs, but also includes other documents subject to version and issue control, such as guidelines, working practices, policies, instruments of work, etc. Different sponsors use different kinds of controlled documents and there are no rules or regulations covering them, although it is important to remember that you will be inspected for all of those documents, not just SOPs.

GCP[1] specifies what must be done; for example, section 5.16.1: 'The sponsor is responsible for the ongoing safety evaluation of the investigational product(s).' However, it does not specify *how* this should be done, how frequently, by whom, how it should be documented, etc. Standard operating procedures should contain this level of detail. They are an important tool for quality control and in controlling the many small parts, the overall quality of the complex clinical trial should be assured.

The use of various controlled documents reflects the fact that SOPs are rigid documents. In some cases, it may be more appropriate to take a flexible approach and put some information in a guidance document instead of within the SOP. In contrast, work instructions often contain very detailed information specific to a particular country and so add detail to SOPs. It is important to write and implement controlled documents that are fit for purpose, and in particular, to avoid documents that are overly complex and above the required standards. Inspectors will make inspection findings if there was a failure to follow SOPs, even if regulatory requirements were met.

Care must also be taken to ensure that uncontrolled documents are not used in place of SOPs. There is flexibility around guidelines, instruments of work, work instructions, etc., which may be used in addition to SOPs, but they should still be controlled documents.

All controlled documents should be issued in advance of their implementation date thus allowing time for training and familiarization. They should also be reviewed and, if necessary, updated on a regular basis or in the event of new legislation.

What makes a good SOP?

SOPs should contain instructions—the 'how', rather than the 'what'— which are already available in the GCP guidelines. A good SOP is as simple as possible whilst still making the instructions clear and unambiguous. Care should be taken to avoid duplication and unnecessary cross-referencing between SOPs. The SOP should include a glossary of acronyms and keep their use to a minimum. And a picture, as they say, can paint a thousand words: while illustrations may not be practical, a process diagram, flow-chart, or process map can give a very valuable overview of the procedure.

Manufacture and provision of investigational medicinal product

The sponsor is responsible for the manufacturing, packaging, labelling, and coding of investigational medicinal product (IMP). This may be delegated, but the responsibility of course remains with the sponsor. IMP includes any active comparator or placebo required for a study, as well as the actual product under study. ICH GCP[1] defines investigational product as 'a pharmaceutical form of an active ingredient or placebo being tested or used as a reference in a clinical trial, including a product with a marketing authorization when used or assembled (formulated or packaged) in a way different from the approved form, or when used for an unapproved indication, or when used to gain further information about an approved use'. The EU Clinical Trials Directive[2] uses the term 'investigational medicinal product': 'a pharmaceutical form of an active substance or placebo being tested or used as a reference in a clinical trial, including products already with a marketing authorization but used or assembled (formulated or packaged) in a way different from the authorised form, or when used for an unauthorised indication, or when used to gain further information about the authorised form'.

In general, the principles of good manufacturing practice (GMP) are followed for IMP, together with specific requirements applicable to investigational products, for example labelling requirements are very different for IMP compared to normal medicinal product. In addition, labelling should comply with applicable regulatory requirements.

It is very common for the production method and the formulation of a medicine to change over the course of a clinical trial programme. A medication may be made up in very small quantities as an injection for initial pharmacokinetic/pharmacodynamic studies, then in slightly larger quantities as plain white capsules in a bottle with a separate sachet of desiccant for the first studies in patients. As the clinical studies become larger, the process used will be scaled up and, where necessary, modified, and this may involve moving production from a specialist research manufacturing facility to a normal commercial manufacturing plant. During a large phase 3 study programme, supplies will generally be produced at the manufacturing plant that is intended to produce commercial supplies so that the site gains experience of making the product to be ready for regulatory inspection. By the end of phase 3, clinical trials may be using what is intended to be the commercial formulation, for example, coloured capsules supplied in a pot with desiccant built into the lid. Any changes of formulation or of manufacturing site or process will need to be reflected in the manufacturing authorization and the study documentation and may necessitate a protocol amendment.

The sponsor is responsible for supplying IMP to the investigator or institution conducting the study, and this should happen only after the sponsor obtains all required documentation (e.g. approval from IRB/IEC and regulatory authority). The sponsor should ensure that written procedures include instructions to follow for the handling and storage of IMP and for documentation. The procedures should include receipt, handling, storage, dispensing, retrieval of unused product from study subjects, and return of

unused IMP to the sponsor (or alternative disposal arrangements if applicable). The sponsor should:
- ensure timely delivery of IMP
- maintain records of shipment, receipt, disposition, return, and destruction of IMP
- maintain a system for retrieving IMP and documenting this (e.g. expired IMP)
- maintain a system for the disposition of unused IMP and documenting this

Does the sponsor have to manufacture the IMP?

The sponsor may manufacture the IMP, including providing comparator medication and placebos where appropriate. However, the sponsor may opt to delegate some or all of the manufacturing and/or packaging of the IMP, whilst of course retaining overall responsibility.

What is a manufacturing authorization?

The manufacturer must obtain a licence to manufacture and/or import IMP unless a marketing authorization has been granted for the product. In the UK, for example, an authorization may take up to 90 days to obtain. An application will include information such as the address of the premises where the manufacture will take place, the product specification, the manufacturing operations, facilities, and equipment. Batch numbers will be required and samples of each batch need to be tested for quality control. In the UK, full details of requirements for manufacturing and importation authorizations may be found in Schedules 6 to 8 of the Medicines for Human Use (Clinical Trials) Regulations 2004.[3]

Who is a qualified person?

This is a specific requirement to meet the EU Clinical Trials Directive and EU Regulation.[2] A qualified person of appropriate qualifications and experience must carry out a review of batch documents and ensure quality control.

What information is required around IMP in a protocol?

The protocol should contain the information required, including:
- name and strength of IMP, including any comparators
- blinding procedures and requirement for placebo
- design of the study (e.g. parallel group or cross-over)
- dosage form (e.g. tablet, capsule)
- doses and duration of treatment
- number of centres and in which countries located
- approach to distribution of IMP (e.g. a centrally based approach)

In addition, further detail may be required around stability data, the time frame for the study, site addresses, QA/QC procedures, and regulatory approval status. The study packaging will need to be agreed (e.g. blister packs or child-resistant bottles), as will the wording for the labels; Annex 13 of the GMP guide[12] gives details around labelling (e.g. sponsor details, study or protocol identifier, period of use (expiry or re-test date), etc.). The style of label must also be agreed; for example, for studies involving a number of countries, separate supplies may be labelled in a number of different languages or a multilingual or booklet style label used that covers every country.

Generally, the protocol will not contain detailed information around the manufacturing process, blinding, etc. for commercial reasons and because this may well change over time; this would be found in the manufacturing authorization. However, the sponsor is required to keep full documentation for GMP reasons and in the event of a regulatory inspection.

How should IMP be documented?

The sponsor is responsible for written procedures including instructions for the handling, storage, and documentation of IMP. This includes documentation of adequate and safe receipt, handling, storage, dispensing, retrieval of unused product from subjects, and return of unused investigational product(s) to the sponsor, or alternative disposition if authorized by the sponsor in compliance with applicable regulatory requirements (e.g. it may be more appropriate to authorize disposition of hazardous material locally rather than returning to the sponsor). The sponsor should maintain records that fully document the shipment, receipt, disposition, return, and destruction of the IMP, and these records are often an area of focus by regulatory inspectors.

What about conditions of storage and expiry dates?

The sponsor should have information about the medicinal product appropriate for its stage of development; thus, for example, the sponsor may have full information around the manufacturing process but may have only preliminary information around the shelf-life of the product and appropriate expiry dates at the start of a study. The sponsor must determine acceptable storage times, conditions (e.g. humidity), and temperatures, as well as processes for handling IMP (e.g. for reconstituting and administering), and ensure that those involved in the clinical trial are appropriately notified (e.g. pharmacists storing and dispensing the IMP). IMP must be packaged to prevent contamination and deterioration during transport and storage.

The sponsor should ensure the IMP is stable over the course of the study. This will generally involve retaining samples from every batch of IMP for analysis to confirm the characteristics of the IMP. Samples should be retained if possible until the analysis of the study data is completed, and as required by applicable regulatory requirement(s), whichever represents the longer retention period.

In the UK, the Guideline on the Requirements to the Chemical and Pharmaceutical Quality Documentation concerning Investigational Medicinal Products in Clinical Trials (CHMP/QWP/185401/2004 final)[11] allows shelf-life extensions to be made without the need for a substantial amendment to a protocol, if this has been planned and included in the initial regulatory application. The MHRA also accepts shelf-life extension proposals as part of a subsequent substantial amendment to allow for further extensions of the shelf-life. This also applies to biologicals.

What if things change during the course of the study?

If significant formulation changes are made during a study, the results of any additional studies of the formulated product(s) (e.g. stability, dissolution rate, bioavailability) needed to assess whether these changes would significantly alter the pharmacokinetic profile of the product should be available prior to the use of the new formulation in clinical trials.

What are the labelling requirements for clinical trial supplies in the UK?

The labelling requirements for IMPs are provided in Annex 13 of Volume 4 of The Rules Governing Medicinal Products in the EU: Good Manufacturing Practices.[12] A sample of the labelling is required as part of the clinical trial authorization (CTA) application. This should include the text of the labelling to be used and be representative of the size of the label to be used. Samples of the actual labels may be provided but are not required. Where labelling is not included as part of the CTA application or where the labelling to be used does not contain all the items required by Annex 13, this should be justified.

Are there any exceptions to the labelling requirements?

In the UK, Regulation 46 of the Medicines for Human Use (Clinical Trial) Regulations 2004[3] allows an exception for studies of marketed products being used within the terms of their marketing authorization, when dispensed to a study subject through a prescription from an authorized healthcare professional and labelled in accordance with regulations for relevant medicinal products. Other countries often have similar exceptions. This can cover provision of relief medication, specified in the protocol and intended to supplement study medication that is not providing sufficient efficacy, for example, provision of paracetamol for additional pain relief should study medication be insufficient to control pain.

Regulations for IMP usually specify that medication labels should include an expiry date, but generally regulatory authorities permit an exception when a centralized process is being used for expiry date handling.

In the UK, manufacture and assembly (including packaging and labelling) of IMP can only be undertaken by the holder of an authorization for the manufacture of investigational medicinal products. However, Regulation 37 of the Medicines for Human Use (Clinical Trial) Regulations 2004[3] does allow for an exception when assembly is carried out in a hospital/health centre by a doctor, pharmacist, or person under supervision of a pharmacist, exclusively for use in that hospital/health centre or another hospital/health centre and trial site. This allows flexibility, for example, for preparing trial chemotherapy based on a patient's weight or surface area, or for dose titration within a study protocol.

What is different about blinded IMP?

Most IMP is blinded and hence must be coded and labelled to protect the blinding, as blinding is a key strategy to reduce bias in clinical studies. If study medication is blinded, there should be a process for emergency unblinding. There have been instances where a patient enrolled in a study has taken an overdose of study medication and clearly in this situation, healthcare practitioners treating the patient need to know urgently exactly what medication has been overdosed and where to find information on appropriate treatment.

Most IMP is now controlled through a centralized process but in some cases a batch of medication will be shipped to a study site along with emergency code break envelopes. These are generally stored in a pharmacy for access in the event of an emergency. The monitor must check the integrity of code-break envelopes or similar materials on a regular basis as any breach of the study blinding is a serious deviation from protocol. There is usually an emergency contact phone number for the sponsor or other contact printed on the medication and study subjects will be provided with a card giving brief details of the study and how to find out more information. These should be used if the subject experiences a medical emergency and cannot contact anyone at the investigational site, perhaps during travel. Any arrangements for out-of-hours contact or emergency unblinding should be checked on a regular basis to ensure that they are working correctly.

How is comparator IMP obtained?

Comparator products will need to be sourced either directly from the regulatory licence holder or purchased from a commercial wholesaler. Sourcing directly has some advantages; for example, the licence holder will have all the required documentation for shipping such as certificates of analysis, packaging will be appropriate for the medication and placebo may be available. However, a protocol and study results will need to be provided (which may cause issues of commercial confidentiality), and provision of medication for a potential competitor may not be high on the priority list, leading to unacceptable delays. A charge would generally be made for provision of IMP. This approach would be preferred if the use of combinations of medication is established, for example, in the area of HIV treatment, where licence holders may collaborate over IMP provision. This approach would be required if access was required to an unlicensed comparator.

Perhaps more commonly, comparator medication will be purchased through a commercial wholesaler. This can often be quicker and more straightforward. One issue is with obtaining an appropriate placebo for blinded studies. The licence holder will have copyright around the product (e.g. on the colour, appearance, and markings on a tablet) and production of a placebo that matches this would infringe copyright. In this case, it may be necessary to coat or encapsulate the medication so it appears a plain white tablet or capsule that may easily be copied as a placebo, but it would be necessary to check the stability and dissolution of the treated product to ensure that it had not altered significantly. Modified-release products and devices such as inhalers present particular challenges. Sponsors may have the specialized knowledge and capability to handle this to GMP standards, or may choose to delegate to a specialist supplier of clinical trial IMP.

The regulatory and documentation requirements around the comparator IMP may be onerous; for example, regulatory approval for the medication may vary between countries which could be an issue for a multicentre study and again, a specialist supplier of clinical trial IMP may be delegated to handle this by the sponsor.

When should medication be held centrally for a study?

For small studies involving only one or two centres, all the medication for a clinical study may be delivered and held at the centres as the simplest and most straightforward approach. This centre-based approach will minimize effort, time, and shipping costs. Arrangements will need to be put in place for emergency unblinding if appropriate. This approach may also be appropriate for multicentre studies where there can be delays in shipping medication, perhaps related to local regulations or for practical reasons (e.g. a remote area of a developing country). Phase I studies generally will also use this approach even if multicentre, as studies tend to be short and involve a small number of subjects; this approach is also more flexible if changes are required for practical reasons around the administration of the medication.

For large, multicentre studies, a centre-based approach may cause issues. It is necessary to ship large quantities of medication to sites which may not then use the medication, if their recruitment does not reach target, and for GMP reasons IMP generally cannot be transferred to other sites for reuse. In the event of a product recall or changes to the expiry date, procedures may be complex to ensure that GMP standards are met and the issue dealt with correctly. The expiry date of the medicine in its current formulation and packaging may not have been established and may be subject to revision. There may simply not be sufficient medication available at the start of a study due to limitations on manufacturing the IMP to fully stock all centres for the duration of a study. In general, for large, multicentre studies, medication will therefore be held centrally and labelled and shipped as required to centres as this prevents these issues arising, although the cost of central IMP handling will then need to be budgeted. This centralized approach permits more efficient management of the IMP inventory and more effective project management.

There are two main approaches to managing centrally held medication. For studies requiring medication immediately on enrolling a patient, a small supply may be held at site. For studies where medication may be supplied the next day, a pack will be sent by courier destined for a specific patient enrolling in the study. Either way, when a patient enters, the site staff interact with a computer database using an interactive voice-recognition service (IVRS) which uses pre-recorded voice messages (in different languages if appropriate) and responds to the answers given using the telephone touch-tone keypad.[13] Alternatively, an interactive web-response system (IWRS) may be used, either instead of or in addition to an IVRS.

The computer database randomizes the patient to the study and the IVRS/IWRS then indicates which pack of medication should be dispensed or will trigger its shipment to site. The medication pack allocated will have an appropriate expiry date. This approach has the advantage that the database ensures appropriate balance in treatment allocation and provides an accurate record of study progress; some systems will integrate with the sponsor's clinical trial database and will provide accurate and up-to-date information about screening, enrolment and early drop-outs. In addition, expensive or scarce medication will be sent to exactly where it is required with a minimum of wastage. Centrally held medication managed by an IVRS was first available around 1990 and employed telephone and fax, but IWRS is now more commonly used. The IVRS/IWRS and computer database may also now be linked to other aspects of the study such as electronic patient diary cards.

A centre-based approach may be preferred for a single centre study and a centrally based approach for a large multicentre study. But which approach is appropriate for small multicentre studies, for example? This will depend on circumstances; for example, if it is known that the expiry date is likely to change or if the IMP is in very short supply then a central approach would be preferred. Other factors to take into account are the availability and cost of the comparator medication and the issue of stopping a study at a specific point; recruitment may be closed immediately where a central approach is used and this may save time and expense. A centralized approach may also be particularly valuable if it is necessary to balance treatment groups within the study for specific prognostic factors, rather than relying on balance being achieved by chance alone. An IVRS/IWRS can be programmed with a number of questions (e.g. patient age, sex, severity of disease, smoking status, red blood cell count, etc.) and can take these into account when allocating the patient to a particular treatment.

Studies with an adaptive design will almost certainly require the more flexible centralized approach. This is because by definition, it is not known at the start of the study how many patients will be recruited to each study arm and hence will require each type of medication.

Can the sponsor charge for IMP?

Generally, no charges are made for the provision of IMP and indeed, UK regulations require sponsors to ensure that IMP is made available to study subjects free of charge. Occasionally, sponsors may make a charge to cover the cost of providing follow-on or named-patient supplies to bridge a gap between completion of a trial and licensing and commercial supply of a product.

What are common issues around IMP?

Common audit and inspection findings around IMP include:
- missing or unsigned documentation (e.g. shipping records, accountability records, receipts)
- insufficient records for the chain of custody (from purchase to destruction) for marketed products used as comparators or as relief medications
- inadequate provision for storage of IMPs; for example, unused IMP may not be separated sufficiently from that returned unused by patients or from non-trial medication
- inadequate recording of conditions of storage (e.g. records of temperature/humidity); this may also apply when IMP is in transit
- emergency code-break procedures were not in place when trial supplies were delivered or when the study started

Safety information

Good clinical practice (ICH guideline E6) is supplemented by the E1 and E2 series of ICH guidelines which specify standards for safety information and reporting. GCP specifies that the sponsor must put in place appropriate systems that enable collection, analysis, interpretation, and reporting of pharmacovigilance information, but E2A for example gives detailed guidance on mechanisms for handling expedited (rapid) reporting of adverse drug reactions in the investigational phase of drug development.[14]

Collection of adverse events

Although definitions are standard, within the protocol, study-specific information may be added by the sponsor as part of a robust pharmacovigilance system. For example, many cancer chemotherapy agents predictably cause myelosuppression as a result of their mechanism of action. A protocol for a study of such a medication may exclude, for example, low white blood cell counts from the requirement for expedited reporting, unless unexpected in some way, such as more severe or more prolonged than expected. The low white blood cell count will still be routinely recorded during the study and will be analysed and reported with all trial data, but there will not be a need to report it as a serious adverse event, even if it results in, for example, hospitalization. This is because (unless the event is unusual in some regard) it will never meet the definition of unexpected and hence never require expedited reporting. Expedited reporting of expected and well-defined adverse reactions would unnecessarily take up investigator, sponsor, and regulatory authority resource and could divert attention away from new and significant safety concerns.

Conversely, relatively minor adverse events may be upgraded if they are known to indicate or predict events of concern, so in the protocol it may be specified that certain minor adverse events are treated as serious adverse events. For example, if it is known that a skin rash may indicate development of a life-threatening adverse reaction to the medication, all skin rashes may be specified as requiring expedited reporting to the sponsor.

The protocol may also provide additional information and clarification from the sponsor around specific study-related situations; for example, in a study of elderly patients, it may be specified that admissions to hospital for respite care are excluded from expedited reporting requirements as they are not due to an adverse event.

In addition to active questioning and assessment in clinic resulting in the recording and reporting of adverse events, many studies involve measurements of blood parameters, blood pressures, peak flows, and other physical characteristics that may all indicate adverse events.

When conducting early phase studies, there is relatively little safety data available to provide context and aid interpretation. A single serious adverse event generally indicates only a need for heightened vigilance, unless it is known to commonly be linked to adverse drug reactions (e.g. Stevens Johnson syndrome).

Once phase 3 studies are underway, there may be a large amount of data available for pharmacovigilance analysis. Techniques are being developed and refined by pharmaceutical companies and regulatory authorities that aim to compare the average rate of occurrence of a particular adverse event to the rate seen in a particular study or trial programme. It may then be seen if the rate is significantly higher than average, and hence a potential safety signal. Conversely, if an adverse event is relatively low, then it may indicate some protective event or even an unintentional beneficial effect.

What responsibilities does the sponsor have according to GCP?

The sponsor is responsible for:

- ongoing safety evaluation of the investigational product(s)
- promptly notifying investigator(s)/institution(s) and regulatory authority(ies) of findings that could affect adversely the safety of subjects, impact the conduct of the trial, or alter the IRB/IEC's approval
- expedite reporting to investigator(s)/institutions(s), to IRB(s)/IEC(s) and regulatory authority(ies) of all adverse drug reactions (ADRs) that are both serious and unexpected
- submitting to the regulatory authority(ies) all safety updates and periodic reports, as required by applicable regulatory requirement(s)

What should go in to the protocol?

The protocol may specify procedures for obtaining reports of adverse events and for recording and reporting them, as well as investigator and sponsor responsibilities in this area. Alternatively, the protocol may contain a statement that the study is being done in accordance with ICH GCP, national or local regulatory requirements, or the EU Clinical Trial Directive, as appropriate.

When should an independent data monitoring committee be used for reviewing safety data?

The sponsor may use an independent data monitoring committee (IDMC) to review unblinded study data to assess progress, and this includes reviewing the safety data. It may recommend that the sponsor continues, modifies, or even stops a study, depending on the risk to benefit balance. The IDMC may, for example, recommend additional assessments of study subjects if there is some evidence of an emerging safety issue.

What responsibilities does the investigator have?

The investigator must report any serious adverse event (SAE) which occurs in a subject immediately to the sponsor, either orally or in writing. This should be followed by a detailed written report. Where the event involves the death of a subject, the investigator should supply the sponsor and/or IRB/IEC with any additional information they require.

What responsibilites does the sponsor have according to the EU?

The sponsor's responsibilities entail:

- recording of adverse events
- reporting of suspected unexpected serious adverse reactions (SUSARs) to the national competent authority (be it directly or through the EudraVigilance Clinical Trials Module) and the ethics committee

- informing the investigators
- annual safety reporting to the national competent authority and the ethics committee

The sponsor should continuously weigh anticipated benefits and risks of the clinical trial, which includes ongoing safety evaluation of IMPs.

The sponsor must ensure that all relevant information on SUSARs that are fatal or life-threatening is reported as soon as possible and no later than seven days after the sponsor was first aware of the reaction. Any additional relevant information should be sent within eight days of the report. A SUSAR which is not fatal or life-threatening must be reported not later than 15 days after the sponsor is first aware of the reaction.

A sponsor therefore needs to collect sufficiently detailed information to determine whether an event meets the definition of a SUSAR, that is:

suspected—the IMP is suspected of being linked to the event. This may involve unblinding, usually by the sponsor's pharmacovigilance function, to determine what medication the subject was taking and hence whether the IMP should be suspected.

unexpected—the reference safety information for the IMP (usually contained in the investigator's brochure) does not include adverse event
serious—the event meets the criteria for serious, for example, involving hospitalization
adverse reaction—there is at least a reasonable possibility that the event is linked to the medication the subject was receiving. Adequate analysis of causality is therefore crucial in identifying SUSARs.

Further information is available in the following European Commission document: Detailed guidance on the collection, verification and presentation of adverse reaction reports arising from clinical trials on medicinal products for human use—2011.[15] The key points relating to pharmacovigilance are included in Part 5 of the Medicines for Human Use (Clinical Trials) Regulations 2004: SI 2004/1031.[3]

What are the legal responsibilities concerning safety reporting in the UK?

Legally, the sponsor's main responsibilities under the UK Regulations are to:
- keep records of all adverse events reported by investigators
- ensure recording and prompt reporting of SUSARs
- ensure investigators are informed of SUSARs
- ensure all SUSARs, including those in third countries, are entered into the European database
- provide an annual list of suspected serious adverse reactions and a safety report

How should the sponsor report SUSARs to the regulatory authority?

Some regulatory authorities require reports to be submitted by fax or a preliminary notification by telephone and then submission by post or fax. However, most regulatory authorities require reporting through an electronic web-based system.

There is ongoing development of the EudraVigilance system for EU clinical trials and currently, there are different systems in operation for submission of relevant reports to the central European database. 'Relevant' includes:

- SUSARs originating in a particular country
- SUSARs originating outside the country but where the sponsor has an ongoing trial in the country with the same IMP

Reporting to EEA Member State Competent Authorities must be carried out in accordance with each individual Member State's requirements. For example, in the UK, SUSAR reporting is to the MHRA through an eSUSAR website.[16] This website may also be used to report SUSARs originating in other EEA Member States to the MHRA and can also produce a record of reports submitted for each of an Institution's clinical trials, for the IRB/IEC. The MHRA website then forwards UK and relevant third-country (i.e. outside the EEA) reports submitted via the MHRA's eSUSAR website to the European Medicines Agency (EMA). SUSAR reports originating in the UK should not be submitted directly to the EMA by the trial sponsor, to avoid duplication. Some other EU countries submit SUSARs to the EMA via their national regulatory authority (Competent Authority) and some report directly using the EudraVigilance Gateway.[17] The EudraVigilance Gateway allows marketing authorization holders (MAHs), applicants, and sponsors to report to a common reporting point within the EEA from where the transactions are re-routed to the Competent Authorities and the EMA.

What are development update safety reports (DSURs)?

The Development Safety Update Report (DSUR) Guidance (ICH E2F)[18] was published in the EU in September 2010 and implemented in September 2011. In addition to the expedited reporting required for SUSARs, sponsors are required to submit a safety report to the regulatory authority and IRB/IEC once a year. Full details can be found in Section 5.2 of Detailed guidance on the collection, verification and presentation of adverse reaction reports arising from clinical trials on medicinal products for human use—April 2006.[15]

The reference safety information (RSI) for an IMP must remain consistent during each annual reporting period. At the end of the reporting period the sponsor should assess the new safety information that has been generated and is found in the DSUR, and submit any proposed safety changes to the IB as a substantial amendment to the study. Examples of changes include the downgrading of reactions from unexpected to expected.

What about urgent safety measures?

The sponsor and investigator may take appropriate urgent safety measures to protect clinical trial subjects from any immediate hazard to their health and safety. The measures should be taken immediately and it is not necessary to wait for regulatory approval. However, regulatory authorities and IRB/IECs must be informed as soon as possible (the MHRA, for example, expects full documentation within three days).

Similarly, when a sponsor halts a trial temporarily it should notify the regulatory authority and IRB/IEC as soon as possible (the MHRA, for example, allows 15 days from when the trial is temporarily halted). Details of what has been halted (e.g. stopping recruitment and/or interrupting treatment of subjects already included) and the reasons why will be required. If a trial is prematurely terminated, the sponsor should notify the regulatory authority and IRB/IEC as soon as possible (the MHRA, for example, allows 15 days for notification).

The regulatory authority may also make amendments or suspend or terminate a trial, for example if there are doubts over the safety or scientific validity of the study.

Are requirements different in the US and other countries?

Requirements for clinical studies are based on GCP, so are similar to those in the EU. For example, the FDA requires annual Investigational New Drug safety reports, in the same way that DSURs are required in the EU, although there are some differences in the content.

How should reactions associated with active comparator or placebo treatment be handled?

Sponsors must report reactions associated with active comparator or placebo to either the manufacturer of the active control or to appropriate regulatory agencies, and ICH guidelines state that it is the sponsor's responsibility to decide which body this should be. Events associated with placebo will usually not satisfy the criteria for an ADR and so will not require expedited reporting.

What common inspection and audit findings are made in this area?

The sponsor has a duty to notify to all relevant bodies any event 'likely to affect the safety of subjects'. It is therefore expected that the sponsor has appropriate quality systems for recording, assessing, reporting, and managing adverse events and these systems will be inspected and audited. Common findings include:

- Failure of the sponsor to monitor increased severity or frequency through trend analysis
- Failure to ensure that events are followed up until outcome (e.g. pregnancies, very long-term SAEs)
- Failure to ensure annual safety reports (DSURs) are reported within required time frames; anniversary dates should be tracked to signal when annual reports are due
- SAEs not being unblinded by the sponsor to check whether they are drug related and hence meet the definitions for an adverse reaction before they are reported as a SUSAR.
- Out-of-hours rotas and systems for cover may be in place, but auditors and inspectors will check that these systems actually work, and for evidence that they have been tested
- Lack of involvement of principal or chief investigator and of awareness of legislative requirements for 7- and 15-day reports
- Investigational site staff unable to distinguish AEs and ADRs, identify 'serious events' or consider event expectedness, and hence identify events which require IMMEDIATE reporting

Conclusion

Sponsor responsibilities are very broad, encompassing overall responsibility for many different trial-related activities, and these are detailed in GCP guidelines, the EU Directive national regulations, and the EU Regulation. Key areas include authorizations/approvals (including indemnity, insurance, and compensation), financing of the study, conduct of the study to GCP standards, provision of quality systems including SOPs and auditing, manufacture, and provision of investigational medicinal product and safety information. Sponsors will therefore require systems to cover these key areas. While activities may be delegated, the sponsor retains overall responsibility, so adequate oversight is required to ensure that these activities are completed to appropriate standards.

References

1. International Conference on Harmonisation of Technical Requirements for Registration of Pharmaceuticals for Human Use. ICH Harmonised Tripartite Guideline. Guideline for Good Clinical Practice E6 (R1).
2. Directive 2001/20/EC of the European Parliament and of the Council of 4 April 2001 on the approximation of the laws, regulations and administrative provisions of the Member States relating to the implementation of good clinical practice in the conduct of clinical trials on medicinal products for human use.
3. UK Medicines for Human Use (Clinical Trials) Regulations 2004 (SI 1031).
4. United States Food and Drug Administration Code of Federal Regulations Title 21 Parts 310 and 3125 NHS Research and Development Forum. Sponsorship: Frequently Asked Questions ॐ www.rdforum.nhs.uk/
5. EU Commission Regulation 536/2014.
6. Universities UK and DH Joint Statement, May 2004 ॐ www.ct-toolkit.ac.uk
7. NHS Research and Development Forum. Indemnity Arrangements within Primary Care - who is responsible for what? A paper prepared by the NHS R&D Forum, Primary Care Working Party ॐ www.rdforum.nhs.uk
8. ABPI Clinical Trial Compensation Guidelines ॐ www.abpi.org.uk/our-work/library/guidelines/Pages/ct-compensation.aspx
9. British Medical Association Private Practice Frequently Asked Questions. ॐ http://bma.org.uk/practical-support-at-work
10. EUDRALEX volume 10 'The rules governing medicinal products in the European Union', Chapter IV 'Guidance for the conduct of GCP inspections—Sponsor and CRO, Annex IV' ॐ http://ec.europa.eu/health/documents/eudralex/vol-10/
11. Committee for Medicinal Products for Human Use (CHMP). The Guideline on the Requirements to the Chemical and Pharmaceutical Quality Documentation concerning Investigational Medicinal Products in Clinical Trials (CHMP/QWP/185401/2004 final) ॐ http://ec.europa.eu/health/files/eudralex/vol-10/18540104en_en.pdf
12. European Commission Enterprise and Industry Directorate-General, Brussels, 03 February 2010. Document number ENTR/F/2/AM/an D(2010) 3374. EUDRALEX The Rules Governing Medicinal Products in the European Union Volume 4 EU Guidelines to Good Manufacturing Practice Medicinal Products for Human and Veterinary Use Annex 13 Investigational Medicinal Products ॐ http://ec.europa.eu/health/files/eudralex/vol-4/2009_06_annex13.pdf
13. Byrom B. Using IVRS in Clinical Trial Management. Applied Clinical Trials October 2002: 36–42.
14. International Conference on Harmonisation of Technical Requirements for Registration of Pharmaceuticals for Human Use. ICH Harmonised Tripartite Guideline. Clinical Safety Data Management: Definitions and Standards for Expedited Reporting E2A.
15. Communication from the European Commission — Detailed guidance on the collection, verification and presentation of adverse event/reaction reports arising from clinical trials on medicinal products for human use ('CT-3') (2011/C 172/01) ॐ http://ec.europa.eu/health/files/eudralex/vol-10/2011_c172_01/2011_c172_01_en.pdf

16. MHRA eSUSAR reporting website ⌕ https://esusar.mhra.gov.uk/
17. EMA EudraVigilance Gateway ⌕ http://eudravigilance.ema.europa.eu/human/evGateway01.asp
18. International Conference on Harmonisation of Technical Requirements for Registration of Pharmaceuticals for Human Use. ICH Harmonised Tripartite Guideline. Development Safety Update Report (DSUR) Guidance E2F .

Monitoring

Review of the responsibilities of the monitor

Evolution of the monitoring role

The role of the monitor has evolved over the decades. The role was created in the 1960s in response to the thalidomide tragedy. The acronym CRA (clinical research associate) was a generic term for any non-medically qualified persons working in a clinical research department. The responsibilities were diverse, ranging from protocol writing to report writing.

Until the 1980s, the CRAs working for pharmaceutical companies would have included CRF design, site evaluation and selection, organization of investigator meetings, data validation and verification, as well as protocol generation and writing the study report.

The role narrowed considerably during the 1990s with the introduction of source data verification (SDV). This process ensures that the source documentation matches the case report form. There was a simultaneous rise in the use of contract research organizations (CRO). The CROs took on many of the tasks, leaving the CRAs with the more administrative aspects of the study.

Changes in paradigm

In 2013 the Food and Drug Administration (FDA) released its guideline, Oversight of Clinical Investigations—A Risk-Based Approach to Monitoring (August 2011), finalized in August 2013. These risk-based approaches to monitoring are most likely to ensure subject protection and study quality and facilitate more effective monitoring. The guidelines state that patient protection and data integrity must be maintained. The FDA states that the focus of monitoring should be on critical data. It encourages a hybrid approach to monitoring activities and encourages reliance on centralized monitoring practices where appropriate. The role of the monitor has therefore changed; site visits will only be required where there are concerns about the safety of the subject or data quality.

What type of person makes a good monitor?

An experienced CRA has a wealth of knowledge. He or she is appointed by the sponsor.

CRAs have to be appropriately trained and have scientific or clinical knowledge needed to monitor the trial adequately. They have to be familiar with drug/product, protocol, written informed consent, and any other written information to subjects, sponsor's SOPs, good clinical practice (GCP), and applicable regulatory requirements.

ICH GCP E6 guidelines state: 'The act of overseeing the progress of a clinical trial and ensuring that it is conducted, recorded and reported in accordance with the protocol, standard operating procedures (SOPs), Good Clinical Practice (GCP) and the applicable regulatory requirements.'

The monitor must have the following attributes:
• Good communication skills—the monitor is the main line of communication between the sponsor and the sites
• Professionalism

- Organization skills
- Business-like approach to work
- Confidence
- Enthusiasm
- Assertiveness
- Empathy
- Tact
- Diplomacy

The dynamics of the working relationships between the CRA, site, and sponsor are complex. The CRA needs to maintain current information on each site he or she is responsible for, including data on site performance, current enrolment status, and outstanding actions and queries. A study may not have as much status at a site as it does at the sponsor company so part of the CRA's role must be to motivate and coach the site personnel as well as act as the 'enforcer'. With the advent of centralized monitoring many of these checks may be done centrally and the CRA will spend more time resolving issues or addressing safety or quality concerns.

The CRA must have an understanding of the therapeutic area in which he or she is working. The CRA should be familiar with the scientific methods and regulatory environment around the conduct of the study. He or she must be able to recognize errors and omissions that could bias the study and invalidate the data. The CRA should be able also to judge whether a site has the expertise, experience, patients, and facilities to conduct a study well, the ability to identify high-calibre investigators, and be able to generate accurate data in a timely fashion.

The current role of the monitor

Fortunately this is not just one of SDV; 'multi-tasking' is still a key feature. The CRA needs to cultivate good relationships with the study site staff, sponsor representatives, and study vendors, acting as the main line of communication between the sponsor and the investigators. The monitor also has to be thoroughly familiar with the investigational product(s), the protocol, written informed consent plus any other written information to be provided to the subjects, the sponsor's standard operating procedures (SOPs), GCP, and the applicable local regulatory requirement(s). All of this amounts to a great deal of information that a CRA should not just be aware of but should know well. Consequently the monitor role is perceived as both more complicated and more restricted than it once was, and, unfortunately, as offering less opportunity for scientific creativity/interest than other roles.

At a time when concerns about drug safety are growing throughout the industry, monitors find themselves on the front line of adverse event reporting. They must ensure that investigators comply with adverse event reporting requirements. They also review initial and follow-up adverse event data to ensure accuracy and also review all other study data to detect any unreported adverse events.

A positive relationship between the monitor and the study site, particularly with the study coordinator/nurse and the clinical trials pharmacist, is vital for maximizing cooperation. A monitor can make all the difference to a study's success. The constructive approach of a good CRA should be different to that of an auditor.

CRAs should be proactive and resolve issues that could adversely affect a study such as speaking to investigators about getting help for overworked staff, noticing problems which could have an impact on data integrity, and helping to solve patient recruitment problems. The monitor's role is key to ensuring the speedy and smooth running of a trial.

It is acknowledged that there are limitations to the current practice, hence the focus is now on risk-based or centralized monitoring.

The next section of this chapter deals with the impact of electronic data capture (EDC) on the monitor's role in ensuring data quality.

EDC has changed the nature of site visits. EDC allows the monitor to check patient enrolment, view actual data, review data queries, run reports, and check the status of data entry before visiting a site. In-built edit checks instantaneously alert data entry staff to out-of-range values. Queries can also be raised remotely by data management staff involved in the study (sometimes based in another country). It has also facilitated the growth of centralized monitoring.

Central monitoring practices mean real-time analysis of data by an application running on a server in data management. This means that the CRA does not necessarily have to be the person to review the data, In fact, many companies have a central site based in a single country where all data are deposited. The data are reviewed for trends and outliers, etc., and many things may be picked up that would have not been seen via traditional monitoring.

Good use of EDC should mean that the 'e-enabled' monitor is free to work more flexibly and that the mundane tasks of query generation and resolution are made less onerous.

EDC gives the CRA the opportunity to input into eCRF design, to create supporting documents such as monitoring and eCRF completion guidelines, and to conduct work remotely.

The adoption of EDC and the transition from paper to electronic data entry and processing is discussed later in this chapter. Mention is made of new technologies, notably point-of-contact data collection systems.

It is estimated that nearly half or more of all clinical trials today are run partially or completely on EDC systems, most of which are browser based with many operating on a 'Software as a Service' (SaaS) model, with remote hosting capabilities. EDC delivers accurate and up-to-date information, offering researchers and sponsors the opportunity to analyse ongoing data, to respond swiftly to findings, and to derive clear and accurate conclusions from the final results. However, implementing EDC is not easy. Training and supporting remote sites in the use of the technology is expensive for sponsors and not always welcomed by site personnel.

Electronic health records (EHR) and EDC

Since 2000 there has been revolutionary change in both clinical research and healthcare, with clinical documentation tasks in both industries moving from paper to electronic data entry and processing. In healthcare, electronic health records have been extensively adopted in some healthcare settings (mostly in Scandinavia—85% of all Danish records are electronic—the UK, and parts of Asia). The trajectory is clearly towards full adoption in many parts of the world.

Some of the driving forces for change are shared between the two industries; for example, efficiency, cost, patient safety, and quality of data. Since both EHR and EDC collect patient data, it would be useful if a standard, usable process could be devised for combining EHR and EDC for multicentre trials. However, significant differences make the sharing of data and the integration of systems quite a complex undertaking.

EDC and/or paper?

Increasing the efficiencies of clinical trial data collection through EDC is important but it is not the only consideration. User preferences, ease of use, content, quality, and overall synchronicity with other components of the process also need to be considered. The cost and lead times needed to develop the original eCRF plus the impact of protocol amendments need to be considered.

According to one survey, 46% of clinical trial staff reported having to spend more time working on trial data due to EDC in 2009, compared to 23% of respondents in 2001. Another problem in the use of EDC systems, noted in this survey, was 'that EDC systems typically don't have the trial data until 48 hours to a week after it is written down by hand or collected in some other system, despite contractual obligations to provide the data entry within shorter time windows'.

Data entry can also sometimes be outstanding for much longer periods of time, for a variety of reasons. Notably, it is imperative to have paper back-up of serious adverse event (SAE) forms (with instructions for use in the investigator site file), in case the EDC system is 'down' at a crucial time.

New technologies and their service delivery

Part of the reason for late data entry could be that it is the normal practice of healthcare professionals to capture data on paper while in front of patients. This aversion to keyboard-based entry has been addressed to some extent in recent years by the development of point-of-contact data collection systems such as the digital pen and tablet PCs. These devices allow the user to input data using a natural pen-based workflow; the data can then be integrated with the data repository and management function of an EDC or clinical trial management system (CTMS).

Another problem is that as more and more technology and solution providers deliver more diverse systems, there is a danger that personnel will suffer from 'e-overload'. An improvement in technology should lead to a decrease in the number of contact points for users who need help with their IT solutions, and ideally there should be provision of a single accessible point of contact and support for study sites, regardless of the query or request.

In this way sponsors, CROs, and sites can continue to benefit from the products and services of multiple vendors via a single helpdesk. It should be noted that EDC systems have been enthusiastically adopted in phase I studies where interfaces between the eCRF and other software prove their worth (e.g. barcoding to track documents and samples; electronic import of laboratory, vital signs, spirometry results, etc., from data recording devices).

With the advent of eClinical trials, the role of the CRA may include an even greater computer-based component.

With centralized monitoring there is no prescribed software but there needs to be robust computer validation in place and integration of existing software and systems.

There are companies that provide sophisticated computer sampling techniques which facilitate centralized monitoring.

What do the guidelines say about monitoring?

ICH GCP E6 guidelines state 'that in general there is a need for on-site monitoring before, during, and after the trial, however in exceptional circumstances the Sponsor may determine that central monitoring in conjunction with procedures such as investigator training and meetings and extensive written guidance can assure appropriate conduct of the trial in accordance with GCP. Statistically controlled sampling may be an acceptable method for selecting the data to be verified.'

Whatever monitoring system is used the sites have to be selected in an appropriate way. Before site selection can take place the CRA has to prepare.

Study preparation

CRAs are involved in the numerous tasks that are required before a study can start. These include applying for ethics and regulatory approvals (plus R&D approval at sites in the UK), preparation of grants and contracts, study supplies, pre-initiation documents plus investigator and pharmacy files, organization of pre-study visit(s) and investigator meeting(s). Some of these topics are discussed in detail elsewhere in this book, notably in Chapters 10, 17, and 22. Topics of particular relevance to CRAs are the types of investigative sites, identifying and evaluating potential investigators, pre-study visit(s), pre-initiation documents, and investigator meetings.

Types of study sponsors

Commercial sponsors are pharmaceutical and biotechnology companies plus medical device manufacturers who usually hold the marketing authorization or licence for the drug or product under investigation. Academic sponsors are either universities or charities such as Cancer Research UK, or (in the US) Federal agencies such as the National Institutes of Health (NIH).

Pharmaceutical and biotechnology companies often operate internationally, have extensive SOPs, and provide the investigational product and medical oversight. CRAs employed by such companies are generally very well supported by in-house staff. However, since the diversity of roles required particularly for phase 3 and 4 trials may exceed the resources of the sponsor, such companies usually hire one or more contract research organizations (CROs) when managing large-scale clinical trials.

CROs tend to be smaller organizations but they also have extensive SOPs. Support to CRAs is usually good but can be variable. Budgetary constraints are more evident.

Clinical trials designed by a local investigator and (in the US) federally funded trials are almost always administered by the researcher(s) who designed the study and applied for the grant. In the UK, hospital R&D departments are relatively new to the role of sponsor. Such departments are generally understaffed and are using SOPs in their infancy. CRAs employed by R&D departments need to be able to operate independently and to be confident in their experience and knowledge to provide advice to the sponsor when necessary.

Types of investigative sites

There are several types of investigative sites conducting studies:
• Academic sites
Sites in universities and teaching hospitals tend to be involved in their own research as well as industry-sponsored trials. Sometimes the industry trials provide a source of funding to allow the sites to pursue their own research. It is desirable for a study sponsor to involve some academic sites in its development programmes as this allows 'opinion leaders', the top specialists in their fields, to become familiar with new compounds and, hopefully, to support the compound when it is marketed. For the CRA, this can add an additional challenge of managing the availability of busy lecturers and clinicians.

• Dedicated sites

At these sites no other medical practice is carried out. They are generally very experienced and productive and aware of their competence. Such sites are unlikely to accept studies unless they think full recruitment of subjects on time is achievable. These sites are usually easy to monitor, being both accommodating and compliant. Almost all phase I studies are conducted at such sites.

• Part-time sites

Here investigators maintain their regular clinical practice as well as participating in research studies. These sites usually have less experienced investigators than dedicated sites and they may need more training.

Site management organization (SMOs)

SMOs bring together a group of sites and manage them centrally, standardizing procedures and materials to each site. Working with multiple sites in an SMO can be advantageous because of the consistency of study practices.

Identifying and evaluating potential investigators

There are several ways to find potential investigators. The best way is via databases maintained by study sponsors and these may also have useful statistics on enrolment rates and performance.

Websites that list investigators and their areas of specialty are also useful. In addition, clinical trial registers allow access to information on investigators who are current or recent participants, and can be searched by location and therapeutic area at ℗ www.controlled-trials.com

Networking is another valuable tool, either via CRAs, who may have contact with investigators, or centres, or via other departments, companies, professional organizations, etc.

Once a list of potential investigators has been compiled and contact made with an appropriate site, then before protocol details are supplied the investigator must return a signed confidentiality agreement (by e-mailing a scanned copy or by fax or mail).

Some sponsors and CROs have now opted to have all start-up activities performed by a dedicated start-up team of CRAs who are submission and contract specialists. This can dramatically reduce the number of days between final protocol and first site initiation.

Although this makes the process faster, it does introduce another party and excludes the CRA from a project's start, which may affect relationships with site personnel.

Pre-study visit(s)

Pre-study activities vary according to the study and may involve one or more site visits. During a pre-study visit, a CRA would expect to:
• verify site personnel qualifications and collect all relevant *curricula vitae* (CVs).
• evaluate the investigator's experience, expertise, and interest in the trial. Conversing in person will allow the CRA to assess research activity in the therapeutic area of interest, to determine if the investigator has conducted trials similar to the one being proposed, or has worked with similar types of investigational product (drug, biologic, or device).

- establish the investigator's satisfaction with the proposed remuneration.
- review investigator/site staff availability for conducting the study plus any training requirements.
- discuss background information on the study drug (biologic or device, as appropriate), key aspects of the protocol (including study objectives, inclusion and exclusion criteria, time and events schedule) and study specific requirements.
- assess if the investigator is willing to follow the protocol as it is written, including differences between routine clinical practice at the site and the protocol requirements. It is better to find out about potential problems and conflicts at the first site visit than later in the process!
- discuss general study requirements, notably obtaining consent, and investigator/institution responsibilities.
- ensure that the investigator has access to a properly constituted ethics committee in compliance with ICH GCP to ensure that local regulatory requirements are met.
- review screening and recruitment strategies/processes/targets and timelines.
- review subject safety reporting and site emergency contact procedures.
- tour the site facilities to check suitability of facilities, particularly requirements for handling and storage of investigational product (IP) and biological samples, record keeping, and arrangement for collection/disposal of any unused IP. Check for maintenance of a temperature log, manual or automated. If a central laboratory is involved, clarify who is going to prepare the samples.
- obtain a copy of the local clinical laboratory current certification/quality assurance document.
- check availability of and access to study specific equipment (such as spirometer, centrifuge, refrigerator, −20 °C or −80 °C freezer, ECG machine).
- verify secure storage facilities and enquire about long-term archive facilities after study completion.
- check technical capability for EDC (if appropriate).
- ensure site has adequate facilities for monitoring activities and will provide direct access to all source data.
- if any subject source data will be stored on a site computer system, assure features include security and data retrieval capability, data storage capacity, plus access to historical data.
- ascertain whether a UK site wishes the study to be network adopted.

UK studies—in particular patient populations (such as those involving children and young people)—can access support from the NIHR by applying for adoption into a portfolio of studies. Network staff have been aware that improved performance can lead to increased funding (and poor performance may lead to resources being withdrawn). This means that network staff are motivated to maximize recruitment once studies have started and to undertake careful feasibility studies in order to ensure that agreed targets are realistic.

Enrolling sufficient appropriate patients/subjects within the allotted time frame is of course a key requirement. The CRA will want to assess whether the subjects will come from the investigator's current patient population or if they will be referred from elsewhere, possibly other physicians in the same hospital or clinic, or from other hospitals. It is usually easier to assess enrolment potential for chronic (rather than acute) diseases such as diabetes or kidney impairment, since the investigator should already have appropriate patients on the hospital/clinic database. However, many of these patients may not qualify for or may not want to participate in a clinical trial so estimates of patient enrolment are usually overestimates. It is also important to ascertain whether the site is running other studies which may compete for the potential patient population.

It is advisable to place a study at a site which has a research coordinator/ nurse/administrator. He or she coordinates patient enrolment and visits, manages the study documentation, completes the case report forms, and is the primary contact for the CRA throughout the study. The CRA has a vested interest in making sure that the site personnel are motivated. It is also useful to ascertain which (if any) team members have experience with any proposed central laboratory, EDC system, central ECG vendor, interactive voice recognition systems (IVRS), etc. Availability of back-up staff in the event of absence, such as illness or holiday, should also be checked.

After the pre-study visit, a report is prepared. This will document any concerns or deficiencies at the site so that the sponsor can see how these can be addressed and decide whether or not to proceed with study set-up at a particular site.

Pre-initiation documents

Before a study can begin, a number of documents must be collected for each site.

If possible, two originals of each document should be obtained, one for the trial master file (TMF) and one for the investigator site file (ISF). If there is only one original of a particular document, it should be kept at the investigator's site and a copy sent to the TMF. Since the CRA is the person who visits the site, he or she will be involved in the collection and maintenance of documents even if the sponsor has assigned the primary responsibility to other internal staff such as clinical trial administrators (CTAs). Most sponsors will not ship any study drug to a site until all the relevant documents have been received (see Chapter 22, Documents required before the trial starts). Some companies do provide the case report forms/organize eCRF training (as appropriate) and deliver other non-drug supplies before receiving all the documents in an effort to speed up the process.

Curricula vitae

CVs should be on file at the site for all staff involved in the study, including those responsible for obtaining informed consent, clinical aspects, pharmacy matters, laboratory procedures, and any study-specific assessments such as performing radiological assessments, computed tomography (CT) or magnetic resonance imaging (MRI) scans, or reading pathology slides. CVs should be collected for the TMF for all medically qualified investigators, the study coordinator, and pharmacists. The CRA should check that each

CV is up-to-date and includes details of the individual's current position and GCP training. Sponsor SOPs normally define 'up-to-date' as being a maximum of two years old.

Ethics committee and regulatory authority approval

As discussed in Chapter 10, ethics committee approval must be obtained prior to study initiation. The final approval letter from the ethics committee must be on headed paper showing the name and address of the committee, the study, and investigator(s) approved. The approval should clearly identify the version numbers and dates of the documents reviewed so that there can be no ambiguity in document or version control. A list of the ethics committee members who approved the study should also be obtained.

Given the diverse range of documents which must be submitted to the ethics committee and regulatory authority (including protocol, patient information, informed consent documents, and investigator's brochure), it is clear that a lot of preparation is needed prior to study initiation. A signature from the investigator on the final approved protocol (and any amendments) is needed.

Financial documents

The financial agreement will require approval not only by the investigator(s) but also by representatives of the NHS/hospital Trust (or phase I unit, as applicable), as well as personnel within the sponsor company plus any involved CRO. Involvement of the CRA in grant negotiation and investigator contracts varies considerably among sponsors. Generally, the larger the company, the less the CRA is involved. This is because large companies generally have a separate department which handles the financial aspects of trials. Chapter 12 includes a section on financing and compensation of trials. A CRA should have a good understanding of how funding is determined in applicable countries.

For UK studies conducted within the NHS, the unmodified Model CTA (Bipartite or Tripartite) should be used, and together with the National Institute for Health Research (NIHR) costing template, will reduce contract negotiating timelines.

Since 1999, FDA regulation regarding financial disclosure (FD) has required that sponsors of studies with a US component certify the absence of certain financial interests of clinical investigators, disclose these financial interests, or certify that the information was impossible to obtain. This applies to any study of a drug, biologic, or device that is used to support a marketing application. Financial disclosure became an issue with small biotech companies in their start-up phases, as sometimes investigators and companies had closely tied financial interests, leading to a conflict of interest in the testing of potential new products. Having a financial interest in a company or product does not mean that an investigator cannot be involved in a trial; it just means that all parties must be aware of the potential for bias based on an investigator's financial interest.

Evidence of study training

In addition to face-to-face training at the site by the CRA, there are several ways by which site staff can be trained in preparation for a study:

- Online eLearning modules, hosted via a learning management system
- eLearning modules via a CD-ROM
- Remote meetings via webcast or teleconference
- Face-to-face meetings

Whatever the method, evidence of training completion should be generated and filed.

Investigator meetings

For a clinical trial with six or more sites, most sponsors hold an investigator meeting for investigators, their coordinators, appropriate sponsor personnel (notably the project manager, CRA, medical monitor, data manager, biostatistician, and a regulatory representative), plus personnel from any involved CRO and/or vendor. The purpose of such meetings is to allow the participants to get to know each other, to review the study in detail, and to facilitate subsequent communication. If well organized, such events can be important motivational and training opportunities. More recently these meetings may be conducted online.

Study initiation

The study initiation visit (sometimes known as the 'start-up' or 'kick-off' visit) is held at the investigator's site after all the approvals are in place and just before the study begins. The CRA (and often additional sponsor and vendor personnel) will meet with the investigator and study site team. The purpose of the meeting is to review the study protocol, processes, and procedures to ensure that all site personnel understand what is necessary to perform the study.

The delivery of clinical trial supplies to the site should be arranged to coincide with the initiation visit. This is done to prevent the possibility of subjects being enrolled in the study without all the necessary documentation and to ensure that the clinical trial supplies will have the maximum possible shelf-life. Sponsors and CROs have strict 'green light' procedures in place to ensure the study starts with all the documentation in place.

It is important that the maximum number of people involved in the study attend the initiation meeting, in order to provide an opportunity for everyone at the site to become familiar with the study and to appreciate each other's role in the study.

Preparing for the initiation visit

The CRA assigned to the site is normally in charge of the initiation meeting. Sometimes, particularly for a single centre study, the sponsor project manager will run the meeting.

The items to be covered are:
- Detailed discussion of the study protocol, notably:
  - Study background
  - Study objectives
  - Study design
  - Inclusion/exclusion criteria
  - Study flowchart (also known as the time and events schedule)
  - Study procedures on a per-visit basis
  - Efficacy assessments
  - Protocol compliance
  - Expected recruitment rate and study duration
- Study drug (IP)
  - Background information
  - IP administration
  - Randomization process and/or use of an IVRS
  - Emergency unblinding/code-break system(s)
  - Storage, dispensing, and accountability plus re-order, return, and destruction procedures/documents
- Study procedures: laboratory, ECG/Holter, imaging, spirometry, etc., as applicable; courier procedures
- Study supplies, reagents, laboratory kits, as applicable
- Informed consent (IC)
  - General and study-specific requirements
  - Documentation of IC procedure in source records
  - Retention of IC forms

- Safety data
  - General rules on AE/SAE recording
  - SAE reporting: timelines and forms
- Ethical and regulatory requirements
  - PI responsibilities
  - Communication with ethics committee
- Source records and case report form completion (or EDC usage)
  - Source records upkeep and filing
  - Data entry time frames
  - Queries resolution process
  - Maintenance of the audit trail
  - How to avoid errors
- Monitoring
  - Visit frequency, what should be ready, procedures
  - Availability of investigator/site staff during visits
- Site team
  - Study personnel roles and responsibilities
  - PI's obligations to conduct the study according to ICH GCP
- Inspection of clinical facilities not assessed previously
- Purpose and value of subject participation in pharmacogenetics (PGx) research, if applicable
- Any other study-specific or sponsor-specific items such as publication policy

In preparation for the visit the following supplies should have been sent to the site: ISF and pharmacy files, study drug if the drug release has been approved plus the applicable study-specific supplies (central laboratory kits and manual, ECG/Holter machines, paper CRFs, patient diaries, patient cards providing emergency contact details, etc.). If a study instruction manual—a quick reference guide including practical hints and tips which would not be found in a protocol—has been prepared, the CRA should be familiar with what is in it and how the site is expected to use it.

During the initiation visit

The CRA is responsible for organizing the meeting whose main purpose is for everyone to have a clear understanding of what is involved in the study and to give attendees the opportunity to ask questions.

If any of the study procedures involved are at all unusual, it may be helpful to take a 'dummy' example for demonstration purposes. It may also be helpful to provide laminated subject inclusion/exclusion criteria or instructions for sample preparation, for ease of reference.

Good source documentation is the key to high-quality data and the method, location, and forms for recording study data should be discussed. The site may need to generate source document sheets to assist with this process if more information than usual is required in the patient notes.

All those attending the site initiation meeting must sign a training attendance log.

At this visit, the CRA needs to make some additional checks in order to ascertain that the study drugs and equipment and necessary documents are correct.

After the meeting, the CRA completes an initiation visit report summarizing what was discussed, recording questions, concerns, actions, or issues, and detailing site-specific logistics procedures, storage conditions, and other issues. If questions that needed further follow-up arose during the meeting, the CRA must relay responses to the site as soon as possible. The report confirms that initiation activities have been completed and a copy should be included in the ISF.

The purpose of the follow-up letter to the site is to thank study staff for attending the initiation training and summarize any outstanding topics. Good working relationships and lines of communication established at this meeting will be invaluable as the study progresses.

Investigator study files

If the study site is new to clinical trials, the CRA should recommend how the ISFs should be maintained. If the site is experienced, this will be a routine activity. Details of documentation and retention requirements are given in Chapters 22 and 23. There are only two items of information which should not be kept in the site files and therefore made available to regulatory auditors: the contract and any report(s) from sponsor QA audits.

Monitoring visits

Good study monitoring and management are essential prerequisites for 'good, high-quality' study data. This has been defined as having certain characteristics (Box 13.1).

Many of the tasks may be done centrally now and may highlight trends across sites that traditional monitoring techniques may not have picked up.

In summary, the aim of monitoring clinical studies, is to collect good, high-quality data which can produce results that are reproducible and that support valid conclusions.

Usually the first monitoring visit takes place as soon as practicable (usually within two weeks) after the first subjects have entered the study.

Box 13.1 Description of good data characteristics
- Can be evaluated and analysed
- Allow valid conclusions to be drawn
- Are complete and accurate
- Do not need to be queried
- Are consistent across subjects and sites
  More specific characteristics are:
- Subjects meet the entry criteria
- All fields are complete
- Entries are legible (paper CRFs) and understandable
- Values are within range (or out of range: this may be the point of the study!)
- Entries make logical sense
- The units (for measurements) are correct
- There are no extraneous comments (paper CRFs)

For inexperienced sites, the first monitoring visit may be planned for when the first subjects are screened to check eligibility prior to drug administration. Any problems identified and rectified at this stage will save considerable time, resource, and cost.

If the first subject is not enrolled within a reasonable time after site initiation, a visit may be planned anyway to investigate the reason why. In the case of sites which are clearly underperforming (or not performing at all), the contractual agreement should allow for early closure of the site.

The monitoring plan

Since 2013, the monitoring plan has to have a risk assessment component and identify 'triggers' that would facilitate escalation to an on-site monitoring visit. No single monitoring approach is appropriate or necessary for every trial. The sponsor has to have a monitoring plan ensuring protection of subjects and data integrity and must identify the risks of the trial. A risk-based plan would include a mix of centralized and on-site monitoring practices and the plan should identify the methods used and the rationale for their use.

The monitoring plan should NOT just specify visits every X weeks, 100% SDV, etc. The monitoring plan should:

- List all types of monitoring to be performed and identify the risks being managed by them
- List the actions comprising each type of activity
- Detail the criteria for determining the timing and frequency of monitoring activities
- List events or results that should trigger changes in planned monitoring activity

A risk-based monitoring plan should outline what checks will be applied on reviewing CRF data and site meta-data before deciding which sites to visit. Past experience can be used to decide which sites represent minimal risk to the study and hence do not need attention. Use knowledge of current issues to prioritize monitoring type and/or SDV percentage, etc.

Examples of things to address:

- Disproportionate AEs
- Disproportionate DCF
- Anomalies in distribution of data and meta-data (e.g. re-signing consent forms)
- Lab data consistently out of range for one site
- Delayed data transfer

The requirements of the monitoring plan are to address the following:

- Type of monitoring to be used on-site or centrally
- Standards and written procedures to be followed
- Frequency of monitoring
- Monitor site capacity (max number of sites per monitor)
- Ancillary departments to be visited (such as pharmacy, labs, imaging)
- Data to be reviewed (percentage of SDV required and on what data)
- Considerations for unblinded monitors and reviewers (if required)
- Expectations for availability of the principal investigator during monitoring visits
- How non-compliance will be recorded and circulated
- Oversight of the investigator and ancillary department site files

- Escalation process:
  - For central monitoring, what triggers will be used for escalating to on-site monitoring
  - For both central and on-site monitoring how unresolved issues or serious non-compliances are handled
  - Management of supplies (IMP and ancillary materials)
- SAE reporting and associated monitoring responsibilities
- Query management:
  - Data queries
  - Protocol queries
  - IMP (including temperature excursion management)
- Documentation and review of monitoring activities:
  - Types and formats of reports (such as monitoring visit reports, central monitoring metrics, statistical monitoring)
  - Responsibility and timelines for preparing and reviewing the reports
- Training of monitors:
  - Specific protocol or therapeutic area training
  - Co-monitoring considerations
  - Handover of monitors

It is recommended that the monitoring plan is considered along with the risk assessment data management and data validation plans where appropriate.

How and how often to monitor

Centralized monitoring has been widely used by non-commercial sponsors. However, an increasing number of commercial organizations and sponsors are adopting a centralized approach as part of their monitoring strategy, moving away from the traditional way of monitoring trials where on-site visits are made four to six weekly irrespective of site performance and quality. The traditional visits incorporate 100% SDV (although some companies have other methods of SDV) believing that this is what the regulators require.

To attain optimal market success, new therapies must be supported by data-driven evidence that demonstrates greater value than the currently accepted standard therapy, a concept that encompasses safety, cost, convenience, treatment outcomes, and quality of life, as well as meeting regulatory requirements for efficacy. To meet the growing requirements for data from evidence-based health outcomes research, companies need information about their products that is not available from most phase 3 trials.

This data can be gathered from a variety of studies, including peri- and post-approval (phase 3b, 4, and PASS) clinical trials, patient registries, and retrospective/prospective observational studies using administrative or electronic health records.

This approach generates large volumes of data, and sponsors and commercial companies have relatively quickly introduced centralized monitoring techniques to handle this. Today, with increasing opportunity to apply technology and enhance visibility to data, clinical trials are shifting to hybrid monitoring models (mix of centralized and on-site) and risk-based triggered monitoring across earlier phase studies. Remote or centralized monitors collaborate with their field monitor counterparts to shift the burden of administrative support, site support, and data/document management.

With a risk-based approach more monitoring tasks are performed centrally. With the advent of eCRFs (electronic case record forms) and other eDCT (electronic data capture tools) it is easy to check things centrally or remotely from the site. Remote CRF review can be used to monitor performance at the site (data not being recorded in a timely manner), to identify missing data, and to check inclusion/exclusion criteria in order to ensure only eligible patients are entered in real time.

Using reports from databases, or statistical sampling methods, centralized monitoring can be used for validation checks of data and help identify triggers or signals that may highlight areas of non-compliance. Centralized monitoring could allow a direct comparison across sites and show trends in data or outliers that may not be identified by a monitor using a traditional approach.

In order to implement a centralized monitoring system there are pre-requisites: robust and validated computer systems are required and very well-defined criteria or triggers for high-risk sites, and data have to be identified and justified in the monitoring plans.

Statistical techniques and modelling to identify patterns or trends may be used. These can pick up incorrect or implausible data. For example, it may compare the number of adverse events at sites and identify outliers, odd distributions, or unusual variability in the data.

It is acknowledged that not all current monitoring tasks may be performed centrally and a 'one-size-fits-all' approach is not the answer. Trials that use a hybrid approach can be a means of directing visits to sites when required, therefore making best use of the resource available without compromising patient safety or data integrity.

The monitoring plan should identify under what circumstances an on-site visit is to be performed.

Traditionally, a suggested sequence of monitoring activities during a site visit would include the following but now, as shown, many of these tasks can be done centrally only, deploying CRAs to sites where there are issues to be addressed.

- Scrutiny of recruitment rate
- Review of informed consent
- SAE review
- Protocol adherence check
- Review of CRF and source documents
- Queries and error correction
- Study drug accountability
- Check of laboratory samples

Scrutiny of recruitment rate

Central monitoring will highlight if the recruitment rate is behind schedule and the reasons for this should be determined. The subject screening log will indicate the main reasons for screen failure and the site's recruitment effort to date. It may be possible to be improved either by changing the way in which the site operates or, by protocol amendment. A site visit may be required to review the practice at site.

- If recruitment rate is faster than anticipated, centralized monitoring will look closely at the eligibility criteria and ensure that ineligible patients are not being recruited. Similarly, reasons for premature withdrawal of any subjects should be reviewed centrally, distinguishing between withdrawals due to safety issues and withdrawals for other reasons, such as lack of efficacy. If there are unusual patterns in withdrawal rate for one site compared to others, this may act as a trigger to facilitate an on-site visit.

Review of informed consent

- Consent forms for all subjects must be checked to ensure that the correct form has been completed in full, and that it has been personally signed and dated by the subject or by the subject's legally authorized representative and any others involved in the informed consent process (such as the investigator or a witness). The date (and time, if available) of signature should precede study entry and any trial-related procedures. It is suggested that some elements of informed consent checking may be done centrally but due to data protection issues, the regulatory authorities (in some EU countries) will not sanction the transfer of consent information to a central location. The FDA, however, does allow transfer of forms and it is also suggesting there could be a portal where site staff could upload consent forms for checking. The FDA states that it is the sponsor's responsibility to maintain data protection although the Health Insurance Portability and Accountancy Act (HIPAA) aims to ensure data are used appropriately.
- If the consent form for a study has changed, for example because of a protocol amendment, it may be checked centrally that all newly enrolled subjects are signing the current form and that subjects who signed the old consent but are still on study, have signed the new consent.
- Except for a file copy, copies of the old consent should be destroyed so that they are not used inadvertently.
- If a study involves pharmacogenetic sampling, the form must indicate how long samples will be kept.

SAE review

SAE review can be done centrally but the CRA should examine the information about SAEs and check that the information provided to the sponsor tallies with that in the patient chart and supporting documentation. If additional information is available that has not been relayed to the sponsor, the CRA can collate and ensure that this is rectified during the visit. Concomitant medications should also be reviewed carefully, both for routine use and for the treatment of SAEs/AEs. It is useful if the CRA can be provided with an electronic tabulation of SAEs, to serve as a prompt with regard to any follow-up required. Source documents should be meticulously checked for evidence of AEs, particularly SAEs which have inadvertently not been reported. If a study patient was admitted to another hospital, there may be a delay in obtaining the requisite details. SAE reporting is discussed in detail in Chapter 19.

Protocol adherence check

This function may be performed centrally and can include comparison against other sites.

- In particular, the eligibility criteria should be checked to ensure that all the inclusion and exclusion criteria have been met. Any ineligible subjects must be brought to the attention of the investigator and a plan of action must be agreed for handling such subjects. There is the possibility that it might not be in the best interests of the patient to remain in the study and there may be issues with the sponsor insurance/indemnity. The site contract should clearly stipulate that payment will not be made for ineligible subjects.
- For randomized studies, it is important to confirm that the correct randomization procedures have been followed and that subjects have been randomized at the correct time in relation to the timing of other study assessments. Each subject should have been given the appropriate dose of the appropriate drug and, during each visit, returned any unused drug so that compliance can be assessed. Any cases of study drug non-compliance as defined by the protocol may have to be investigated. This may not require a site visit, but instead a telephone monitoring call or checklist may be completed by the site.
- If paper CRFs are being used the CRA will need to confirm that each subject attended for each visit during the appropriate time period. If using eCRFs, an autoquery will alert the site and CRA to any visits which occur outside of the visit window. Also to be noted as deviations are any missed or incorrect assessments at each subject visit.

Review of CRF and source documents

- Many of the traditional CRA validation checks conducted on paper CRFs will be done automatically when using eCRFS. Traditionally in the past 100% SDV has been performed. Thorough CRF (or eCRF) and source document review is the most time-consuming aspect of each monitoring visit and requires concentration and attention to detail. A suggested approach is to start with the subjects enrolled since the previous monitoring visit, to check that they qualify for the study. Once a CRF has been reviewed, the contents can be checked against the source documents
- After completing CRF review for a subject, the CRF should also be checked against the source documents, a process usually called source data verification (SDV).
- The purpose of SDV is to confirm that the subjects exist and to confirm that data in each CRF are consistent with the source data—the place where the data are first recorded—so verifying the integrity of the data.
- It is not necessary for every entry in a CRF to have a matching entry in a source document, but where the data appear in both, they should agree. On occasion, the original collection of data may be done directly on the CRF; in effect, the CRF becomes the source. This is frequently the case when capturing data needed solely for study purposes and not essential to the clinical care of subjects. Examples are psychiatric rating scales, visual analogue scales, repeated vital signs, ECGs, lung function

tests. The sponsor may require documentation to record when the 'CRF is source'.

- If the source data include electronic data, direct access to the relevant electronic subject data is preferred to allow the CRA to check that CRF data are supported by information in the computer records. If it is not possible for the CRA to have read-only access to the relevant subject data, printouts (signed and dated by an authorized investigator) are required. It is one thing, however, to request blood results to be printed from an electronic system if we know they exist. But how is it possible to monitor adverse events when we may not be aware they have occurred? There is a need for a definitive process for monitoring of electronic source data, especially since the amount of electronic healthcare data is increasing.

- The source data normally takes precedence if there is a discrepancy between the CRF and the source data, but the CRA should always ask site personnel to determine which is correct and to make the appropriate corrections. If the source data needs to be corrected, the site staff making the change should sign and date the document, including an explanation for the error.

- Some companies require 100% source data review. However with large-scale studies this activity can prove extremely time-consuming. Other sponsors have a sampling scheme, and these also vary considerably. Whatever the scheme, as a GCP requirement the key or critical documents and/or information in Box 13.2 must always be verifiable from source records other than the CRF.

Queries and error correction

Perhaps the most important errors a CRA might discover are those that result in protocol violations. These include such findings as a subject not fulfilling the inclusion or exclusion criteria, a wrong diagnosis, a subject taking prohibited concomitant medication, problems with visit windows, a subject not returning unused medication and not maintaining a diary card, etc. Usually these errors are found during SDV. Other less significant errors include missing data, out of range values, and transcription mistakes.

Box 13.2 FDA definitions of critical and less critical data

The FDA 2013 guidelines state:

Critical data (for monitoring focus) include:
- Subject eligibility
- Data that support primary and secondary end points
- SAE data and treatment discontinuation data
- Informed consent and agreement to extra visits
- Randomization/blinding and specific event adjudication data

Less critical (less monitoring/reduced SDV)
- Age
- Concomitant medications
- Concomitant illnesses

When potential errors are identified in paper CRFs or source data, the CRA should note them in a corrections/queries log and discuss them with the study coordinator. When they are resolved, the coordinator (never the CRA) should make the necessary corrections to the CRFs. Corrections are made by drawing a single line through the incorrect entry, making the correct entry, and initialling and dating the correction. If the reason for the change is not obvious a comment should be added for clarification. Anyone reviewing the forms must be able to see what was changed, when, and why. With centralized monitoring, data queries are raised by data managers or the centralized monitoring teams either when the data is entered onto the study database in the case of paper CRFs or on reviewing the data in the EDC system in the case of eCRFs. Sometimes the CRA is involved in the correction process, sometimes it is solely the site and central monitoring site. It is ideal if data management staff can enter data from the first few subjects' paper CRFs as early as possible in order to give timely feedback to the site. This is especially important in the case of consistent errors which are usually due to misunderstanding. Fast turn-around on edits and queries should then eliminate repeat errors.

Errors should decrease as the study progresses as a result of feedback and training by the CRA and central monitoring team, and experience on the part of site personnel. If during central monitoring a site has a high error rate, the CRA may be required to make an on-site visit to discuss this with the investigator and coordinator. Errors are very costly, both in terms of money and people-hours to correct.

As discussed in early sections of this chapter, EDC is now being used for many studies and has changed the nature of site visits. For studies involving eCRFs, the CRA needs to encourage prompt data entry by site personnel. It is particularly important for data entry to be as up-to-date as possible. The centralized monitoring team may review internal logic checks and any other tool built into the eCRF as a means of ensuring internal consistency, completeness and logic. Both CRA(s) and central monitoring team can often enter remote queries into an eCRF, allowing site staff to respond to these without the need for an on-site visit.

Study drug accountability

IP accounting is an important task for the CRA. A complete and detailed paper trail needs to exist to account for movement of IP from the sponsor/supplier to each study site, with documentation of use and eventual destruction (whether performed at the study site, by the sponsor/supplier, or by a third party).

The central monitoring team can check that the subjects are being dispensed study medication according to the protocol and any randomization scheme, but it will require a site visit by the CRA to check secure storage, ensuring that any special conditions such as refrigeration are being met. Integrity of the treatment blind should be checked, if appropriate. Any discrepancies between the records and actual site supplies must be investigated and recorded. It is best if IP is stored and dispensed by a pharmacy as they are routinely required to keep meticulous records. Dispatch and disposal of supplies is discussed in Chapters 17 and 18.

Check of laboratory samples

Any blood or other samples taken during a study should be obtained correctly and labelled, stored and delivered for analysis. The timing of collection, plus any storage and batching for shipping, should be checked by the CRA at initiation to ensure that protocol requirements are met. Sometimes this information is detailed in a separate laboratory manual. The shipping must be done according to all applicable laws and regulations, and each delivery of samples to an analytical laboratory should be documented.

The CRA should be aware of servicing/calibration requirements for any equipment or analytical processes. This is particularly important where a biochemical value is a primary end point and where analytical reagents or tubes have expiry dates.

Additionally, a change to a biochemical method might alter the normal range for a measured end point and this may have significant consequences during a study. If changes in equipment or methodology are unavoidable, a measurement with the new and the old equipment/assay at the same time point would identify potential problems.

Any such changes must be reported to those who will be involved in interpreting the data.

Review of investigator site file and study materials

If the CRA has not compiled/checked this file at the initiation visit, it should be checked at the first monitoring visit. With the advent of centralized monitoring, it is advisable for sites to use a checklist to ensure that current versions of documents, notably the protocol and consent, are being used and to check for missing documents. The correspondence section, the subject screening/enrolment log, subject identification log, and the monitoring visit log should be up-to-date. Safety reports issued since the data cut off for the most recent version of the IB should be filed. If there have been any changes in site staff, the delegation log should be updated to reflect this and the site file should include evidence of their qualifications and study training.

Older versions of documents can be removed from the site files and kept separately.

Ensuring that the site has sufficient materials (e.g. CRFs, copies of the protocol, subject ID cards, blood sampling kits, etc.) to ensure smooth running of the study may be coordinated centrally.

Verify continuing investigator oversight

It is important to ensure that the PI is actively involved in the study and is maintaining oversight of the study. Delegation to unauthorized or untrained individuals is not allowed.

During monitoring visits, the CRA must ensure the confidentiality of all study subjects. No study record other than the consent form and the subject identification log should identify the subject. The study documents are also confidential and should be kept in a secure location. Careful checks for personal details should be made prior to sending subject information, notably SAE follow-up details, to sponsors.

In the US, the HIPAA covers a wide swathe of all personally identifiable information both in the clinical and research arenas. One standard directly affects clinical research and relates to how unique patient-identifying information can be transmitted electronically, possibly over the Internet. A full explanation of the HIPAA can be found at ℘ www.hhs.gov/ocr/hipaa.

Before concluding a monitoring visit, the CRA should check the last site visit report for any unresolved issues. If the CRA is involved in grant requests, this should be discussed with the investigator.

The CRA should relay pertinent monitoring findings, which should be recapped in a follow-up letter or e-mail to be kept in the site file

Preparation of visit reports will be discussed in the last section of this chapter.

Serious findings

On occasion, the central monitoring team or the CRA may uncover a serious finding that requires urgent action. The MHRA guidelines (Serious Breaches Guidance) include a useful appendix of examples showing what qualifies as serious enough to be notified. This topic is discussed in detail in Chapter 19. Any suspicion of a serious breach, fraud, or any other concern during monitoring should be immediately reported to the study sponsor and would undoubtedly result in an on-site visit by the CRA or possibly require an audit.

Close-out visits

When a study is over, each site must be officially closed by the CRA. Usually, the main reason to close a study is because enrolment has completed, all study-related assessments have been completed for all subjects, and the data are complete and correct. Sometimes, however, studies may be terminated prematurely, generally for negative reasons; for example, the study medication was not safe, not effective or problems arose regarding manufacture or stability; the protocol was too difficult to execute; the sponsor ran out of funds or decided that the potential product was not viable for marketing; compliance or other problems at the site.

Positive reasons for early site termination include: target patient numbers in a multicentre study were achieved sooner than planned; interim analysis showed that the study medication is so effective that it would not be ethical to conduct a trial in which subjects might not be receiving active treatment; statistical stopping criteria, defined in the protocol, were met.

If the study should need to be stopped abruptly whilst subjects are still taking study medication, the sponsor will need to plan for discontinuing each subject. The CRA should be prepared to explain the plan and ensure that it is correctly followed.

When a study is being closed for a negative reason, the CRA will be responsible for informing on-site staff.

Whatever the reason for closing the study, the main items which need to be addressed finally during a close-out visit are:

- CRFs and data queries
- accountability and reconciliation of study drug
- investigator's site file including the end-of-study notification to the ethics committee (MHRA and local R&D in the UK), plus acknowledgement of receipt letters
- administrative issues including provision for archiving
- any follow-up of SAEs

CRFs and data queries

Outstanding CRFs or eCRFs that have not already been reviewed and final corrections made must be completed before the close-out visit.

All SAEs, any pregnancy or medical device incident and other adverse event follow-up should be complete. The CRA must ensure that all CRFs, as well as any corrections or query forms, are complete, well organized, and ready for storage/archiving. Any original diary cards and other subject-completed forms should remain with the other source data where possible.

Accountability and reconciliation of study drug

- If there are still IP supplies at the site, the CRA should complete a final inventory at the close-out visit. IP should then be packaged for return to the sponsor/supplier or destroyed on site, according to company policy.
- Prior approval for local IP destruction should be obtained from the sponsor. Confirmation of destruction should be documented and should include an inventory of all IP destroyed. Destruction should

only be carried out by personnel who are aware of possible hazardous effects.
• If the study was randomized, both the unopened and any opened randomization envelopes should be collected and returned to the sponsor.

Investigator's site file including the end-of-study notification to the ethics committee

The investigator site file needs to be finally reviewed for completeness, in particular to confirm that any recent e-mail correspondence or notifications to the ethics committee have been added. If there were protocol amendments during the study, or amendments to the informed consent form, all versions should be in the file, including their dates of use. Original informed consent forms for each subject must be present. If any documents are missing, the CRA should help the site to obtain copies. If at all possible, consistency should be verified between the sponsor trial master file (TMF)—an eTMF may be accessible by the CRA—and the investigator file.

Responsibilities for checking the ISFs and TMF contents are usually specified in the study monitoring plan.

Other administrative issues

• Often the sponsor will loan equipment (such as ECG machines, Holter monitors, centrifuges) to sites; such equipment will need to be retrieved and appropriate receipt/return documentation completed, and any contracts/equipment rental agreements will need to be terminated.
• The CRA should check that all laboratory samples have been received by the designated analytical laboratory and that final transmissions have occurred for all data collection tools (eDiaries, ECGs, etc.).
• A variety of administrative issues, notably records retention, should be discussed with the investigator. Not only do the records need to be stored and maintained, but there must also be a record of where they are stored. Most sponsors expect the investigator to retain all study records until notified by the sponsor that they may be disposed of. Sponsor companies may provide labels for patient notes to state that a subject has taken part in a clinical trial. It is recommended that the boxes of files be labelled on the outside 'DO NOT DESTROY', with the names of both the investigator and the sponsor as contacts for questions about them. The important topic of records retention and archiving requirements is discussed in Chapters 22 and 23.
• After study close-out, the possibility of regulatory audit remains, especially for pivotal studies and high-recruiting centres. Even if an audit has already taken place, the investigator should be advised of the possibility of audit from another authority. The timetable for preparation of the clinical study report and any publications/conference presentations must be outlined. This is also the time to reiterate the publication policy already discussed at the initiation visit.
• In the study close-out report (normally prepared using a sponsor specific close-out visit template), the CRA should ensure that the report is clear and confirms any outstanding follow-up actions.

How to report monitoring visits

Most sponsors have three standard visit report templates and checklists used to document visits to investigative sites: pre-study/initiation, monitoring, and close-out. Should a sponsor not already have these, refer to the generic example checklists given at the end of this section.

The visit report is a business document that will stay in the sponsor trial file for many years and can be accessed by the regulatory authorities in case of a sponsor inspection. The investigator is provided with a copy of the initiation visit report (but not subsequent reports). The language used in visit reports should be business-like and factual. The ICH GCP Guidelines (5.18.6) summarize the requirements for monitoring reports as follows:

- The monitor should submit a written report after each monitoring visit.
- Reports should include the date, investigative site, name of the monitor, name of the investigator, and any other individual(s) contacted.
- Reports should contain a summary of what was reviewed and statements concerning significant findings/facts, deviations and deficiencies, conclusions, actions taken or to be taken, and/or actions recommended to secure compliance.
- Monitoring reports are only for review by the study sponsor and so are confidential to the study sites.

The CRA should communicate any serious issues to appropriate management personnel, as soon as possible, during or after a site visit. Examples of significant findings/issues might include: PI unaware of study progress; ineligible subjects enrolled; improper delegation of responsibility to site staff; CRFs not completed; failure to report SAEs within the required timelines or update the ethics committee regarding safety issues, etc.

It is advisable for the CRA to make notes during the site visits and to write up the report as soon as possible. The CRA's manager should submit evidence of report review within the agreed time frame and request clarifications/corrections from the CRA, if necessary. A copy of each report including evidence of review is maintained in the TMF.

Example checklists

Site evaluation visit

- Protocol ....
- Sponsor ....
- Investigator..
- Site address..
- Attending personnel..
- Date ....

Investigator

- Qualifications
- Licensure (if appropriate) and GCP training
- Specialty
- Clinical study experience
- Number of previous and similar studies
- Enrolment in previous studies
- Any audit findings

Staff

- Study coordinator
- Other specialist personnel: pharmacists, MRI operators, etc.
- Training and clinical study experience
- Turnover

Facility

- Appropriate for studies
- Ample storage for study supplies
- Appropriate study medication storage
- Study specific equipment available
- Technical capability for EDC (if appropriate)
- Tour

Ethics committee

- Central ethics committee
- Local ethics committee
- Frequency and timing of meetings
- Average time to approval

Laboratory/tests

- Necessary tests can be done at local laboratory
- Local laboratory certification/quality assurance document
- Local laboratory normal ranges
- Experience with the central laboratory
- Staff able to process central laboratory samples

Protocol feasibility

- Interest in participating
- Availability of sufficient potential subjects in requisite time frame
- Competing studies
- Study staff availability/capacity
- Able to attend investigator meeting

Study documents (based on ICH GCP)

- Protocol . . . .
- Sponsor . . . .
- Investigator . . . .

Pre-study

- Investigator brochure
- Signed protocol and amendments (if any)
- Informed consent form
- Any other information to be given to subjects
- Any advertising materials for recruitment
- Ethics committee (plus MHRA and R&D in the UK) approvals for
  - Protocol   Date:
  - Amendments (if any)   Date:
  - Consent and any subject information   Date:
  - Advertising (if any)   Date:
- CVs for investigators
- Financial disclosures (if required)
- Any forms required to meet local regulations (e.g. FDA 1572 form)
- Laboratory certification and normal ranges
- Study manual, if available
- Shipping records
- Decoding procedures for blinded studies
- Contract
- Sponsor's insurance statement
- Sponsor specific documents

During the study

- Investigator brochure and safety updates (superseded versions to be marked as such and filed separately)
- Protocol amendments and/or revisions
- Consent versions
- Local ethics committee approvals for
  - Protocol amendments   Date:
  - Consent versions   Date:
  - New or revised subject information   Date:
  - New or revised advertising   Date:
- CVs and training records for new investigators
- Updates to laboratory certification and/or normal ranges
- Shipping documentation (receipt of study materials)
- Monitoring visit log
- Communications with sponsor
- Signed consent forms
- Source documents
- Protocol deviations—recorded in a protocol deviation log/file note
- Other relevant file notes
- CRFs and audit trail for CRF corrections
- Communications with sponsor (letters, e-mail, telephone reports)
- Notification to sponsors and ethics committee of SAEs
- Safety reports received from sponsor

- Interim and/or annual reports to ethics committee
- Subject screening log
- Subject identification code list
- Subject enrolment log
- Study drug accountability
- Study staff signature sheet/delegation log
- Record of retained body fluids and/or tissue samples (if any)

After study completion
- Drug (device) accountability
- Documentation of drug/device return or disposal
- Completed subject identification code list
- Copies of Declaration of End of Trial forms sent to ethics committee (MHRA and local R&D in the UK), with acknowledgements of receipt
- Final study report to ethics committee   Date:

Site close-out visit
- Protocol ....
- Sponsor ....
- Investigator ....
- Site address ....
- Attending personnel ....
- Date ....

- Study documents file is complete
- Final report has been made to ethics committee
- All CRFs are complete and have been submitted to the sponsor
- All source documentation is in order—location to be noted in the document file, if not with the study files
- Study staff signature sheet/delegation log is complete
- Subjects' signed consent forms are filed
- Drug dispensing, accountability, and disposal forms are complete
- Study drug/device has been returned or destroyed as per sponsor instructions
- All other study materials (unused paper CRFs and diaries, etc.) have been returned to the sponsor
- Investigator brochure and safety updates are stored together with the study files
- Reminder of investigator obligations

Conclusion

Successful monitoring requires experience, people skills, management ability, and knowledge of the protocol, GCP, CRFs, study drug/device, therapeutic area, regulations, and SOPs. The guidance presented in this chapter does not claim to be exhaustive and will need to be supplemented by individual sponsor procedures. However, it should help CRAs perform their essential role in encouraging good, high-quality research, and provide an insight into the CRA role to those whose work is being monitored. It also describes the role of risk-based and centralized monitoring which will ensure that resources are deployed where safety and data quality indicate on-site visits are needed.

Further reading

FDA Guideline 'Oversight of Clinical Investigations—A Risk-Based Approach to Monitoring' August 2013.

ICH Guideline (1996). Topic E6: Good Clinical Practice—Consolidated Guideline. International Federation of Pharmaceutical Manufacturers Associations, Geneva (Issued as CPMP/ICH/135/95.

Guidance for the notification of Serious Breaches of GCP or the protocol (updated in January 2014) www.mhra.gov.uk

Clinical trial design

Phases of development

The clinical development of a drug is classified into four phases, each requiring a different approach to trial design. Development programmes are based on what has been discovered about the drug in the pre-clinical testing phase and commence with phase 1 studies in a small population to evaluate the pharmacology in humans. They then move into phase 2 to evaluate whether there is an efficacious dose/dose range that is safe enough for further testing in a larger population, which takes place in phase 3. There is further investigation in phase 4 if the drug is approved for marketing. Since the development programme may not always move directly from phase 1 to phase 4 (e.g. phase 1 pharmacokinetic studies in children are usually conducted after adequate safety is available in the adult population), the International Conference on Harmonisation (ICH) has defined these phases according to the purpose of the clinical trial (ICH E8).

Phase 1 (ICH terminology: human pharmacology studies)

The initial administration of an investigational new drug into humans is the start of phase 1. Although human pharmacology studies are typically identified with phase 1, they may also be conducted later in the development sequence in different populations (e.g. human pharmacology in paediatric populations are normally carried out after information has been gained in adults). Studies in this phase of development usually have non-therapeutic objectives and may be conducted in healthy subjects or patients; for example, drugs with significant potential toxicity (e.g. cytotoxic drugs) are studied in patients.

Studies in this phase are exploratory and conducted in small subject populations who are selected by narrow criteria, leading to a relatively homogeneous population which is closely monitored. Subjects are often admitted to specialized phase 1 units where adequate medical back-up is available should a clinical emergency arise. Study designs are generally open-label and baseline controlled.

Studies conducted in phase 1 typically involve one or a combination of the following objectives, as follows.

Evaluation of initial safety and tolerability

The initial administration of an investigational new drug into humans is intended to determine the safety and tolerability of the drug and to determine the nature of adverse events or reactions that can be expected as development proceeds in later studies. These studies typically include both single- and multiple-dose administration.

Define and describe the pharmacokinetics

Characterization of a drug's absorption, distribution, metabolism, and excretion (ADME) usually starts as part of phase 1 studies and may continue throughout the development of the drug. The preliminary pharmacokinetic (PK) characterization is an important goal of phase 1 and PK data is used as the basis for decisions about the dose regimen or schedule to be used in later studies. Pharmacokinetics may be assessed via separate studies or as a part of the early safety and tolerability studies. It is particularly important to assess the clearance of the drug and to anticipate possible accumulation of parent drug or metabolites. Some PK studies are conducted in later phases to answer more specific questions such as the PK in special populations (e.g. the elderly, children, ethnic subgroups, or patients with renal or hepatic impairment which may impair elimination depending on the excretion pathway).

For many orally administered drugs, especially modified-release products, the study of food effects on drug availability is important. Drug–drug interaction studies are important for many drugs; these are generally performed in phases beyond phase 1, but results of the pre-clinical studies in animals and *in vitro* studies of metabolism and potential interactions may lead to such studies being conducted earlier in the drug development programme.

Define and describe the pharmacodynamics
Depending on the drug and the end point studied, pharmacodynamic (PD) studies and studies relating drug blood levels to response (PK/PD studies) may be conducted in healthy subjects or in patients with the target disease in phase 1. In patients, if there is an appropriate measure PD data can provide early estimates of activity and potential efficacy and together with PK data may be helpful for estimating the dose and dose regimen to be used in later studies such as in phase 2, when the end points are usually therapeutic.

Preliminary evaluations of activity or potential therapeutic benefit are usually secondary objectives in phase 1 studies. More definitive assessment is generally performed in later phases but may be appropriate when drug activity is readily measurable with a short duration of drug exposure in small numbers of patients at this early stage.

Phase 2 (ICH terminology: therapeutic exploratory)

The initiation of studies in which the primary objective is to explore therapeutic efficacy in patients is considered to be the start of phase 2. Initial therapeutic exploratory studies may use a variety of study designs to try to establish whether there is a dose and dose frequency that could be of therapeutic benefit in a particular therapeutic indication.

As in phase 1, studies in phase 2 are typically conducted in groups of patients who are selected by relatively narrow criteria, leading to a relatively homogeneous population and these individuals are closely monitored. An important goal for this phase is to determine the dose(s) and regimen for the phase 3 confirmatory trials. Early studies in this phase often utilize dose escalation designs (ICH E4) to give an early estimate of dose response, and later studies may confirm the dose–response relationship for the indication in question by using recognized parallel group designs comparing different doses and dose regimens. Confirmatory dose–response studies may be conducted in phase 2 or be part of the phase 3 programme.

Decisions about the doses used in phase 2 are based on the results of the phase 1 studies and doses are usually lower than the highest doses used in phase 1. Additional objectives of phase 2 clinical trials may include evaluation of potential study end points, therapeutic regimens (including concomitant medications), and target populations (e.g. mild vs severe disease) which will help later study design. In phase 2 studies, exploratory analyses of subsets of data and multiple end points is a valid and important approach in these exploratory studies, unlike the more formal approach required in the later confirmatory studies of phase 3.

Phase 3 (ICH terminology: therapeutic confirmatory)

The initiation of studies in which the primary objective is to confirm therapeutic benefit is considered at the start of phase 3. Studies in phase 3 should have a formal hypothesis and they are designed to confirm the preliminary evidence accumulated in the exploratory studies, that is, to confirm that a drug is both effective and has an acceptable safety profile in the intended indication and target patient population. These studies are aimed at providing an adequate basis for a submission for marketing approval. Studies in phase 3 are conducted in a wider patient population than in previous phases and should include a population representative of the intended target population that will use the drug. Study designs are commonly randomized, parallel group, active and/or placebo-controlled comparisons. For drugs intended to be administered for long periods, trials involving extended exposure to the drug (for up to one year in chronic diseases, ICH E1) are ordinarily conducted in phase 3, although they may be started in phase 2. These studies carried out in phase 3 are often known as the 'pivotal' studies and complete the information required to support the proposed product information for use of the drug in the marketing authorization application (MAA).

Phase 4 (ICH terminology: therapeutic use)

Phase 4 begins after the approval of the drug. Therapeutic use studies are designed to investigate the use of the drug beyond the prior demonstration of the safety, efficacy, and dose definition. Phase 4 studies (other than routine surveillance) are all performed after drug approval and related to the approved indication. They are studies that were not considered necessary for approval but are often important for optimizing the drug's use. They may be of any type but should have valid scientific objectives. Commonly conducted studies include additional drug–drug interaction, dose-response or safety studies, and studies designed to support the commercial use under the approved indication; for example, cost-effectiveness, patient acceptability/quality of life, mortality/morbidity studies, epidemiological studies.

Sources of bias

For a trial to make a credible contribution to the clinical development of the drug, the results must not be biased by any outside influence. All clinical trials should be designed to avoid bias so that the results achieved are robust and credible and clearly representative of the drug's effect. Ensuring that the chosen study design avoids various forms of bias and generates data that can answer the scientific questions being asked can be difficult.

One of the causes of bias in the interpretation of a drug's activity is when the people involved in the clinical trial hold preconceived expectations of that activity. The way that this will introduce bias may be reflected in the investigator's **choice of subjects to be treated with the trial product**. For example, concerns about a potential adverse effect may lead the investigator to select a study population that may have a lower risk of experiencing the adverse effect in question. In the case where an investigator is unconvinced of efficacy, the population selected may be those subjects who exhibit a less severe form of the target disease. In the case of a comparative study, an investigator may select which participant will receive which drug, perhaps on grounds similar to those previously cited. Such a selection strategy may yield results that cannot be transferred to a real patient population. This could be particularly dangerous if the basis for selection is not documented.

Another source of bias relates to the **nature of the target indication**. Many diseases are cyclical in nature, having periods of flare-up and remission (e.g. rheumatoid arthritis). Other diseases that are self-limiting will improve even without treatment (e.g. some skin infections or injuries). The result of a trial for a new treatment of these diseases will be biased by the stage of the disease at which the treatment is introduced. This makes it difficult to separate the effect of the test treatment from the natural history of the disease.

The **choice and method of use of clinical measurements** is also a potential source of bias. This is illustrated particularly where the measurement method is subjective (e.g. in the assessment of pain). The individual subject's response to a question about a sensation will be influenced by the way in which the question is asked and by the choice of words available. Both these influences may be affected by the observer's and the subject's preconceived idea of the trial or treatment, and may be further compounded by existing relationships between the interviewer and the subject. A willingness to please can bias the result towards efficacy, or some other concern may lead to a more negative response.

The most frequently used design mechanisms for eliminating bias are:
• definition of the study population (including the disease severity) to avoid bias in selection of the subjects
• use of a comparator treatment (control) with randomization to avoid bias in treatment allocation, and
• blinding to avoid bias in the study assessments.

Ways of eliminating bias
Definition of the study population
Eligible study subjects are defined by the inclusion and exclusion criteria. These criteria specify the demographics of the desired population, disease

and medical history requirements, and any treatments or medical conditions that the subject cannot have in order to be eligible for inclusion in the study. The inclusion criteria often include a baseline assessment of the disease using the evaluation criterion to be used in the study; for example, in a hypertension study a certain diastolic blood pressure measured in the same way as described in the protocol (which is usually a more accurate method than used in daily practice), or in a pain study, a baseline severity assessed using the relevant pain rating scale could be specified. For a cyclical disease, the phase could be specified to ensure subjects are at the same disease stage when they start treatment (e.g. the criteria for flare-up of the disease could be specified because that is when treatment would usually be initiated in clinical practice).

The subject population must be defined in all clinical studies but additional sources of bias must be eliminated in studies that compare more than one treatment. In these cases it is important that the different treatments are allocated to groups of subjects which are similar and also that the assessment methods are standardized and not subject to bias so the comparison is fair. This is ensured by two techniques: randomization to ensure fair allocation of treatment, and blinding to ensure that the assessment is fair.

Randomization

Despite the definition of subject characteristics there will still be variability. For example, ages may range from 18–65 years, both men and women may be included, and more than one grade of severity may be allowed. This will provide an opportunity for the introduction of bias because an investigator may consider that only subjects with milder disease should receive the new drug and allocate the new drug accordingly so that those with greater disease severities would be on the control drug, especially if this was an established treatment. This would mean that the different treatment groups may not be comparable; the group on the new drug would have more subjects with mild disease and any difference in efficacy or safety may be due to this rather than the drug. Another important example of randomized controlled trials (RCTs) includes behavioural interventions in general practice (e.g. the effect of a multi-component intervention to increase physical activity vs only brief verbal advice). In this case, an investigator may consider that those with higher levels of education would be more likely to change their behavior in response to the multi-component intervention and allocate this intervention to more educated subjects, which would in turn limit the comparability of the groups being compared. To overcome this, subjects are allocated to treatment using a method called randomization. In a randomized trial, successive subjects are assigned to a treatment in a predetermined but random manner.

The most common practice when randomizing subjects is to assign equal numbers to each treatment group which is called simple randomization. However, there are situations where unequal randomization may be appropriate. By allocating more of the subjects to a new treatment, more experience of its effects can be gained, particularly if the comparator is a well-known standard. Since fewer subjects are needed for a placebo/active comparison than for an active/active comparison, unequal randomization so that fewer subjects receive placebo could limit the ethical objections arising from subjects getting 'no treatment'.

In cases where there are differences in the nature of the disease (e.g. relating to severity or anatomical site), there may be different responses to treatment. Randomization should ensure that each treatment group contains similar number subjects with the same extent of variability. However, if it is known that a markedly different response is expected because of a prognostic factor in the disease (e.g. subjects with stage 1 or 2 tumours are likely to respond better than those with larger stage 3 or 4 tumours), a method called stratification (sometimes known as stratified randomization) can be employed.

Separate randomization lists are prepared for each of the different prognostic factors (covariates) or strata, and patients will be assigned to a stratum and then randomized to treatment. This ensures that there will be an equal number of subjects receiving each of the treatments within each of the disease categories and the comparison of the treatments will be fair. Examples of the use of stratification might be to separate subjects with mild or severe pain in an analgesic trial, where the response might be different, or to separate subjects with a first or second renal transplant in a study of an immunosuppressant drug because the risk factors for rejection might be different. Analyses can be conducted to compare the different treatments (or other interventions administered to the subjects), but each stratum may then be analysed separately, if deemed appropriate. Advice is required from the medical expert to identify the relevant prognostic factors and then the statistician must ensure that use of stratification is appropriate. Stratification may be particularly important in small trials in which known clinical factors may have a major influence on prognosis, hence affecting treatment outcome, and also in large trials when interim analyses are planned which contain smaller numbers of subjects.

Another method that can be used to produce treatment groups that are well matched for several variables is adaptive randomization or minimization. In adaptive randomization subjects are assigned to treatment in order to minimize the differences between the treatment groups on selected prognostic factors. The method starts with a simple randomization method for the first subjects and then adjusts the chance of allocating a new subject to a particular treatment based on existing imbalances in those prognostic factors. For example, consider if treatments A and B are to be compared with age as a prognostic factor (aged < 20 or ≥ 20 years). If treatment A has more < 20 subjects than ≥ 20, then the allocation scheme is such that the next few subjects aged < 20 years are more likely to be randomized to treatment B. This method is used when there are many prognostic factors to be considered, thus allocation is aimed at balancing the subtotals for each prognostic factor.

With the increasing availability of interactive randomization systems via the telephone or Internet, sophisticated randomization methods may be easily incorporated into clinical trial designs, but statistical advice should always be taken.

Blinding

To avoid the bias from the investigator and subjects having preconceived ideas about the expected treatment efficacy, the majority of clinical trials are carried out in a 'blind' manner so that comparisons are fair. Studies can be conducted single-blind or double-blind (sometimes known as double-masked). In a single-blind study the person responsible for the main assessment of the disease (e.g. the subject if the disease assessment is a symptom such as pain, or the investigator if the disease assessment is a clinical measurement such as blood pressure) does not know which treatment has been administered. In a double-blind study neither the subject nor the assessor knows which treatment has been given.

If the treatments being compared have different formulations or dosing regimens then the double-dummy technique is required to maintain the double-blind design. For example, if a capsule given twice daily is being compared with a tablet given once daily, to maintain the blind each group will receive both capsules twice daily and tablets once daily but some will be inactive dummies as follows:

- capsule treatment group:
  - active capsule twice daily
  - dummy (placebo) tablet once daily
- tablet treatment group:
  - dummy (placebo) capsule twice daily
  - active tablet once daily.

A double-blind study design is generally recommended to eliminate possible bias in assessment and is preferred especially by the regulatory agencies. However, there may be decision points for which the investigator in clinical practice would need to know the identity of all drugs administered (e.g. in cases of serious adverse events). Contingency must be built in to accommodate this, either by disclosing the treatment by means of code breaks (e.g. code-break envelopes or online), or by providing some type of decision tree. An example of such a contingency in the event of failure might be the use of a specified rescue medication that is known not to interact with either of the blinded treatments, to avoid breaking the blind.

Maintenance of the blind nature of the study is vital to preserving the impartiality of the investigator and consideration must be given regarding how the blind will be maintained, especially if there are differences in the presentation or effects of the various treatments that are apparent to others. It is conceivable that representatives of the sponsor may unwittingly influence the investigator if they become aware of the treatment allocations. This may become apparent to the investigator because of a particular focus at monitoring visits. It is therefore appropriate that monitoring staff should not become aware of treatment allocation, and it may be necessary to consider the use of an independent committee to monitor safety reports. In some disease areas (e.g. oncology studies) blinding of the investigator can be impossible because of the variable regimens, different routes of administration, and range of toxicities involved. However, if a laboratory test or other test (e.g. radiography, ultrasound, etc.) is the primary end point, assessment blinding can be accomplished by blinding the staff who make that assessment and thus blinding the investigator may be good practice but not critical.

Elements of trial design

The design of any given clinical trial will be dependent on many contributing factors. The fundamental factor in the design is clearly the target indication, the influence that this will have on the objectives of the trial, the options for clinical measurement, and the circumstances in which the trial is to be carried out. Bearing in mind that the individual trial is part of a larger clinical development plan, some of the influencing factors such as target population, primary end points, etc., may already be defined, and there may be standards set by the programme plan that must be included in the design. These must be considered, where appropriate.

Although this chapter is too short to provide an account of all possible clinical trial designs, Box 14.1 summarizes those elements of trial design that need to be considered in some detail. It is important to obtain input from all available sources, and in particular, to be aware that not all designs are appropriate to all situations. A particular therapeutic area or study phase of development may have specific trial designs that have become standards of practice.

Box 14.1 Summary of elements to be considered in clinical trial design

- Types of trial design
  - Non comparative (open, open-label)
  - Comparative—between subjects (e.g. parallel group) or within subject (e.g. cross-over)
- Patient population
  - Indication being treated
  - Concurrent diseases
  - Concomitant medication
- Types of control for comparative studies
  - Active control
  - Placebo control/no treatment
- Sources of bias
- Randomization
- Levels of blinding
- Duration of dosing
- Methods of clinical measurement

Type of control

To enable a robust conclusion to be drawn from the results of a scientific study, there must be a control group. The purpose of the control group is to allow discrimination of patient outcomes (e.g. changes in symptoms, signs, or other morbidity) caused by the test treatment from outcomes caused by other factors such as natural disease progression. The control may be an untreated group, a group receiving an active treatment (which could be standard care or another dose of the same drug), a placebo group (or vehicle in the case of topical treatments), or comparison can be with a group external to the study.

Most of these control treatments are used as concurrent controls in the same clinical study. However, external control compares a group of subjects receiving test treatment with a group external to the study. This can be concurrent (e.g. in a different geographical location or social or political environment) or treated at an earlier time (historical control). Historical controls are employed in retrospective studies, which utilize data from medical history, either from the literature or from records of the same institution or from a previous but similar trial. These studies are mostly used in phase 4 and a good example is the case-control study. In this type of study groups of cases (or individual cases) with the disease and controls with similar demographics and history but without the disease are chosen and the comparison is conducted between the case subjects and control subjects. As an example, the link between lung cancer and smoking was discovered using case-control studies.

Most studies are carried out prospectively. In a prospective study, the control group is studied as part of the trial in question; all subjects are entered into the study over the same time interval and experience the same conditions of treatment with either study drug or control treatment. The comparator group therefore 'controls' sources of variability due to the situation so that any differences between the groups can be attributed with confidence to the difference between the treatments.

Factors affecting the choice of control group

When there is no established (standard) treatment for a disease, the Food and Drug Administration (FDA) states that a placebo control is often the design of choice. Indeed, a placebo-controlled clinical trial is generally considered to be the most scientifically valid study to evaluate efficacy and safety. Although placebo is a frequently used control, it is increasingly commonplace to compare an experimental intervention to an existing established effective treatment. Indeed, some regulatory agencies (e.g. in Europe) require comparison versus an active treatment that is already marketed. These types of studies are called active control (or positive control) studies and they are designed to answer one or more of the following:

- Whether the new drug will be superior to the active control
- Whether the new drug will be equivalent to (i.e. no better and no worse than) the active control
- Whether the new drug is non-inferior to (i.e. at least as good as) the active control.

ICH efficacy guideline E10 'Choice of Control Group and Related Issues' provides guidelines for choosing controls. Although trials using any of the control groups described and discussed in the guideline may be useful and acceptable in clinical trials that are the basis for marketing approval in at least some circumstances, they are not equally appropriate or useful in every case. The general approach to selecting the type of control is outlined in ICH E10 which has a very useful system for choosing the type of control in various situations (Box 14.2), and Figure 14.1 provides a decision tree for choosing among different types of control groups.

Although Box 14.2 and Figure 14.1 focus on the choice of control to demonstrate efficacy, some designs also allow other comparisons of test and

---

Box 14.2 Usefulness of specific concurrent control types in various situations

- Placebo control
  - Measures 'absolute' effect size
  - Shows existence of effect
- Active control (testing for superiority)
  - Shows existence of effect
  - Compares treatments
- Active control (testing for non-inferiority)
  - Shows existence of effect
  - Compares treatments (possible only if disease is still sensitive to the active control; if in doubt then include placebo to confirm both are superior to placebo and have an effect)
- Both active and placebo control (testing for superiority vs placebo and non-inferiority or superiority vs active)
  - Show existence of effect
  - Measure 'absolute' effect size (vs placebo)
  - Compare treatments
- Different doses
  - Show existence of effect
  - Show dose–response relationship
- Different doses and placebo
  - Show existence of effect
  - Measure 'absolute' effect size (vs placebo)
  - Show dose–response relationship
- Different doses and active
  - Show dose–response relationship
  - Show existence of effect
  - Compare treatments (possible only if disease is still sensitive to the active control; if in doubt then include placebo to confirm both are superior to placebo and have an effect)
- Different doses and active and placebo
  - Show existence of effect
  - Measure 'absolute' effect size (vs placebo)
  - Show dose–response relationship
  - Compare treatments

Data from Table 1, ICH E10

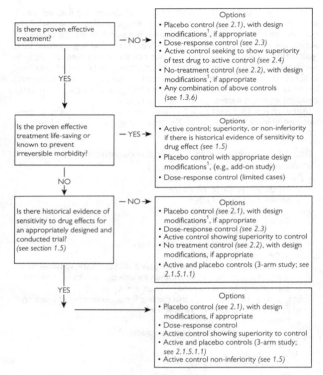

Figure 14.1 Choosing the concurrent control for demonstrating efficacy. (The references in brackets refer to the relevant sections in the ICH E10 guideline.)

Reproduced from ICH-10, Choice of Control Group and Related Issues in Clinical Trials (E10), 20 July 2000) with permission from ICH (http://www.ich.org/products/guidelines/efficacy/article/efficacy-guidelines.html).

control agents. The choice of comparator can be affected by the availability of therapies and by medical practices in specific regions.

In placebo-controlled studies, comparison against a non-pharmacologically active compound will undoubtedly provide data to show whether the new drug has an effect. However, the use of placebo is fraught with ethical issues and practical trial-management issues, the comparative importance of which will depend on the disease being treated and the treatments currently available. Placebo control would be unethical if it would pose undue risk to the patient's health or well-being. For example, in serious or life-threatening diseases (e.g. cancer, heart failure, etc.) the patient must be assured of receiving effective treatment so the only way a comparison with placebo can be conducted is if the new drug or placebo is added to normal standard care. Similar considerations are relevant to no-treatment control. The difference between placebo-control and no-treatment control studies is that the placebo-controlled studies can be double-blinded whereas no-treatment controls can only be single blind. No-treatment control is therefore only used when it is difficult or impossible to double-blind (e.g. for treatments with easily recognized toxicity, or when comparing non-invasive treatment such as radiography with an invasive procedure such as surgery). However, blinding of the assessor may be possible in cases where the study outcome measure is unlikely to be influenced by observation (e.g. a laboratory parameter, radiograph, scan, etc.).

In active-controlled trials, both the objective of the study and the strategy of statistical testing should be considered when selecting the control groups. If the objective is to determine whether the new drug is superior to the active control, then only the active control is required. If the objective is to evaluate whether the new drug is equivalent to the active control, again, only an active control is required because the effect of the new drug must be within the predefined equivalence limits (i.e. above the lower equivalence limit and below the upper equivalence limit).

However, in some therapeutic areas due to the presence of many really effective active treatments (e.g. antibiotics in chest infections), it is difficult to show superiority of a new drug to a clinically relevant extent. In these situations the strategy used would be to show that the new drug is at least as effective as the active control but that it may have an advantage of a better safety profile or more acceptable to patients. Thus, in these situations whether the new drug is only at least as effective as the active control (i.e. non-inferior to the active control) is evaluated. The active control must be chosen carefully because it must have a proven established effect on the disease being studied and must be proven to also be still currently active against the disease in order for the results to be valid. An active control that no longer has an effect on the disease (e.g. in an antibiotic study, choosing an old antibiotic to which resistance has developed over the years) is not acceptable. Indeed, in non-inferiority studies ICH 10 and the current regulatory guidelines recommend that a placebo arm is included to confirm that the active control chosen has an effect on the disease (i.e. is superior to placebo), and then any comparisons of whether the new drug is as effective as the active control are valid.

Another situation where the addition of a placebo control arm is useful is where the natural history of the disease varies with time and from patient to patient (e.g. depression), and it is difficult to prove that an active treatment has had an effect. So studies of antidepressants usually include both an active control arm and a placebo control arm. In both these situations where a placebo control arm is added for validation of the results it is important to limit the numbers of patients assigned to placebo for ethical reasons. Unequal randomization is often used with fewer patients randomized to placebo because the differences in response between active and placebo is expected to be greater than differences between the active treatments.

Different doses of the same treatment can also be considered to be active control treatments. In addition to the considerations previously stated there are other practical considerations when choosing the control treatment. The following are some of the points to consider.

Objective of the study

In simple terms, the objective of most studies is to investigate the efficacy and safety of a test treatment. In order to maintain clarity of design it is paramount that every study has one primary objective that is stated in the protocol. In cases where efficacy has not yet been established it may be that a placebo is the most appropriate control in early phase studies. Assuming that the compound has been shown to possess efficacy, the objectives of later phase studies (phase 3 onwards) will be to compare the extent of efficacy and safety with that of currently used therapies. These studies will be used as a major component of the regulatory submission and therefore input from regulatory colleagues is most important. They will be able to provide information as to what is accepted as the best current treatment against which all new treatments must be compared, as well as the latest regulatory guidelines and thinking on clinical trial design in a particular thera-peutic area. Further sources of valuable input are marketing colleagues who can provide information as to the most widely prescribed current treat-ment. It will be valuable for future marketing to have a comparison against such treatment(s).

Countries where the study is to be conducted

This is an area where thorough research is needed, particularly in multicen-tre, multinational, or global studies. The vagaries of the regulatory process may mean that a drug that has been suggested as a potential comparator may not be approved for sale or, if approved, may not be marketed in countries scheduled for participation in the clinical trial. In these cases there may be regulatory obstacles to running the study in that country. A further source of variation between countries can be found in the different formu-lations and dosing instructions that are registered in different countries. This may be particularly true for older drugs that have many generic forms or older non-standardized marketing licences. Differences in clinical practice are more difficult to tackle than these regulatory issues. For example, the standard treatment in one country may not be considered efficacious or safe in another, and therefore it is disqualified from use as a standard com-parator. The suitability of a placebo control may also be an ethical issue in some countries and must be clearly addressed in the earliest stages of study preparation.

Registration status of the potential comparator

For the reasons stated previously, when discussing the objective of the study, regulatory and marketing considerations suggest that it is most productive to choose an active comparator that is established and marketed. To use an unlicensed comparator as well as the new drug in a study increases the complexity of study set-up for two reasons. From the regulatory point of view, full information about both drugs would have to be submitted to the licensing authority in an IMPD (investigational medicinal product dossier), and it would be highly unlikely that a competitor company would make their pre-clinical information available to another company. From the practical point of view, it would be very difficult to obtain supplies for use in a comparative study from the manufacturer of a future potential competitor.

The status of the drug in terms of exclusivity

While a patent is still current for any drug, it is likely that the drug will be available only from the original manufacturer or its licensees. Since the ideal study design may be considered to be double-blind and marketed formulations are often identifiable, perhaps by unique markings on a tablet, it is difficult to ensure a double-blind supply of medication. Sometimes a simple encapsulation of a tablet may be possible, but any manipulation (e.g. grinding a tablet to fill a capsule) will mean not only extra work for the clinical trial supplies department but also, as a minimum, dissolution studies to ensure that this manipulation has not affected the characteristics of the formulation such as bioavailability. Blinding might necessitate the use of a double-dummy design. Placebos matching the active treatment must be obtained and this will undoubtedly be from the patent holder, will take time, and sometimes mean revealing your protocol to the other company. When a patent is no longer current, generic forms will be available and the manufacturers will frequently supply their active formulation with matching placebos, perhaps more quickly than if the patent is still in place.

Dosing regimens of the potential comparator

It has already been stated that for a study to have value for both registration and marketing, the study drug should be compared with a known and established active treatment. The active comparator should be used in the way in which it is known to be effective. Therefore, it is not advisable to use a dosing regimen different from that registered or in common use. To do so would create specific problems that would need to be taken into account in the trial design. Examples of such problems might be that the comparator has a once-daily dosing regimen while the new drug has a twice-daily regimen; alternatively, one of the two may be formulated to be long-acting or slow-release. Differences in dosing frequency may reflect a difference in the pharmacokinetic properties of the two drugs. A further, more complex situation related to pharmacokinetics might arise if one of the drugs has a very long or a very short half-life; this may affect how a subject is withdrawn from the drug, a factor that is of particular significance in a cross-over trial where a wash-out period is required between treatments.

Populations

The patient population from which the study participants will be drawn must be carefully defined to avoid the bias that derives from a non-defined, perhaps investigator-specific, selection strategy. In early phase 2, the entry criteria for a study may be very restrictive, and throughout the development programme these criteria will be adjusted to be more inclusive to reflect the intended target population as the drug's characteristics are discovered. For example, phase 1 trials may have studied healthy subjects, probably with a restricted age range, usually between 18 and 45 years. As further studies are completed in older (and possibly in younger) subjects, the patient population may be extended to include these age groups. In phase 3, the studies should include a population that is representative of the wider patient population who will potentially receive the drug when approved so that the results can be generalized to the intended target population.

Within one study the protocol should clearly define which subjects are eligible for entry, so that the differences between groups may be reliably ascribed to treatment differences, and not to variability between subjects.

The following are some of the points to consider when preparing the inclusion and exclusion criteria:

• Indication being treated (nature and history of the disease)
• Concurrent diseases
• Concomitant medication

In the effort to achieve uniformity in the population of study participants there is a risk of limiting the selection criteria to such an extent that the trial may not be feasible. Therefore, it is helpful to consult with some investigators, usually using a feasibility questionnaire, before finalizing the protocol.

Indication being studied

Certain elements that are considered when designing a trial will be influenced by the natural history of the disease being treated. For example, the onset and progression of the disease will affect the duration of the trial, the timing of each subject's treatment, and the number and timing of assessments.

A neat classification of disease might be between acute and chronic, each having implications for trial design. Acute indications (e.g. infections or musculoskeletal injuries) will require a short treatment period, and during that period it is expected that a cure (or at least an improvement) would be observed. These types of disease also display spontaneous remission within a certain time after onset. Additionally, the signs and symptoms are not constant, and indeed may initially increase in severity. Therefore, the known profile of the disease may dictate that the study treatment period is one week, that subjects should enter the study within one day of onset, and that assessments be carried out daily for the first four days, to detect any signs of efficacy in the early stages. In comparison, the signs and symptoms of some chronic diseases will be stable over long periods of time. This may dictate, for example, a study of six-months' duration, with monthly assessments carried out for efficacy although more frequent assessments at the start of the treatment period may be necessary in early phase studies to monitor safety.

This rather simplistic approach to chronic disease may be confounded when study participants are already receiving treatment that may necessitate a wash-out period. Any withdrawal of previous therapy must be carefully considered so as not to destabilize the subject without clinical justification. If a wash-out period is used, the trial design should incorporate repeat assessments of the variable under study (e.g. blood pressure) to provide a stable baseline against which to assess efficacy.

The nature of the disease may, however, dictate that withdrawal of any current therapy is not clinically justifiable. There are several ways to continue clinical development despite this hurdle. The first is to use only subjects who are newly diagnosed with the condition. This will mean that the number of subjects available for the study may be small compared with the total population suffering from that disease. One implication is that a longer trial period may be needed to find treatment-naïve subjects and the response in this population may be different from those who have previously received treatment which may be the intended target population. Thus, another study in these subjects will be needed. Alternatively, the need to withdraw treatment can be avoided by designing a trial where the test treatment is added to the current treatment. This implies that current therapy is inadequate and that there is still measurable improvement to be gained, either in terms of efficacy or safety. This type of add-on trial may be used (e.g. in epilepsy). There is a need for adequate knowledge about the potential for interaction between treatments. In this situation, a placebo may be the most appropriate comparator. Following a trial that proves efficacy and safety of the combination treatment, it may be appropriate to design trials that investigate the potential for decreasing the dose of the standard medication, while still maintaining efficacy. This is a particularly appealing approach when the standard therapy has an adverse event profile that is clinically undesirable. This type of trial is frequently referred to as a 'sparing' trial, and examples appear in the use of systemic corticosteroids, anti-rejection treatments, and narcotic analgesics.

Some diseases may be cyclical in nature, exhibiting periods of exacerbation and remission; one example in this category is rheumatoid arthritis. The anticipated length of the cycle between the two extremes of disease will influence the time at which subjects can be entered into the study in order to ensure a standardized baseline population. It will also influence the treatment period within the study because the remission of the disease itself may inflate the apparent treatment effect.

Some diseases are seasonal; obvious examples are allergic rhinitis and influenza. To complete a study within one season will require careful planning, with particular consideration given to sample size and the necessity for many centres. A back-up plan to roll over to the other hemisphere could be considered.

Variability is inherent within any population or subpopulation. In a study of an antihypertensive therapy, simply enrolling any subject with elevated blood pressure will introduce a wide range of variability into the trial. This may have consequences for the response that is being measured, as this will also be variable. Expressed in terms of the actual blood pressure, subjects with severe hypertension could display improvement of a greater magnitude than those with mild hypertension. Therefore, the disease severity should be specified. In particular, terms such as mild, moderate, or severe must be clearly and objectively defined. Using the example of hypertension, this may be expressed in terms of a diastolic blood pressure between X mmHg and Y mmHg. Continuing with this example, caution must be exercised to ensure that information is gathered for all three grades of severity to avoid unnecessarily limiting the final licence of the drug to one of these categories only. This can be done in one study by stratifying for severity (mild, moderate, severe substrata), or separate studies for each severity may be appropriate. A large variability in disease severity will necessitate a greater sample size. Other sources of variability due to disease may derive from the time since disease onset or diagnosis, and response to previous treatment.

Concurrent diseases

It is unlikely that the patient population suffering from the target disease will present with no concurrent diseases. This will undoubtedly affect the interpretation of trial results and therefore must be considered in the criteria for selecting study participants. In the early phases the decision to include or exclude subjects with specific diseases will be based on pre-clinical pharmacology; the knowledge base can then be extended in the light of the results of phase 1 and 2 trials.

Concurrent diseases may influence the efficacy and safety of the drug through, for example, metabolic interaction, but the necessity for medication to treat a concurrent disease may confound the interpretation of the result. Hence concurrent diseases and concomitant medication need to be considered together.

Concomitant medication

While concurrent diseases may be easy to control by excluding certain subjects, the use of concomitant medication is difficult to standardize. Different formulations and different dosage regimens will be used and often entirely different treatments. To address this issue, it must be clear what influence any concomitant medication will have on the primary assessment in the study and subjects taking such medications should be excluded. In multicentre, multi-country studies it may be impossible to change a treatment protocol that is well established and a valuable way to resolve clinical differences is to arrange a meeting of the investigators to discuss ways to compromise, where necessary.

Patient populations in multi-country trials

Differences in clinical practice may emerge when discussing the population of study participants in multi-country studies. There may be differing opinions as to what defines a particular disease, and also what severity of disease demands which type of treatment. Clarity in defining the study population is most important. This may require prolonged discussion in order to identify sufficient numbers of subjects according to a common definition.

Types of trial design

There are many different designs for clinical studies and the choice of an appropriate design depends on why the trial is being conducted (e.g. for a submission dossier or for market support), the phase of the study, and the study end point (subjective or objective).

There are two main types of study design, comparative or non-comparative (sometimes known as non-controlled or open-label as blinding is not required). Comparative designs are used when comparing treatments.

Non-comparative study designs

Non-comparative designs are used when safety, PK, and tolerability data are required (e.g. in phase 1 studies). Some phase 3 studies are also non-comparative; for example, in chronic diseases such as rheumatoid arthritis where the treatment will be used continuously or intermittently for a number of years and safety data are required for the regulatory filing. ICH E1 recommends that data should be available for at least 100 subjects treated for one year.

Non-comparative design is often employed for pilot studies. Pilot studies may be used to give justification for developing larger RCT studies at a reduced cost as they are simple to conduct, there is no development cost of a placebo or blinding procedures, and unlike RCT there is no need to enrol large numbers of subjects.

Other examples of non-comparative studies are case studies of single cases or a series of cases. A case study is a brief description of a single case that an observer feels should be brought to the attention of colleagues, such as an unusual episode of poisoning or an atypical rash developing after administration of a new drug. Case series are several case reports of similar observations or procedures that may be grouped together, usually in consecutive patients. Case series may be an important way to establish a new surgical procedure. The advantage of this type of study is that they are simple to perform and can be written up and published rapidly. The disadvantage is that there is limited insight about the disease or treatment efficacy and retrospective case series may contain incomplete data.

Comparative study designs

Comparative study designs are either 'between subject comparisons', when the response is compared between groups of subjects treated with the different treatments, and 'within subject comparison', which compares the response to the different treatments administered to the same subject. The most commonly used 'between-subject' comparative design is the 'parallel group' design, and the most commonly used 'within-subject' design is the so-called cross-over design.

Parallel group and cross-over designs

In a parallel design each subject receives only one of the treatments for a predetermined time and the response between the different groups of subjects are compared (Figure 14.2). Parallel group designs are usually the design of choice for most therapeutic exploratory and therapeutic

Parallel Group (between patient comparison)

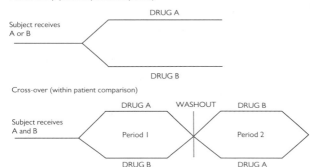

Figure 14.2 Schematic diagram of parallel group and cross-over designs.

confirmatory (phase 2 and 3) studies intended for regulatory submissions, where an objective scientific assessment of the relative efficacy and safety of two or more treatments is required. Subjects enter the trial and are randomized to one of the treatments to be compared, and the between treatment group responses are analysed. These trials are often conducted blind, especially where the primary end point is a subjective one. If there are two treatments to be compared then this is referred to as a two-arm parallel group study, three treatments will mean three-arms, etc.

In a parallel group study each subject is assigned to receive one or other of the treatments, and the subjects are studied 'in parallel'. The advantage of this design is that bias can be kept to a minimum (e.g. no sequence effects), but the disadvantage is that variability between patients and therefore the treatment groups can affect the results. This between patient variability can be accounted for by using an accurate standard deviation (SD) in the sample size calculation which usually minimizes this disadvantage by ensuring sufficient subjects are included.

In a cross-over design each subject receives one treatment then crosses over to receive the other treatment. The response within each subject is then compared (Figure 14.2). The advantage of a cross-over study is that each subject receives all treatments to be compared, and the variation of the measurement is within each subject which will be less than in a parallel group study, where the variation of measurement is between groups of subjects. The disadvantage of the cross-over study is that it can only be used for efficacy trials if the disease is such that an adequate wash-out period can be included to avoid a different baseline when the second treatment is given (the effect of the first treatment could be carried over). Therefore the disease must be stable and the wash-out period long enough to ensure no carry over effect. This sort of design is not used in diseases where there is marked disease progression, or in studies in diseases where it would not be ethical to withhold treatment, or if the safety of the subject would be at risk during wash-out, or the wash-out period would be too long to be practical (e.g. acute studies on antibiotics).

Cross-over studies are often used in episodic conditions such as migraine where the subject's disease status returns to baseline after each episode.

Cross-over designs are used in phase 1 studies to evaluate the effect of food or drug interactions and in later phase studies destined for marketing use, where the aim of the study is to assess subject acceptability of the treatments being compared. As every subject receives every treatment, acceptability of use by the subject can be compared.

The choice of one of these two designs over the other demands careful consideration. Selection of the cross-over design may be appealing because fewer subjects are required because each subject acts as his/her own control. In the context of clinical treatment this may be helpful in identifying which treatment is best for that particular subject. However, the application of that result to the general population cannot be extrapolated from the results of that particular subject.

One practical issue to consider is subject (and perhaps investigator) compliance with the protocol. A typical cross-over study may have two treatment periods of four weeks each, with one wash-out week at the beginning and one in the middle (a total of ten weeks). For a comparable parallel study, each subject will be in the trial for five weeks (one wash-out week plus four treatment weeks). The cross-over study will clearly necessitate more subject visits, invariably more than they would make in the normal course of treatment. This increases the probability of subjects not entering the study due to the additional commitment or of them dropping out between treatment courses which make any within-subject comparison impossible.

The choice of a comparator for a cross-over study must be made carefully. For example, the safety profile is an important factor. A cross-over comparison between drugs with different adverse event profiles, such as a beta-blocker (bradycardia) and a calcium channel blocker (tachycardia), may cause a double-blind study to become unblinded, leading to the potential for bias.

Careful consideration of such issues will ensure that the cross-over design is used in an appropriate way. Statistical advice is of paramount importance at the design phase, and the final analysis must investigate the possibility that differences observed between treatments may be due to 'period effects' rather than to genuine treatment differences.

Alternative between-group comparative designs

Sequential design

Ethics are a prime consideration in the design of clinical trials. It is a basic principle that no subject should be harmed by receiving a drug that is known to be inferior. Hence, it may be considered appropriate in some instances to review the incoming data to avoid prolonging a trial where efficacy may have already been established beyond doubt.

The sequential design is a type of parallel group design that uses repeated analyses conducted at predefined time points to evaluate between-treatment differences while a trial is ongoing. The advantage of this design is that the total trial length may be reduced, as fewer subjects would be needed. This type of trial is useful for rare diseases, particularly where a rapid response to treatment is likely to be shown by each subject. Certain practical problems are posed when planning a sequential trial if the interim analysis is conducted after completion of each subject so a group sequential design, where analysis is carried out after completion of blocks of subjects, may be easier to conduct. The analyses must be carried out at predetermined intervals usually based on patient numbers until a difference is shown between treatments or it becomes clear that there is no difference. This design is ethically sound as the number of patients is reduced and the length of time in a trial is reduced. There are practical complications to be overcome such as getting the data back and cleaned for multiple database locks so that each interim analysis can be conducted, and this leads to time delay for the study and interruption of recruitment. There are also major statistical complications to be overcome if interim analyses with significance testing are required in a trial. The use of repeated significance tests increases the chance of multiplicity, that is, detecting a treatment difference at the conventionally accepted level of 5%, and the possibility of reporting a false-positive error is increased. As a consequence, a method for correcting for multiplicity using a significance level that is more stringent than $p < 0.05$ must be chosen. This will influence the sample size in the study, and statistical input is vital in this context. Most importantly, interim analyses should always be planned from the outset, blinding of the study staff must be ensured and stopping rules should be developed at that time.

Factorial design

Sometimes in a trial a comparison of a number of treatments is required. To complete multiple comparisons would require complex multiple-arm parallel group designs or could result in the possibility of having to conduct several separate studies to evaluate each treatment. The factorial design allows evaluation of several treatments within the same trial by using various combinations of the treatments.

For example in a balanced 2×2 factorial design of 12 patients, 6 receive drug A, 6 are randomized to receive no A and correspondingly 6 receive B, or 6 do not receive B. Thus overall, 3 receive no intervention, 3 receive intervention A only, 3 receive intervention B only, and 3 receive A + B simultaneously. Thus, of the 12 subjects, 9 receive some form of treatment and only 3 receive no treatment.

The main advantage of a factorial design is cost saving. A comparison of multiple treatments in a single study instead of separate studies is an advantage and fewer subjects are required than in multiple-arm parallel trials. Factorial designs can study whether combinations of treatments are effective and can identify the best dose of two treatments used together as well as evaluating any interactions. Factorial designs are often used in oncology studies to find the best combination of treatments. For example, for treatments A, B, C, and placebo, there are eight possible combinations:

A+B+C	A alone
A+B	B alone
A+C	C alone
B+C	neither A, B, or C

Alternative within-subject comparative designs

Left/right comparison

In some disease areas where the disease presentation is symmetrical, a left/right comparison of topical treatments can be used. Examples would be comparison of two topical treatments for psoriasis, or two eye drops for glaucoma or allergic conjunctivitis. The disadvantage of this design is that if a systemic adverse event is reported then it cannot be ascribed to the specific treatment. Thus it is important to establish that there is no systemic absorption of active compound prior to using this design.

A further variation on this type of design is the matched-pair design where pairs of subjects are treated with the alternative treatments. The pairs will be matched for the age, sex, and those prognostic factors appropriate to the indication.

The considerations thus far have dealt with the RCT but there are other trial designs that need to be considered.

Outcomes research

Traditionally, the focus of clinical research has been on the end points employed to define success or failure of a treatment or intervention (i.e. does a treatment work in ideal conditions). Nowadays, outcomes of a new drug or intervention are considered more broadly looking at changes in patient quality of life but also on the health service in terms of numbers of inpatient days in hospital.

Outcomes research, which encompasses clinical, economic, and social outcomes of treatment, is therefore becoming increasingly important to ensure that a drug once approved by the regulatory authorities can be marketed and reimbursed in different countries. Thus, frequently outcomes research measures are added into later phase (3 and 4) trials. Examples include quality of life (QoL) assessments and other pharmaco-economic measures such as 'willingness to pay' questionnaires. There are advantages to including extra measurements in a study, but it is unwise to attempt to achieve too much with a single trial. Extra measurements are often time-consuming, and the clinical setting of the original trial may not be appropriate for gathering this additional information.

The assessment of QoL is becoming common in clinical studies and may be used to identify benefits of one treatment over another when their effect on the disease is equal. These studies measure the physical, emotional, and social aspects of an illness and its treatment. A treatment which improves clinical status but reduces QoL may not be a positive outcome, but a treatment which has little effect on illness severity but improved QoL may be useful to patients with certain diseases. An example of this is the comparison of a beta-blocker and an angiotensin-converting enzyme (ACE) inhibitor in the treatment of hypertension. The two drug classes generally do not differ in any clinically significant extent in terms of lowering blood pressure, but subjects receiving the ACE inhibitor feel better. Assessment scales have been developed to assess what 'feeling better' means, in an attempt to quantify apparently subjective end points. In some cases the scale may identify which drug displays the most acceptable adverse effect profile.

As with all measurement methods, the scale (or instrument) chosen must be appropriate for the situation. It should be meaningful for the disease being studied, and should be practical to administer in the given trial situation. There are a number of quality of life scales; some are disease specific, like the Dermatology Quality of Life Index (DQLI) for dermatology studies, and some generic to assess general health, like the SF-36 scale. Quality-of-life scales are often added to pivotal studies to gain additional information that may be useful to the prescriber.

Pharmaco-economic studies

Pharmaco-economic studies allow comparison of health resource implications. They do not focus just on the efficacy of a drug but also on effects of the length of hospital stay, doctor's time, the use of hospital beds, and also on consequences (e.g. avoidance of an event such as heart attack).

There are four main types of study:

- Cost-effectiveness: examines the cost of treating a patient. If two antibiotics are compared, the outcome can be measured in the same way (number of infections resolved by the antibiotics) and the costs expressed as cost per unit outcome (i.e. cost per infection resolved).
- Cost minimization: a form of cost-effectiveness analysis where benefits have been proven (or assumed) to be equal so the cheapest treatment is chosen. If a branded drug is compared with a generic drug, the decision is made on least cost (i.e. the generic drug).
- Cost–benefit: compares the costs of treatments with the effects measured in money. This allows comparison across all treatments because effects are measured in the same units and can reveal whether a treatment is worthwhile (i.e. whether benefits outweigh costs). The outcome is the saving made comparing different treatments (i.e. cost consequence).
- Cost utility: a comparative analysis of alternative courses of action; it focuses particular attention on the quality of the health outcome. A quality-adjusted life year (QALY) is a unit of output that combines both quality and quantity of life (QoL). These studies measure the value derived by the patient from the treatment by comparing the cost per QALY of each treatment. This economic evaluation is useful when a health authority has to choose in which patient groups to spend scarce resource or money (e.g. hip replacement or heart transplant).

Dose-escalation and dose–response studies

Single ascending dose studies

The single escalating dose study is commonly used in phase 1 development for first time in human studies to determine the pharmacokinetic profile and safety in human beings. The route of administration should be the intended route to be marketed, and if the route is oral, the pharmacokinetics with and without food need to be investigated. No route of administration that has not been previously tested in animals should be used.

The starting dose in human beings is decided generally based on one or more of the following:

- 1% or 2% of the no observable adverse effect level (NOAEL) dose in animals

- 10–20% of the maximum tolerated dose in the most sensitive species of animal tested
- Examination of animal data to assess the dose which produces the pharmacodynamic action relevant for its proposed therapeutic role in man
- Scrutiny of the effective and safe dose in man of closely related compounds.

Often eight to twelve healthy subjects are used; two to four subjects receive placebo, and six to eight receive the new drug at the starting dose and are then monitored to observe any effects. The effects being monitored are based on the effects observed in animals in the pre-clinical work performed before the first in man studies and it is hoped that the effects observed are consistent. Screening is usually carried out within two to four weeks before drug administration. Meticulous screening is carried out to minimize risk and to facilitate interpretation of results. The drug is then given and blood and urine samples are taken at various time points according to the kinetic properties predicted from pre-clinical work. The next group of subjects should not receive the next dose level until the results of the previous group safety tests are known. The doses in each group may be increased by doubling doses used in the previous stage or by smaller or larger steps depending on response. The increments are stopped by the appearance of toxicity or attainment of the desired activity.

Repeated dose studies

Only when single-dose administration has been investigated can repeated dose studies begin. In this type of study, drug or placebo is given repeatedly for one or more weeks dependent on disease area. Antibiotics, for example, may be tested for a shorter period of five to seven days whereas an anticonvulsant (which is likely to be used for several years) may be tested for four weeks or more.

Doses for the repeat-dose studies are selected based on the results of the single-dose studies. Usually one dose just below the maximum tolerated dose (MTD) and two to three lower doses (e.g. 10%, 30%, and 50% of MTD) are selected. The frequency of the repeated administration is based on the pharmacokinetic profile observed in the single dose studies and is often one half-life. But it is desirable to aim at what can be easily accomplished practically and what will be commercially acceptable.

The effects of repeat dosing on the pharmacokinetic profile and the dose response at the various dose levels are investigated to ascertain the effect of the drug on the disease (pharmacodynamics). A decision is then made as to which dose or doses will be investigated in further development based on the relative effect of each dose level and the associated adverse events. For example, several doses of new drug may have similar efficacy but some doses may be associated with more or severe adverse effects (Figure 14.3). The effects on intraocular pressure (IOP) are plotted for various doses of an anti-glaucoma drug versus the hyperaemia (eye redness) caused by using the drug and the dose of 3 mg is selected for further development.

Once the single-dose and repeat-dose studies have been completed the pharmacokinetics of the test treatment will be known. However, these early pharmacokinetic studies will have been conducted intensively in small

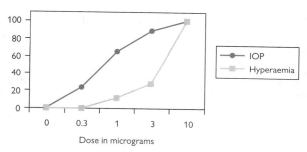

Figure 14.3 Dose response curves for IOP and hyperaemia.
Y-axis represents relative effect (%)

numbers of subjects (often healthy subjects). In parallel with broadening the target population for the safety and efficacy assessments in phases 2 and 3 so that the phase 3 population closely approximates to the target population, there has been a recent development in pharmacokinetics known as population pharmacokinetics.

The aim of population pharmacokinetics is to collect a small number of samples for drug concentration assay from a large number of subjects, in order to identify the extent of variability in the population. This may have implications, for example, in dosing. Basic demographic details of the subjects need to be recorded: age, weight, race, and, depending on the type of drug, metabolic status. The samples, perhaps only two or three, would be collected at target times associated with one dose. The modelling of the pharmacokinetic parameters will take account of variability around the target times, but the accurate times in relation to a dose must be recorded.

The incorporation of such testing into a trial design should ensure that it does not interfere with the primary objective, which is probably an efficacy assessment. Additionally, it must be practically feasible. This type of sampling may be carried out in long-term studies, and if the subjects are outpatients or the trial is carried out in a general practice setting, the availability of adequate time and facilities should be established.

Methods of clinical measurement

The primary assessment method for efficacy must be standardized so that the results from all subjects may be pooled in any regulatory submissions, and therefore the trial design will specify which method will be used and at what time intervals throughout the study. It may appear obvious to state that the measurement method chosen must be relevant, but in ensuring relevance, the following factors should be considered.

The method chosen must have been validated as being accurate and reproducible in the given situation. For a quantitative measurement such as blood pressure, the use of standardized, calibrated equipment (e.g. the sphygmomanometer) is clearly most appropriate. For an assessment of a more subjective parameter (e.g. depression), there may be many rating scales available, or there may be proposals to use a new scale. In such a situation it is advisable to use a scale for which there is documented information about its specificity and reproducibility for depression. Without appropriate assurance of the validity of a new scale in the same population, it could be unwise to use any novel instrument to support claims of efficacy for a new treatment. If it is necessary to develop a new scale then it is advisable to do so in parallel with established scales.

Assessment methods routinely used in clinical practice may not always be appropriate for repeated use in clinical trials. In these situations scales are often developed specifically for trial use. For example, in the assessment of depression, standard clinical rating scales such as the Hamilton Rating Scale for Depression were felt to lack sensitivity in consistently detecting differences between drugs and a new scale (the Montgomery and Asberg scale) was therefore developed and validated for this purpose.

Having confirmed that the method is suitable for assessment of the given parameter, the practical feasibility of the measurement method must be addressed. The time required to carry out the measurement should be determined because clinic visits may be brief. Frequent, repeated inpatient measurements may be very time-consuming; for example, studies of analgesic efficacy following administration of a single dose will require the time of a devoted observer, or a subject in the immediate post-operative period may have difficulty responding. The statistical implications of such repeated measures such as multiplicity should also be considered.

The timing and circumstances of the assessment should be standardized when considering the design of a trial. Even the result of an apparently objective and quantitative measurement such as blood pressure will be influenced by circumstance unless a standard procedure is specified. For example, the subject should have been sitting for 10 minutes before two blood pressure readings are taken, and the mean of the two readings is then recorded. This type of instruction will control many of the biases caused by local circumstances. Additionally, the time of day for the measurement may be standardized to avoid the introduction of additional variability due to diurnal variation. There is a further cause of bias that can be controlled, namely observer bias. In the case of blood pressure, this may be due to number preferences, or 'rounding' when reading the pressure. The use of a device such as a random zero sphygmomanometer is one way to avoid this pitfall. The device introduces a random baseline, which is subtracted from the numbers initially recorded to obtain the true blood pressure.

The choice of measurement method will affect other aspects of the trial design because of the statistical implications. The accuracy of the measurement, reflected by the variability about the mean, will be needed for the calculation of the sample size (see the *Oxford Handbook of Medical Statistics*). Additionally, the statistician will require information about what is considered to be a clinically relevant difference in the primary assessment method. The sample size will then be calculated so that, given the variability, any clinically relevant difference will be detected.

Regulatory authorities such as the European Medicines Agency (EMA), the FDA, and the World Health Organization (WHO), and ICH have published guidelines on preferred and acceptable clinical measurement techniques in many therapeutic areas. Further useful information can be derived from the European Public Assessment Reports (EPARs) if there has been a recent approval of a similar drug in Europe via the centralized procedure. An EPAR reflects the scientific conclusion reached by the Committee for Medicinal Products for Human use (CHMP) at the end of the centralized evaluation process and provides a summary of the grounds for the CHMP opinion in favour of granting a marketing authorization for a specific medicinal product. The EPAR is made available by the EMA for information after deletion of commercially confidential information. In the US there are two ways of getting input to ensure acceptable trial design. A similar report to the EPAR is available as a Summary Basis of Approval (SBA) which details the basis of approval for marketed products. In addition, Special Protocol Assessments (SPAs) provide an expedited evaluation by FDA of certain manufacturing, toxicology and clinical trial protocols to assess whether they are adequate to meet scientific and regulatory requirements. SPAs provide valuable information for sponsors, significantly reducing regulatory uncertainty for submissions in the US.

Reference

1. www.ich.org E10 Guideline 'Choice of control group and Related Issues in Clinical Trials' 2000.

Further reading

International Conference on Harmonisation of Technical Requirements for Registration of Pharmaceuticals for Human Use efficacy guidelines. ℗ www.ich.org

E8 Guideline 'General Considerations in Clinical Trials' 1997.

E4 Guideline 'Dose Response Information to Support Drug Registration' 1994.

E1 Guideline 'The Extent of Population Exposure to Assess Clinical Safety for Drugs Intended for Long-Term Treatment of Non-Life-Threatening Conditions' 1994E10 Guideline 'Choice of Control Group and Related Issues in Clinical Trials' 2000.

℗ www.fda.gov/downloads/Drugs/GuidanceComplianceRegulatoryInformation/Guidances/UCM202140

Clinical trial protocols: study protocol

Definition and purpose of the protocol

The ICH E6 Good Clinical Practice (GCP) guidelines give the definition of the protocol as 'a document that describes the objectives, design, methodology, statistical considerations and organisation of the trial and usually gives the background and rationale for the trial'.

According to these guidelines, the term 'protocol' encompasses any protocol amendments. The protocol usually includes the background and rationale but these sections can be contained in other trial-related documentation such as the investigator's brochure (IB), if this is referenced in the protocol.

In short, the protocol is the reference document which describes why the trial is being done, how to do it, and what to do in any eventuality. The protocol, therefore, is used by many different people involved in the trial and it must contain all the information that is required to conduct the trial. Those using the protocol include all study site staff (investigators, study site coordinators, research nurses, pharmacists and dispensing staff, laboratory staff, and staff from other departments if any special procedures are required, e.g. radiographs, endoscopies, etc.) as well as study monitors, data managers, statisticians, auditors, regulatory inspectors, and ethics committee members. Therefore, the information contained in a protocol must comprehensively cover all aspects of the study.

It should give details to the staff at the study sites such as how the subjects are going to be treated, how the treatments will be assigned, how the treatment will be packaged, and when it will be dispensed, returned, and tracked. Will special storage facilities be required? What biological samples will be required, and who is responsible for the laboratory analyses? What is to be done if an adverse event is encountered, especially if this is in an emergency situation? The protocol must also give information about how the data collected in the study will be analysed; this will be relevant not only to the data managers and statisticians who will be responsible for the data handling and analysis but also to the ethics committees and regulatory authorities from whom permission will be required before the study is started.

The end product of the clinical study is usually a clinical study report which may form part of a submission dossier for approval of the drug. The protocol will be an appendix to the clinical study report (ICH E3), so it is important to keep in mind what the final study report might look like when writing the protocol. Some of the questions that need to be borne in mind when writing a protocol are: what data is essential to collect, what will the data look like? How will the data be analysed and then presented (e.g. in tables and figures)? By thinking about the final report the writer can assess which data are absolutely essential to answer the question posed in the protocol. As a rule of thumb, if the team cannot explain why each data point is being collected and presented, then the importance of collecting that particular data should be questioned.

Writing a protocol

What do you need to know and who should have input?

Writing a protocol is a time-consuming occupation but the time is well spent if a good, sound protocol is the result. Thus, before writing a protocol it is important to do a little research to address the following:

- Why is the protocol needed?
- Where does this study fit into the clinical development for the product?
- What question is the study supposed to answer?
- How will the data be used (e.g. to make a decision about further development, to support a submission for approval of the drug, or support marketing of the drug?)

A good place to start is the clinical development plan (CDP) for the product (ICH E8 and 9) which details all the studies required to develop the product. Writing the CDP for the product is a team effort. The commercial department will usually discuss and define the maximum and minimum prescribing information for a product, and then the clinical and regulatory teams develop a CDP which should map out the trials required. If there is no CDP then these questions will need to be answered by staff from the various departments within the company developing the drug (e.g. the regulatory and marketing departments for studies intended to be included in the submission dossier for drug approval and, for the later post-approval studies, the commercial, reimbursement, or marketing teams).

The protocol writer will also need knowledge of the disease area itself, common treatments for the disease, and methods of assessing the disease in clinical studies. This is available from a number of sources such as medical literature (textbooks and online search), company medical advisors, investigators, pharmacists, etc. If the proposed study is destined for an approval submission and there has been a precedent approval of a similar product, then this sort of information may be available for previously registered products via the Summary Basis for Approval (SBA) for products approved by the US Food and Drug Administration (FDA), or the European Public Assessment Reports (EPARs) published by the European Medical Association (EMA). Posters and symposia at medical congresses and meetings are also a useful source of this sort of information as they often describe the study design, subject population selected and the assessments used and their timings for the reported studies.

If the study is to be multinational or even global then the cultural differences in treating the disease in different countries need to be understood by the protocol writer. A protocol designed to cover a disease area where there are culture differences in treating the disease is always a compromise. Depending on the extent of the cultural differences it may not be possible to design even a compromise protocol so decisions have to be made about the best way forward in these cases. The judgement call as to whether to proceed with a compromise protocol is a difficult one and is not usually made by the protocol writer alone. The situation is discussed with the clinical development team and other involved parties. Frequently, an expert panel or steering committee of investigators/opinion leaders from the countries in which the study will be performed and where it is planned to be registered are consulted for their opinions also.

Conducting multiple separate studies is not ideal in terms of the time and money required to undertake them, but sometimes there is just no alternative. Other challenges present themselves if a single compromise study is undertaken, such as finding investigators who are sufficiently flexible and who can work with and recruit subjects to the compromise protocol, not to mention the task of putting the rationale for the study into context in the submission for approval of the drug.

Knowledge of the drug and its pre-clinical and clinical development are also required. A good starting point to obtain this information is the investigator's brochure if previous clinical studies have been conducted. If not available, then this information must be gathered and an IB will need to be produced in addition to the protocol. A list of the contents required in an IB is given in the addendum to the GCP guidelines (ICH E6).

Before embarking on writing the protocol it is often a good idea to discuss the design options and possible subject numbers with the study statistician. There is no point in writing a protocol only to find that the subject numbers required are so large that the study would not be affordable within the budget provided or that the subject numbers were impossible to achieve.

The main decisions when developing a protocol

The items which must be included in a clinical study protocol are described in the ICH E6 guidelines. In addition, ICH E8 outlines the considerations for individual clinical trials. There are many different ways to go about writing a protocol but sketching out some sort of skeleton protocol outlining the main decisions makes a good starting point. The exact details can be added later.

Suggested contents of an outline protocol are detailed in Box 15.1.

It is a good idea to develop a study schedule as the main decisions are made so that this can be used when expanding into the larger protocol document. An example of such a chart is given in Table 15.1.

The schedule could contain not only the visit timings and assessments to be done but also relevant notes regarding any special ways that assessments will be performed. Key inclusion/exclusion criteria and study phases (screening, dose titration, etc.) and/or eligibility requirements for

---

Box 15.1 Suggested contents of an outline protocol

- **Title and rationale**: Short title and brief rationale
- **Objectives**
  - Primary
  - Secondary
- **End points** (assessments of the disease)
  - Primary (including primary time point of interest)
  - Secondary
- **Subject population**
  - Main inclusion criteria
  - Main exclusion criteria
- **Study design and methods**
- Type of study design
  - Non-comparative
  - Comparative (within-subject or between-subject)
- Treatments
  - Investigational medicinal product (IMP)
  - Control treatment (including any placebo or no treatment or standard care)
  - Doses, regimens, and treatment duration
- Assessments and timings (include any special equipment required)
  - Investigator's assessments
  - Subject's assessments
  - Laboratory
  - Other assessments (e.g. quality of life, tolerability)
- Statistical considerations
  - Randomization and blinding
  - Estimated subject numbers required

Table 15.1 Skeleton protocol example

Assessment	Visit 1 (Day 1)	Visit 2 (Day 7)	Visit 3 (Day 14)	Follow-up
Informed consent	X			
Medical history	X			
Inclusion/exclusion	X			
Vital signs	X		X	
Disease assessment	X	X	X	
Laboratory	X	X	X	X
Adverse events		X	X	X
Dispense/return medication	X	X	X	

Follow-up to be conducted at 14 days if laboratory value abnormal or adverse event ongoing at study exit.
Details of assessments to help protocol writing.
Medical history: specify which medical history will be included.
Disease assessments: specify these here (can be useful to include primary and secondary assessments).
Laboratory: specify which parameters will be assessed.

progression from one phase of the study to another are also useful notes to include.

The exact layout of the final protocol document is usually governed by company standard operating procedures (SOPs) and electronic protocol templates are usually available. These make life a little easier for the protocol writer as they frequently contain instructions for the author and standard wording for the administrative and other 'standard' sections that are included in every protocol (e.g. collecting adverse events, monitoring, data management and data protection, etc.). However, the wording of these sections must be reviewed to determine whether they are applicable to the protocol being developed and appropriate edits made.

Since a complete list of what should be included in the protocol is given in ICH E6, only relevant thoughts about the main considerations which make up the skeleton outline are elaborated here.

Objectives and end points

When writing a protocol it is sensible to simultaneously consider the objective (what question are we seeking to answer) and the end point (what assessment will give us the answer).

The primary objective of any study should be clearly stated and can be exploratory or confirmatory characterization of safety and/or efficacy and/or assessment of PK parameters and pharmacological, physiological, and biochemical effects (ICH E8). Pivotal phase 3 therapeutic confirmatory studies intended for a submission dossier seek to confirm efficacy and safety and thus have confirmatory objectives. Phase 2 therapeutic exploratory studies such as dose finding have exploratory objectives. Exploratory studies should have clear and precise objectives but unlike the objectives of confirmatory trials, they may not lead to simple tests of a predefined hypothesis. Exploratory studies are not considered to form the basis of efficacy for a filing (filing of information to obtain a marketing authorization approval (MAA). The process of sending the information for review is called a filing) and confirmatory studies therefore must be conducted to confirm the results from exploratory studies in the population that will ultimately receive the drug (ICH E9).

The primary objective must be described in exact terms and should have a well-considered rationale behind it. The rationale of why you are doing the trial is very important and needs ample logical elaboration in the protocol. Justification will be examined by the ethics committee who will need to ensure that the objective is appropriate and that it is being answered by the trial in an ethical way with the best interests and safety of the subjects in mind.

It is a good idea to 'keep the objective simple' and have just one primary objective even though it is tempting, for cost, time, or other reasons, to try to answer as many questions in one protocol as possible. However, if one protocol is trying to answer too many questions at once, there is always a risk of answering none of them adequately. This is because the subject numbers are calculated using the primary objective and end point only, and the study therefore may not include sufficient subjects to answer the questions other than the primary objective adequately. Clarity of thought and focus is required. This can be difficult when opinion leaders and advisory boards suggest the latest ground-breaking assessment or test, or wish to measure novel or an excessive number of laboratory parameters because of their personal research interests. It is important to remember that, when a study is being conducted to support a submission for drug approval, the disease must be assessed using a standard and well-established methodology that is acceptable to the regulatory authorities. An idea may be worthy of consideration as a secondary objective or alternatively, as the subject of an additional protocol. However, the ICH guidelines recommend that the number of secondary objectives should be limited and should be relevant to the primary objective (ICH E9).

The most common primary objectives of clinical trials are to evaluate either the efficacy or safety of a drug. Other objectives include investigation of pharmacokinetic parameters, pharmacological effects, or pharmaco-economic measures assessing a subject's quality of life or subject acceptability, etc. Assessment of safety is important and even when it is not the primary objective, safety should always be considered to be an objective, albeit a secondary one.

It is important to word the primary objective correctly because this is the question which dictates the primary end point measurement upon which the statistical sample size is calculated. Some guidance is given in Box 15.2. Generally the objective should clearly state the purpose of the experiment (e.g. to compare, to assess, etc.), not predetermine the outcome (e.g. to show, to prove, to demonstrate). The objective should detail the treatments to be compared over what time period and in what subject population (e.g. the disease, indicating disease severity if applicable).

Box 15.2 Objectives and end points

Objectives

- Start with a verb, 'To' e.g. to compare, to evaluate, to assess, to investigate, etc.
- Indicate which treatment(s) are to be used
- Specify over what treatment duration
- State in which subject population (disease and severity)

Primary end point

- An assessment that is relevant to the objective (i.e. will assess the drug's effect on the disease)
- The primary assessment is the one that is accepted in use to assess changes in the disease
- The primary end point should also state the time point of interest: when the judgement will be made about the efficacy of the treatment

There are many ways to write an objective and some examples follow.

'To compare the blood pressure lowering effect of Drug A with Drug B in mild hypertensive subjects treated for three months.'

'To evaluate the efficacy of Drug A versus Drug B in terms of the percentage of subjects with mild to moderate back pain who are classified as 'responders' (which should be defined) after six months treatment.'

'To assess the efficacy and safety of seven days treatment with Drug A and Drug B in paediatric subjects with acute bacterial conjunctivitis.'

'To assess the pharmacokinetic effects of single ascending doses of Drug A in healthy subjects'

As with the primary objective, the primary end point (sometimes called the primary outcome measure or primary response variable) needs careful thought.

Study end points are response variables that are chosen to assess drug effects that are related to PK parameters, pharmacodynamic measures, efficacy, and safety. The primary end point should assess clinically relevant effects and is based on the primary objective. Secondary end points assess other drug effects that may or may not be related to the primary end point (e.g. quality of life). The end points should be assessed at clinically relevant time points and the most clinically relevant time point overall should be selected as the primary time point of interest. For example blood pressure may be assessed after two, four, six, and eight weeks of treatment. The primary end point could be defined as 'the percentage of subjects with a diastolic blood pressure below 90 mmHg at Week 8' which will include the time point of interest when the primary comparison will be performed.

It is best to use an end point that is objective and not dependent on opinion of either the observer or the subject. Such end points are sometimes referred to as 'hard' end points; common examples are death, blood pressure measurements, laboratory values, etc. Some disease areas lend themselves well to using 'hard' end points, but many do not.

Choice of end points in therapeutic areas where the main disease manifestation involves measuring subjective symptoms such as pain, discomfort, irritation, etc., presents the protocol writer with challenges. In such cases there may be a surrogate marker of the disease which could be used but care must be taken to make sure that this marker does accurately correlate with disease levels and symptoms and is likely to predict clinical outcome (ICH E8). An example of a well-established and accepted surrogate end point is bone density in trials of osteoporosis. Osteoporotic subjects eventually suffer fractures, and bone density has been proven in epidemiology studies to be a good predictor of fractures. The use of bone density avoids having to use the occurrence of a fracture as an end point which is better for the subject and also shortens the time taken to get the study results. Alternatively, symptom-scoring systems can be used in an effort to quantify symptoms. Many scoring systems have been developed and validated in many different disease areas and are regularly used as research tools. Examples of scoring systems are the Psoriasis Area and Severity Index used in dermatology studies, or the Hamilton Rating Scale used in depression studies. It is preferable to use a recognized and validated scoring system and it is well worth searching the literature and consulting experts to decide on the most appropriate one to use.

If the disease area does not have a recognized symptom scoring system that is validated, one can be developed. A panel of experts can be consulted in order to do this, and this will add weight to the appropriateness of the scoring system. In some diseases only the subject can score the symptoms as these are feelings such as itching, pain, or irritation, but sometimes there are related clinical signs such as redness that the investigator is able to score. It is tempting to use only the investigator's score as the primary end point but this decision must be based on the clinical relevance of the clinical sign that the investigator is scoring. In these cases, a score of the clinical effectiveness as judged by the investigator is often an additional measurement rather than the primary one. At the end of the day the protocol writer has to justify the choice of the primary end point in the rationale for the study and clarity of thought is required to ensure that the end point chosen is as objective as possible.

Subject population

The eligibility criteria define the subject population to be studied. They define which subjects are to be included and which excluded. There is always a balance to be struck between a well-defined subject population on the one hand, and the presence of so many exclusion criteria that recruitment of such subjects becomes difficult on the other. In early studies (e.g. phase 1 exploratory studies) these eligibility criteria are very well defined in order to control the subject population tightly so the effect of the drug can be closely studied with minimal between-subject variation. However, as the drug is further developed in phase 3 confirmatory studies, it becomes increasingly important for the subject population to reflect the wider population that will ultimately be treated. Extrapolating the results of a trial conducted in an extremely tightly defined subject population to the general subject population is of questionable validity. So the aim is to get a balance between scientific integrity and final application. For phase 3 studies that are to be submitted to confirm efficacy and safety in a submission dossier, it is important that the subject population reflects as far as possible the target population that is intended to be treated. For example, if the treatment is intended to be used in all severities of the disease, all severities must be included in the phase 3 studies.

In addition to defining the inclusion criteria, there are certain standard exclusions which are often detailed in the SOPs. Usual exclusions are concomitant therapy that could affect the course of the disease or could lead to drug interactions and contraindicated therapies. Informed consent and how to deal with women of childbearing potential, pregnancy, or nursing mothers, or subjects that cannot comply with a protocol (such as alcoholics, drug users, etc.) are also addressed.

Study design

There are many different designs for clinical studies, and the choice of an appropriate design depends on why the trial is being conducted (e.g. for a submission dossier or for market support), the phase of the study, and the study end point (subjective or objective).

There are two main types of study design, comparative or non-comparative (sometimes known as non-controlled or open-label as blinding is not required). Non-comparative designs are used when safety, PK, and tolerability data are required (e.g. in phase 1 studies). Some phase 3 studies are also non-comparative (e.g. in chronic diseases), where safety data are required for the regulatory filing and ICH E1 recommends that data should be available for at least 100 subjects treated for one year. Comparative designs are used when comparing treatments. Chapter 14 describes the different types of study design including parallel group, cross-over, factorial, dose escalation, and fixed-dose response. However, the two most common comparative design types are summarized here.

Comparative study designs are either between-subject comparison, when the response is compared between groups of subjects treated with the different treatments, and within-subject comparison, which compares the response to the different treatments administered to the same subject. The most commonly used between-subject comparative design is the parallel group design where each subject will receive only one of the treatments for a predetermined time and response is compared between the different groups. The most commonly used within-subject design is the so-called cross-over design where each subject receives one treatment then crosses over to receive the other treatment, and the responses are compared within each subject.

The cross-over design at first sight looks a very attractive option in that each subject gets all treatments to be compared which minimizes the individual variation. Thus, the variation in a cross-over study will be less than in a parallel group trial where each group to be compared includes many individuals. The disadvantage of the cross-over study is that it can only be used for efficacy trials if the disease is such that an adequate wash-out period can be included to avoid a different baseline when the second treatment is given (the effect of the first treatment could be carried over). In order to ensure the baseline disease status is the same for each treatment period, the disease must be stable and the wash-out period long enough to ensure that the effects of the previous treatment are reversed. This sort of design therefore is not used in diseases where it would be unethical to withhold treatment or the safety of the subject would be at risk during wash-out, or the wash-out period would be too long to be practical. Cross-over studies are often used where the aim of the study is to assess subject acceptability of the treatments being compared, as in studies to be used for marketing purposes.

The parallel group design is usually the design of choice for phase 2 and 3 studies intended for regulatory submissions where an objective scientific assessment of the relative efficacy and safety of two or more treatments is required. The subjects enter the trial and are randomized to one of the treatments to be compared. Although there will be more variation between subject groups than within each subject, the inclusion and exclusion criteria specify the type of subject that enters. Randomization ensures that the groups are well balanced at baseline so that the response between groups can be compared fairly. These trials are often conducted blindly (i.e. the assessor cannot determine the identity of the treatment). This is especially important when the primary end point is a subjective one. If there are two treatments to be compared then this is referred to as a two-arm parallel group study, three treatments will mean three arms, etc.

Choice of comparator

For comparative studies, the choice of the right comparator is important. Options include placebo, no treatment or standard care, the established (gold standard) treatment or another treatment, or different doses of the drug under investigation. In the early phases of drug development a placebo is used as the comparator if possible to see whether a drug really works. Comparison with placebo is only possible in life-threatening diseases when the active treatment or placebo is added to usual therapy. Some regulatory authorities, such as the FDA, request a comparison vs placebo if possible to prove efficacy because they consider that comparison vs treatments already licensed may not always be clinically meaningful. This is because the response to treatment can change over the years. For example the response to penicillin V has declined due to the emergence of bacterial resistance, and a study confirming that a new antibiotic is as effective as penicillin V would not necessarily prove that the new drug is effective but a comparison versus placebo would. The FDA requires two 'adequate and well-controlled' trials to confirm efficacy and comparison against placebo should be included. The European regulatory authorities require comparison against an active treatment (e.g. the usually used treatment or gold-standard treatment). The 'usually used' active treatment can be different from country to country due to cultural differences, so sometimes a series of studies is required. In practice, most clinical programmes for submission dossiers include comparisons with both a placebo and a standard active treatment. Guidance on the choice of comparator is given in ICH E10 which is described in more detail in Chapter 14. As the drug approaches the marketplace, other comparative trials may be conducted against less well-known treatments for marketing purposes.

Assessments and timings

All assessments used to measure the end points should be validated and meet appropriate standards for accuracy, precision, reproducibility, reliability, and responsiveness (sensitivity to change over time) (ICH E8). In the skeleton protocol, only a broad outline of the assessments for efficacy and safety is needed. But in the final protocol, a full description of the methodology, recording equipment, and its calibration will be required.

The protocol user must be given accurate and detailed descriptions of exactly how all the measurements are to be made so that all observations are done in a standard way. For example, blood pressure can be measured in a variety of ways, taking the mean of three readings, the median of three readings, or taking readings until two are within a certain margin of each other. It can also be measured using a normal sphygmomanometer or a special sphygmomanometer that has a random zero to exclude observer bias. Whatever is used, to avoid variation in the measurements, the same observer and the same sphygmomanometer should be used and this must be stated in the protocol to ensure standardization.

If laboratory assessments are included, then a decision about which tests are clinically relevant and sample collection details must be included in the protocol. It is not always a good idea to report all the automated tests on offer because there is a risk of finding an abnormal result in a clinically irrelevant parameter and having to explain this in the report and/or the regulatory submission. In a multicentre study, use of a central laboratory if possible makes data handling and analysis easier as there are only one set of normal reference ranges. Stability of the parameter to be transported often dictates whether or not a central laboratory is practical from a logistic point of view. Bacteriological and other biological samples can also be transported with appropriate media. The laboratory should be consulted for its advice on transport and stability as well as appropriate assays.

In the case of adverse events, precise definitions (usually as in ICH E6) and instructions need to be available, especially for serious adverse event (SAE) reporting (by whom, to whom, and within what time frame). This adverse event section is usually a company standard one included in the protocol template or company SOPs, and is usually based on ICH E2 and E6. However, the protocol writer is allowed to list certain exceptions for immediate SAE reporting to the authorities in disease areas that predictably will yield many SAEs; for example, deaths in oncology studies are expected so frequently that they are listed as not requiring immediate reporting.

It is a good idea to include in the protocol a list of the source data expected to be recorded in the source documentation such as the patient notes. Source data that are expected to be recorded directly onto the case report form (CRF) should also be described. This sort of data are usually the rating scales or special research scoring systems that are not generally found in patient notes because these assessments are used as research tools only, and not used routinely for the clinical management of the subject.

A schematic representation, such as a study schedule or flow chart giving the timing for each of the assessments, can be generated as part of the skeleton protocol. This chart as a reference makes it easier to write the complete protocol accurately.

Statistical considerations

The number of subjects required (sample size) should be calculated using the primary response variable (i.e. the end point by which success or failure of the treatment will be measured). It is helpful if this is as objective as possible (e.g. complete cure, survival, etc.). For multicentre studies, the numbers expected per site should be included to ensure similar subject populations between sites so that between-centre statistical comparisons (which are often of interest to regulatory authorities) are possible.

All studies should be designed to avoid bias if possible. Sources of bias and how to avoid it are addressed in detail in Chapter 14. In summary, the two most common techniques to avoid bias are randomization and blinding.

Randomization is when a subject is assigned treatment by chance. It is used to try to eliminate the bias which arises if the assessor knows which treatment is which and if he or she may be tempted to give the 'new' treatment to either subjects who have failed on previous therapy, or even to give it to those he or she thinks will do well on it. Randomization to the different treatments can be done in its most simple sense by whether an odd or even number is drawn on cutting a pack of cards, or whether a tossed coin gives a head or a tail. In clinical trials, randomization is more sophisticated and is done using computer-generated random number tables. Balanced blocks of treatment are generated according to the number of treatments being studied and the next subject to be randomized is assigned the next subject number in the block.

Blinding is used to eliminate the bias that can occur if the assessor knows which treatment is the new one and if he or she could score the subjects on the new treatment more optimistically. In a blinded study, the treatments appear identical so the observer does not know which subject is taking which treatment. This is called 'single blind' because only the observer is blind to the treatment. However, subjects often give clues to the observer about what they are taking so many studies are conducted 'double blind' (i.e. neither the observer nor the subject can distinguish one treatment from another). This is possible providing that the treatments look, smell, and taste identical, and have the same dosing regimen. Double blinding becomes tricky when the treatments are presented in different formulations and/or different dosing regimens. In such cases, the 'double-dummy' technique is used which is a form of 'double blinding' to take this into account. For example, if a capsule taken twice daily is to be compared with a tablet taken four times daily, dummy (placebo) capsules and tablets will have to be made. Subjects will take either active capsules twice daily and dummy tablets four times daily OR dummy capsules twice daily and active tablets four times daily to retain the 'blind' nature of the study.

Stratification is another technique sometimes used in comparative studies to avoid bias. This is used when a certain factor is thought to affect the subject response, and an imbalance of subjects with this factor between the randomized treatment groups could bias the trial. Stratification takes place before randomization to ensure subjects with this factor are distributed equally between the treatment groups and treatment allocation is equally balanced. For example, if large tumours and small tumours are thought to respond differently to treatment, then subjects would be 'stratified' (assigned) to a 'large tumour substratum' or 'small tumour substratum' prior to randomization. Separate randomization lists are generated for each substratum to ensure that allocation to the different treatments is balanced within each substratum, and similar numbers of subjects with large and small tumours receive each treatment.

Details of compliance measurements and methods for statistical analysis may or may not be part of the skeleton protocol but they should be elaborated in the full protocol.

Administrative sections

Once these main decisions have been made in the skeleton protocol, the first full draft protocol can be written by elaborating every detail and adding administrative sections as set out in the company SOPs and the ICH GCP guidelines.

A protocol template is often available which should include all the required elements of a protocol as outlined in Chapter 6 of ICH 6. The template often includes instructions to help the protocol writer and proposed text for the 'standard' administrative sections that are present in most study protocols (e.g. reporting adverse events, monitoring, data management, protection of subject confidentiality, and adherence to GCP, etc.). However, any suggested text in the template should be reviewed by the writer to ensure it is applicable for the protocol.

Protocol review and sign-off

The full draft protocol will then undergo review preferably by a team of people representative of those who will ultimately be operationally involved within the sponsor (e.g. clinical, data management, statistics, regulatory, and commercial), and also sites involved outside the sponsor if possible (e.g. investigator sites, central laboratories, contract research organizations, etc.).

Robust review which leads to the best possible protocol usually means that there are several review rounds, and when making any changes it is important that all the relevant sections of the protocol are changed so that all the sections fit together. Eventually a final protocol will result.

Many sponsors will have SOPs on protocol development which include a formal protocol review process which may give guidance. However, if no guidance is available, thought needs to be applied so that the reviewers are appropriate; for example, the team reviewing a study to justify reimbursement may not necessarily include exactly the same functional groups as a study aiming to confirm efficacy and safety for a regulatory dossier. It is helpful for the reviewers to be independent of the team developing the protocol, and often the reviewers are the relevant heads of departments. It is important to ensure that key stakeholders for that particular protocol are not overlooked.

Sign-off should be conducted by the appropriately qualified people who are experts in the methodology and usually include those who are responsible for the clinical and statistical aspects.

Protocol amendments

If sufficient time is allowed and a well thought-out, researched, robust protocol is produced, it is always hoped that changes to the protocol and protocol amendments can be avoided. However, there is always a great deal of pressure to complete the protocol as swiftly as possible so that the study can start. A balance has to be struck between a well thought-out, researched, robust protocol which is unlikely to be amended and starting a study earlier but risking losing time later due to protocol amendments. Amendments not only create extra work for the study team, ethics committee, and competent authority but can also drain motivation from the sites that are waiting to enrol subjects in the study.

A feasibility exercise is often used to try to avoid protocol amendments. This is often run in parallel with the development and review of the detailed protocol either on the skeleton protocol or a later draft. Time allowed for feasibility prior to the finalization of the protocol is time well spent, especially if a multinational or global study is planned and there may be added complexity due to the differences in cultures and medical practice. Input about the practicalities of running the study, such as patient recruitment rates, feasibility of assessments, availability of special equipment, electronic data capture, etc., can be gained early before the protocol is finalized. A robust feasibility can identify aspects of the study which are difficult or even impossible operationally. The issues identified can then be discussed and evaluated and solutions developed. It may be possible to change the protocol slightly, without changing the main study focus, to facilitate recruitment easier; doing this before protocol finalization avoids losing time due to an amendment.

However, amendments can arise due to things which are unforeseen at the time of protocol finalization (e.g. emergence of non-clinical information, new guidelines or advice from regulatory authorities, or even administrative changes such as changes to staff names or site addresses, if they are included in the protocol).

A protocol amendment is defined as a 'written description of a change(s) to or formal clarification of a protocol' (ICH E6), and according to ICH E8 a clear description of the rationale for any change should be provided.

Protocol amendments that affect the safety or physical or mental integrity of the subjects, the scientific value of the trial, the conduct of a trial, or the quality or safety of any investigational medicinal product used in the trial are considered to be substantial amendments and should definitely be submitted for ethical and/or regulatory approval, depending on the local laws and regulations.

If a protocol does need modification, a protocol amendment process should be followed. This is often detailed in an SOP and involves the generation of the amendment (which should include a clear description of any change and also its rationale), and then an evaluation of the amendment by appropriate experts. The evaluation should include an assessment of what impact it will have on the trial and whether it is a substantial amendment or not, which will dictate whether it requires submission to the ethical committee and/or regulatory authority. All protocol amendments that are submitted to the ethics committee and/or regulatory approval should be approved before they are instituted.

Special considerations in healthcare protocols

Ethical issues should always be considered when writing a protocol. In particular, informed consent procedures in the subject groups concerned especially in special groups such as children, females of childbearing potential, mentally ill or incapacitated subjects, should all be considered. Confidentiality, compensation, and indemnity, audit and finance are also important ethical issues.

In addition, ethics committees will be assessing the scientific integrity of the study and will want to know if the results will give a robust answer to the question posed in the objectives. Thus, the rationale for important design features of the study (e.g. end point, duration, sample size, comparators, assessments, changes to study conduct—amendments and deviations), needs to be elaborated in the protocol.

One of the most important considerations is the practicality of conducting the study. The balance of inclusion and exclusion criteria to ensure sufficient subjects can be enrolled has already been considered, but other practicalities also need to be contemplated. For example, there is no point doing a study in a hospital setting when the subjects with the disease being studied are treated only in general practice. Transport of biological samples to a central laboratory can also be challenging to ensure that stability is maintained or that any biological samples are still viable. There may be many other practical issues to consider so when writing a protocol, the question 'is this practically and logistically possible' should always be borne in mind.

Last, it is imperative that all healthcare protocols are ethical and of good quality. During protocol development there is a need to get into great detail and this can lead to lack of focus in the protocol. The one thing that will really add quality to a protocol is to keep the 'big picture' in mind to aid robust decision making: why is the protocol being conducted? What is the objective? If these questions are asked during the many discussions that take place during protocol development, focus should be maintained, a quality protocol should result, and the need for subsequent amendment avoided unless an unexpected change takes place in the marketplace or in the regulatory environment.

Further reading

International Conference on Harmonisation of Technical Requirements for Registration of Pharmaceuticals for Human Use efficacy guidelines. ℘ www.ich.org

E6 Guideline 'Good Clinical Practice (R1)' 1996.
E3 Guideline 'Structure and Content of Clinical Study Reports' 1995.
E8 Guideline 'General Considerations in Clinical Trials' 1997.
E9 Guideline 'Statistical Principles for Clinical Trials' 1998.

Data capture tools: case report form (CRF)

Introduction

The case record form or CRF came into being as a way of regulating the collection of clinical trial data. The traditional paper-based CRF has been a very important tool for the clinical trial team. However, the advent of electronic data capture and remote data entry confronts the CRF designer with fresh challenges.

This chapter will outline the overall design process, highlight the aspects of design that are significant for the success of the CRF, and consider the effects of electronic data capture on the production of electronic CRFs (eCRFs).

Definition and purpose of CRFs

The CRF is the document used to record the data on which the eventual analysis and reporting of the clinical trial will be based. Although the study protocol provides the detailed methodology for running the trial, the CRF is the main day-to-day tool that enables the correct information to be captured at the right time. CRF design must therefore reflect two principal uses of this document in the trial: the collection and extraction of data.

The CRF is significant to the investigator or research nurse who will complete it, the monitor who checks it, and the data manager who will use it to construct the database.

The objective of the CRF is to capture the data specified in the protocol and to prompt the investigator to perform all the necessary assessments.

From the investigator's point of view, the CRF should be clear, unambiguous, and easy to follow and complete. The investigator will be seeing patients as part of a routine clinic day and will not have the opportunity to refer back to the protocol and other documentation so the CRF should contain comprehensive instructions and guidance. It should also enable the investigator to confirm the subject's eligibility to continue in the trial at any given point.

The monitor will review the completed CRF against the protocol requirements in order to validate and clarify entries. The CRF should therefore be designed to minimize uncertainties and to facilitate entry verification; for example, cross-checks between related data.

In a clinical trial in pharmaceutical-sponsored trials, the final recipient of the CRF is the data manager who will use it first to design the database and then as the source of the data to fill the database. By securing clear unambiguous responses, minimizing the amount of free text, and guiding the study team to make correct entries in the correct places, the CRF designer contributes to the creation of a clean database with minimum need for query resolution.

Regulatory requirement

All elements of a clinical trial including the CRF must comply with ICH Good Clinical Practice (ICH GCP) and adhere to the specific regulatory requirements of the regulatory authorities that will review the final clinical trial report as part of a regulatory submission.

ICH GCP (8.2.2) states that the CRF should form part of the protocol, implying that the protocol should not be finalized until the CRF is complete. In practice, this often does not happen and the protocol and CRF go through separate development and editorial procedures, often resulting in discrepancies.

The guidelines have very little to say about CRF design per se. Many companies and institutions including the UK National Health Service (NHS) have standard operating procedures (SOPs) or template documents. The CRF is a critical document and in some cases may be the source data and as such should be carefully constructed to ensure recording of data meets the ICH GCP requirements.

The design and review process

CRF design is very similar to that of protocol design in that there needs to be a team approach. The team would as a minimum consist of:
- CRF designer
- Medical advisor
- Clinical monitor
- Data entry team member
- Data manager
- Statistician

CRF design starts with the protocol. From the protocol, the designer will initially generate a skeleton plan showing the visits and each associated assessment. The assessments are then reviewed to determine which are visit-specific and which are global. Using this information the designer can map out the number of pages required and what will appear on each page. Implicit in this process is the need for the CRF designer to have the final version of the protocol (if possible!), and to be informed of any change to the study design.

Where possible, standard pages will be used to maintain conformity with other studies. New pages designed specifically for the study will follow the standard formats. The designer next distils the requirements of the protocol into clear, simple, unambiguous questions and creates appropriate areas for data to be recorded. The CRF will also include a series of instructions for the investigator as a guide through the various required assessments. Once completed, the first version should undergo quality checks by an independent person to ensure that the CRF matches the requirements of the protocol as well as checking for internal consistency.

This first version is then sent to the individual team for its input. The designer will draw up a second version based on the feedback from the team.

In parallel with this process, the designer will select a printer who will be briefed about the number of CRFs required, the design characteristics, the type of paper and any other specific requirements, and the deadline for distribution.

Comments on the second version will be reviewed and will be incorporated into the final version. This version will be quality-assured to ensure that all changes have been made as indicated.

Once approved, the final version can be forwarded to the printers for designing a proof copy. This should reflect not only the content but also the binding format and should be as close to the final version as possible.

As with all documents, there should be a clear audit trail of the generation of the CRF. All the steps in its generation should be documented, retained, and archived.

Purpose of the information to be collected

The two main purposes of the data collected in the CRF are to answer the hypothesis formulated in the study protocol and provide relevant safety data relating to the study drug. The protocol will have been carefully written and reviewed so that the right questions are asked to obtain the information required. The purpose of the CRF is to ensure the precise collection, collation, analysis, and reporting of these data. The accuracy of the data is very important as any discrepancy between the data required and the protocol and those collected on the CRF will undermine confidence in the findings of the study.

It is tempting when designing a CRF to ask questions that may be of academic interest but are not strictly required in the protocol. These 'nice to haves' are not advisable. They may not be ethical, may make the CRF longer than necessary, and may also mean that the 'need to have' data may be missed. Additional data may also result in a delay at the end of the study with time spent on cleaning unnecessary data.

To avoid pitfalls, the designer must ensure that the CRF:
- requests the data as required by the protocol
- collects only the data required by the protocol
- collects the data in as simple, relatively, and unambiguous way as possible, making assessments straightforward to complete
- presents the information clearly in as logical an order and uniform style as possible
- phrases the questions to minimize queries arising

Identifying and ensuring the integrity of the data

Each CRF page should be uniquely identifiable to the centre conducting the trial, to the trial itself, and identifiable by name. A unique system of codes is needed usually consisting of the subject's initials and identification number within the trial.

Each page of the CRF will usually contain the following information:
- Unique subject ID (subject number, CRF number, and subject's initials (some companies do not routinely collect initials and date of birth as anonymity may be lost))
- Name of the sponsor of the trial
- Trial identifier (trial code or name)
- Centre number
- Visit number for each assessment
- Study day/assessment reference
- Page number (X of Y)
- An indication of distribution of copies in cases where there is no carbon required (NCR)

The data is usually captured using standard headers (Figure 16.1).

These identifying items ensure any loose pages can be confidentially assigned to the correct study centre and assessment. They also allow the data manager to confirm that all pages are present or to establish which data are missing.

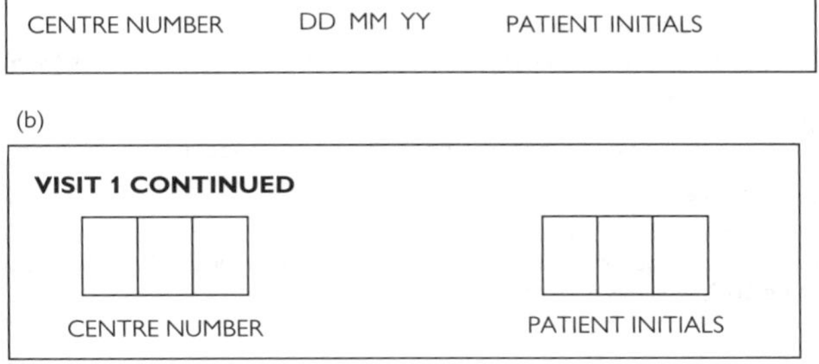

(a)

VISIT 1   DAY 1

CENTRE NUMBER   DD MM YY   PATIENT INITIALS

(b)

VISIT 1 CONTINUED

CENTRE NUMBER   PATIENT INITIALS

Figure 16.1 Standard headers.

Layout and style

A CRF tells the story of what happens to a patient in the study. It should flow from one assessment to the next in a clear, simple, and logical order. The CRF should be aesthetically pleasing; a document that is easy to read and attractive will encourage careful and accurate completion. A wordy and overcrowded CRF will be viewed as a burden by the investigator and is an invitation to error or misinterpretation.

The layout or the form text style and phrasing of questions can all play a part in ensuring data quality.

Here are some considerations.

Formatting and sequencing

The data should be recorded in the sequence that they are performed.

When multiple assessments are repeated at subsequent visits they should appear in the same format and sequence for each visit. This will not only help the investigator to develop a routine but will also assist database building and therefore data entry.

It is easy and quick for the investigator to use tick-box forms but these forms must state clearly if more than one box may be ticked as the database will be constructed on the expectation that only one box will be ticked.

If there is a series of 'Yes or No' options, the boxes should appear in two columns. All 'Yes' boxes should be in one column, and all 'No' boxes in the other. It is advisable to keep the sequence of 'Yes and No' in the same columns throughout the CRF.

For inclusion/exclusion criteria, care must be taken as sometimes shading or emboldening the 'right' answers could lead to incorrect entries!

Investigator comments

White space is conducive to completing the CRF and can guide the investigator from one assessment to the next. However, too much white space encourages the investigator to write notes on the CRF. Handwritten notes cause problems for the data managers who are taught to enter all data from the CRF into the database.

If investigators' comments are required, a text box may be used but the box should not be too big!

Choosing a readable font and point size

Font styles can influence the readability of the CRF. A serif font (Times New Roman) is ideal for text articles. A simpler style (Arial) has a much clearer appearance on a form and encourages a more detailed review.

A 12-point size would appear to be the best, with 10-point for instruction.

Rotated text

If the text needs to be rotated 90 degrees for tab edging or column headers, the text should be turned in complete words and not individual letters—see Figure 16.2; which is easier to read?

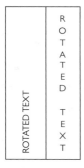

Figure 16.2 Rotated text.

Hyphenation
Hyphenation allows more words to be fitted on the page but may make the text harder to read. Hyphenation should be used sparingly.

Uniformity
Uniformity of layout is very important for a CRF. If a series of studies is conducted in a therapeutic area, it is advisable to develop a uniform standard across all trials. All will be helped if similar information is presented in a standard way. The designer is not reinventing the presentation in every trial, and the investigator becomes used to the format and therefore makes fewer errors, thus the database will require less specification each new study.

Many data fields can be collected on global or standard forms. The demographics, medical history, lab data, vital signs, physical examination, previous medication, concomitant medication, adverse events, and end of study records could each become standard CRF modules. They would require minimal modification from study to study.

There are four types of data collected in most trials:
- Baseline data—inclusion/exclusion, demographics, medical history, etc.
- Efficacy data—assessments that are specific to the objective of the study
- Safety data—adverse events
- Compliance data—treatment accountability, concomitant medication, end of study records

Instructions for CRF completion

Every CRF should provide precise but sufficient information for the investigator to carry out the visit assessments, entry of any additional information, and ensure subjects' continued compliance.

A schedule or calendar at the start of the CRF may help with ensuring all assessments are recorded as required

There should be guidance on how to record data (e.g. dd/mm/yy), how to correct data, and how to deal with missing information.

Prompts should appear throughout the CRF to help the investigator to complete the required fields and actions to be taken.

CRF completion

- Required format (see Figure 16.3)
- Provide an example of the format of text entry required.
- The design should be influenced by the way in which the data would be entered into the database
- If more than one identical assessment is to be taken twice on one day, it is easier for data entry purposes if each is listed on a separate line rather than on one line running across the page

(a)

Date	Time 1 HH:MM	Temperature °C	Time 2 HH:MM	Temperature °C
DD MM YY				
DD MM YY				

(b)

Date	Time 1 HH:MM	Temperature °C
DD MM YY Time 1		
Time 2		
DD MM YY Time 1		
Time 2		

Figure 16.3 Preferred format: blocked list data.

Include units of measurement on the form
For example, the investigator should be in no doubt if the height is recorded in centimetres or inches.

This can be achieved by ensuring that the units of measurement are specified and that the boxes provided for entry are appropriate to the units including the position of the decimal point as shown in Figure 16.4.

Graphic design
Guide the quality of text entries
The interpretation of handwritten entries, especially if they are medical terms, can be very difficult for data entry and data management personnel. This is especially true if the study is multinational as different countries format letters in their own way.

It is easier to read block capitals than script, so simple instruction to print entries may reduce queries.

Providing the correct amount of space is also important; free text boxes should be kept to a minimum. Too much space encourages the investigator to wax lyrical while too little space results in abbreviations or cryptic comments which have to be interpreted (Figure 16.5).

Text justification
The layout of questions and their corresponding answer boxes can greatly affect the ease of CRF completion. There are several ways to align more than one row of questions, as shown in Figure 16.6.

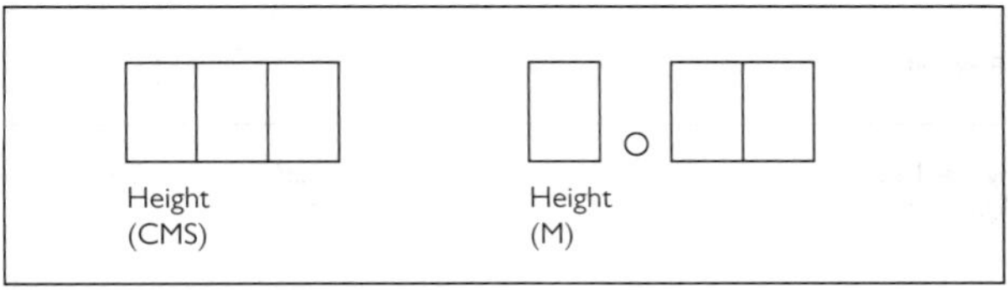

Figure 16.4 Data entry boxes on the CRF showing the required units and the position of the decimal point.

Check boxes

Numeric data box

Text data box

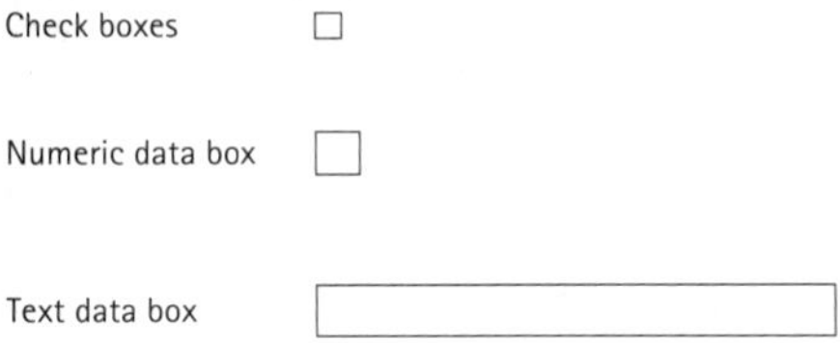

Figure 16.5 Providing the correct amount of space.

Example a)

Informed consent? ☐ Yes ☐ No	
Aged between 18 and 45 years inclusive? ☐ Yes ☐ No	
Any allergies or hypersensitivity? ☐ Yes ☐ No	
Received any other investigational drug within the last 30 days? ☐ Yes ☐ No	

Example b)

Informed consent?	☐ Yes ☐ No
Aged between 18 and 45 years inclusive?	☐ Yes ☐ No
Any allergies or hypersensitivity?	☐ Yes ☐ No
Received any other investigational drug within the last 30 days?	☐ Yes ☐ No

Example c)

Informed consent?	☐ Yes ☐ No
Aged between 18 and 45 years inclusive?	☐ Yes ☐ No
Any allergies or hypersensitivity?	☐ Yes ☐ No
Received any other investigational drug within the last 30 days?	☐ Yes ☐ No

Figure 16.6 Illustration of how ease of CRF completion is affected by different alignments of rows of questions and corresponding response boxes.

Example a) is untidy and difficult for monitors to check, the boxes are amongst the writing, and it is difficult to spot if a box is missed in error. According to Pocock,[1] however, it is the quickest and easiest for the investigator to complete. Example b) is much easier for a monitor to spot any missing ticks. Example c) offers a clear layout for both monitor and investigator. Example b) is the one generally utilized in CRFs.

Typesetting

CAPITALS—USED TOO MUCH CAN MAKE TEXT DIFFICULT TO READ

Underlining text also makes it difficult to read

Use emboldened text sparingly for effect

Use italics for specific purposes, e.g. instructions

Shading and colour, white on black, can help in the design of the CRF.

Too much shading is not to be recommended as if data has to be faxed or copied it takes longer and the ensuing copy is often not clear.

To make something stand out, white on black may be useful (Figure 16.7).

Question formats

If a clinical trial is to be successful it is vital that the CRF questions are formulated so as to be understood and to yield an answer in the correct format. All questions should be worded to eliminate confusion and to ensure that their answer cannot change. Figure 16.8 shows examples of poorly constructed questions.

It is far easier for an investigator to tick a box than write text.

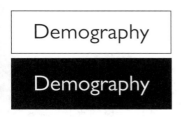

Figure 16.7 Demonstration of how white on black makes things stand out on a page.

Avoid double negatives

e.g.

• Is the patient taking no antihypertensive medication?   Yes No

Is the answer NO they are not or YES they are not?

Avoid ambiguous questions

e.g.

• Has the patient experienced this adverse event before?   Yes No

Why is this ambiguous?

Which event?

Since when? From first visit? From baseline or ever in their life?

For such questions you have to give the term of reference.

Avoid compound questions

e.g.

• Does the patient have ventricular tachycardia with a history   Yes No
of myocardial infarction and one of the following:

a) Syncope

b) Aborted sudden death

This question should be split into three separate questions for ease of completion and for greater clarity.

Figure 16.8 Examples of poor question construction.

There are four things to remember:
- Every question should require a response
- Indicate the format of the response
- Do not record the same data in more than one place
- Use simple language

Other rules of question construction
- For comparative questions, indicate the basis for comparison: e.g. increase from baseline
- If answering a question requiring referral to definitions, put the definitions in the CRF
- Use instructions if necessary (e.g. actions)
- Time—specify a.m./p.m. or 24-hour clock
- Date—specify order (e.g. dd mm yy)
- Avoid mixing time frames on a page
  - e.g. past weekly consumption
  - e.g. current daily consumption
- Calculations—record raw data
- Allow for 'other' or 'none' in checklists
- Do not mix longitudinal and vertical listings
- Put 'Yes' and 'No' in the same order throughout
- With numeric data, state the units and the number of decimal places expected

Printing requirements

The production of artwork for commercial printers to reproduce must satisfy a number of requirements:
• The dimensions must be standard size
• Allowance must be made for margins to ensure binding holes do not go through the text
• If colour graphics are to be used, colour separate copy is required
• If the file is supplied electronically, the printer must be able to access the file so a compatible system must be utilized.

It is important that the printer receives absolute clear instructions on printing and assembling the CRF
• The size and weight of the paper, the colours of the NCR copies, logos, formats, type of binding, position of plastic wallets, etc.
• The printer must be given sufficient time to allow for the printing of the CRFs as described
• Before final print approval is given, the printer should supply a proof copy for review by the study team and this should be signed off

Binding

The CRFs may be presented in ring binders. This allows for pages to be replaced should a printing error occur. However, in the same way as it is easy to remove pages for replacement, it is easy for the investigator to remove the pages required in the clinic without the necessity of carrying around a bulky file. Once pages are removed they could easily be lost.

Glued books are good for keeping the pages together but depending on the environment (heat for example), the pages may become detached.

There is no right or wrong way to present the CRF and much will be dependent on the study and the number of CRF pages to be presented.

It is very useful to use tabs for navigation to split visits or sections so that they may easily be found within the CRF.

If the CRFs are NCR, the way in which the papers are perforated is important so that the information required (two parts of the NCR copies) may be easily torn from the CRF.

Sections for completion by the subject

Some parts of the CRF such as questionnaires and diary cards are intended for completion by the subject rather than the investigator.

These documents should be printed separately. Care should be taken to ensure the layout and wording of questions for subject completion reflects the fact that subjects may have a limited vocabulary.

The following points should be borne in mind:

- Many people struggle to read 10-point text
- Medical jargon should not be used
- All text should be as simple as possible
- Full training and examples should be given to ensure understanding by the subject
- An attractive, easy-to-use format will encourage completion of a diary
- Text entry by subjects should be minimized
- It is better to have several short diary cards (no more than two to four weeks) than one large card as if it is lost, you will have lost a considerable amount of data
- The diary card itself should be robust

Electronic or eCRFs

The management of clinical trial data using paper methods is not efficient in terms of data recording and subsequent data processing. The paper-based system is dependent on legible data recording supported by manual and computer-assisted data integrity checks performed by monitors or data managers.

As IT has advanced, the acceptance of the electronic signature has made it possible for the introduction of eCRFs. These record the data directly into the database from a remote location. This system prevents transcription errors and reduces the time taken to database lock at the end of the study.

Many commercial companies work globally and the eCRF allows access to data in real time wherever the study may be performed.

One of the first elements to be electronically captured was that of laboratory data. Laboratory results now tend to be sent directly to the database. Other data generated electronically include ECG traces, ambulatory blood pressure measurements, and spirometry results.

eCRFs have successfully replaced paper as the interface between the investigator and the database (Figure 16.9).

The merits of the eCRF

The merits of collecting data electronically can be summarized as follows:
- The data can be checked at the time of entry against appropriate field validation criteria thus providing assurance that correct data have been entered.
- The inclusion of traditional monitoring and data-management validation checks in the eCRF should reduce the number and frequency of data clarification forms (DCFs).
- The eCRF can aid compliance by cross-checking key data.

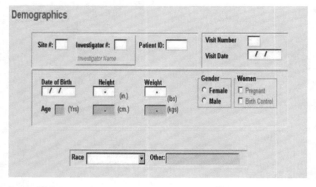

Figure 16.9 Shows a typical interface between investigator and database.

- Instructions for completing the eCRF can be presented on-screen and as validation help messages.
- Moreover, the acceptance of an appropriate electronic signature by the regulatory authorities means eCRF data can be electronically signed by the investigator.
- Finally, if the data is being entered directly to a centralized database, monitoring staff will be able to review data more quickly and remotely.

eCRF considerations

- The provision of adequate support to ensure continuity of data collection if there are technical problems
- Including data validation checks into the eCRF has considerable advantages but only the checks written into the programme will be completed. The monitors will still have to validate the data manually

A number of issues have to be considered:
- The IT infrastructure has to support eCRFs
- The time to design the eCRF

eCRFs and paper CRFs

The design of eCRFs still requires the same skills as the traditional CRF but they also require technical IT support to design the data entry screen, validation checks, and overall system security. Computer systems have to be compliant with CRF 21 part 11, and companies have to demonstrate the robustness of their systems.

Wherever possible, the eCRF should be similar in design to its paper counterpart since the layout and data flow are designed to reflect the traditional data collection sequence and procedures. Many of the design features listed earlier in this chapter will be equally applicable to the eCRF. This continuity of design features will also help in the transition from paper to the electronic version for research staff who are unfamiliar with electronic data-collection methods.

The header information is still critical in the eCRF and electronic checks should be included here. This information is essential to identify the subject specific data records for the corresponding eCRF page and visit when it is stored in the database.

It is used to check the subject's initials, centre number, visit date, and subject number are of the correct data type and format. Where a series of pages are collected during a visit, the header information should automatically be carried over to all pages for that subject's visit.

Where tick boxes are used in the eCRF, validation checks can be set so that only one box can be ticked. Date fields can be checked to ensure that they are in the correct format and fall within expected ranges; for example, date of birth can be used automatically to verify the subject's age and this can be checked against the inclusion/exclusion criteria for the trial.

Numerical fields can be checked against reference ranges or expected answers and values falling outside the limits can be flagged or noted for confirmation.

The eCRF pages for adverse events, concomitant medication, and other across-visit observations need to be designed differently. The form should be designed to retrieve previous observations and records that require a relevant status update for that visit.

Drop-down selection menus can be used for coded fields. There may be the option to incorporate special computer-generated components into the CRF design (e.g. date selection) where standard elements are available.

Thus, while many of the traditional CRF design skills will still be appropriate for the design of eCRFs, there will be a need for understanding and utilization of the computer-aided design components to be included.

The traditional monitoring, checking, and validation elements have to be incorporated into the eCRF design, and the eCRF has to be planned and produced as early as possible in the study lifecycle.

As more commercial organizations provide eCRF systems, their use has increased and many pharmaceutical companies and CROs use them. In academia, the change is not as marked, perhaps because data tend to be collected in single or relatively few sites and the costs of production do not warrant eCRFs.

Conclusion

Good CRF design has an influence on the success of a clinical trial. By asking the right questions in the right way and by providing appropriate space for data to be entered correctly, the designer ensures that the CRF accurately captures the data generated in the trial.

By presenting the data in a clear format, the quality of the transfer of data into the database is assured.

The move to eCRFs has already occurred in the commercial sector. The basic design features are the same as for paper CRFs. However, the increased complexity of the eCRF, with the in-built validation and parallel database development, means the eCRF designer will have to be involved at an early stage of study planning. Also, the eCRF design team will include at least one or more expert such as a database programmer.

The rapid development in mobile technology (e.g. tablet PCs, smartphones, etc.) is creating the opportunity for eCRFs and electronic patient reported outcomes to be designed and used for data collection using these innovative devices. Once again, the same design features and considerations need to be incorporated for use on these mobile devices too.

Reference

1. Pocock, S. *Clinical Trials: A Practical Approach*. Oxford: Wiley-Blackwell, 1983.

Further reading

International Conference on Harmonisation of Technical Requirements for Registration of Pharmaceuticals for Human Use. Guideline for Good Clinical Practice (ICH E6), April 1996. ℰ www.ich.org

Code of Federal Regulations Title 21, (volume 1 revised as of April 2011). Food and Drugs chapter 1—Food and Drug Administration Department of Health and Human Services subchapter A—general. Part 11: Electronic Records; Electronic Signatures. ℰ www.fda.gov

Clinical trial supplies: investigational medicinal products (IMPs)

Introduction

The sponsor is responsible for supplying investigational medicinal products (IMP) to the investigator or institution conducting the study and this should happen only after the sponsor obtains all required documentation (e.g. approval from the institutional review board/independent ethics committee (IRB/IEC) and regulatory authority). The sponsor should ensure that written procedures include instructions to follow for the handling and storage of IMP and for documentation. The procedures should include receipt, handling, storage, dispensing, retrieval of unused product from study subjects, and return of unused IMP to the sponsor (or alternative disposal arrangements if applicable).

In general, the principles of good manufacturing practice (GMP) are followed for IMP, together with specific requirements applicable to investigational products; for example, labelling requirements are very different for IMP compared to normal medicinal product.

The requirements may be found in EudraLex, Volume 4, Good manufacturing practice (GMP) Guidelines, and more specifically in annex 13.

How to source clinical trial supplies

There are many issues to consider when planning where and how to have clinical trial supplies prepared. This section attempts to lead the reader through the necessary thought processes involved.

Insourcing or outsourcing

The first consideration when sourcing clinical trial supplies is whether the supplies should be produced in-house or if some or all of the activities should be outsourced. The answer to this question will be partially dependent on the nature of your organization.

• Large **pharmaceutical companies** will normally have manufacturing, packaging, and storage and distribution facilities of their own and will only outsource when specific expertise or capacity constraints arise.

With the vast growth in biotech and virtual pharmaceutical companies over recent years however, there is a vibrant outsourcing market and a wide range of potential service providers.

• An **academic institute** is unlikely to have the necessary licences of manufacturing and packaging, so will need to work with an outsource provider.

• Working with outsourcing companies requires a technical agreement which outlines the responsibility for aspects of the process. The technical agreement covering manufacturing, analytical, packaging, storage, distribution, returns, and destruction activities is a requirement of GMP and, if your supply chain is complex, multiple agreements with different suppliers will be required.

All clinical trial materials must be manufactured and packaged in facilities and with processes that comply with GMP and, in order to confirm that this is indeed the case, the facility needs to be audited and approved by the relevant regulatory authority. This results in the award of a manufacturing licence or GMP certificate. Continued compliance with GMP is confirmed by the regulatory authority via regular audits of the facility and the processes.

If supplies are to be used within the EU, they will need to be released by a qualified person (QP).

Who is a qualified person?

This is a specific requirement to meet the EU Clinical Trials Directive and the future EU Clinical Trials Regulation. A person of appropriate qualifications and experience must carry out a review of batch documents and ensure quality control.

Considerations when choosing a manufacturing site

Geographical

It is important to think about where the supplies are destined for when determining a supply chain strategy. There will be limited options for the location of the manufacturing operation as this will have been determined earlier in the drug development process.

Phase of trial

The phase of the trial in question will have a fundamental effect on the sourcing considerations for the supplies as the manufacturing and packaging requirements will vary significantly through the development cycle. For early-phase studies, the material may not yet have been formulated so a process of filling active pharmaceutical ingredient (API) directly into capsule shells would be required. This process requires entirely different facilities and expertise to those required for large-scale blistering or bottling of materials for late-phase trials.

Nature of product

Many biotech products require very specialized manufacturing techniques. Thus, the decision on where to source clinical trial supplies may be a relatively simple one as there may be few facilities that have the necessary equipment and expertise required. The importance of the potential issues related to scale-up activities cannot be underestimated.

Manufacture of clinical trial supplies

This section outlines some of the considerations that need to be taken into account when deciding on a strategy for the manufacture of clinical trial supplies.

The nature of clinical trial materials

There are some particular challenges with the manufacture of IMPs. There may be additional risk to subjects participating in clinical trials as opposed to those taking licensed medication because there is often limited information available on the safety and efficacy of the medicinal product. The application of GMP to the manufacture of IMPs is intended to minimize the risk to trial participants and also to ensure consistency between batches of product. Procedures need to be both flexible to provide for potential changes as knowledge increases, and also appropriate to the stage of development of the product.

Many sponsor companies aim to meet GMP requirements by applying very tight specifications to the manufacturing process during early-phase trials. This may lead to issues during the scale-up process and can lead to the necessity to repeat some toxicology work, for example if the level of impurities increases.

Thus, the practical outcome is that detailed risk assessments need to be carried out at all stages of the process to ensure that sufficient controls are built into the system, but that these controls do not stifle development of the product.

Regulatory requirements

IMPs must be manufactured under GMP at an appropriately licensed facility and, as mentioned earlier, since the implementation of the EU Clinical Trials Directive in 2004, any IMPs that are destined for use in Europe must undergo QP release.

A QP is typically a member of the quality assurance department and is formally qualified to meet the requirements of the post. A QP takes *personal* responsibility for the quality of the clinical trial supplies that he or she releases and, should things go wrong, the QP could be held personally liable.

When carrying out a QP release of an IMP, the QP is looking for a number of assurances. Not only should the IMP and the API have been manufactured to GMP standards, but they should also have been manufactured in accordance with the details stated in the clinical trial application and the investigational medicinal product dossier. The QP will also expect to see a statement to the effect that there is no bovine spongiform encephalopathy/transmissible spongiform encephalopathy (BSE/TSE) risk associated with the materials.

Some of the data that the QP will be reviewing will relate to the analytical testing that has been carried out on the material so it is normal for the QP to audit the analytical laboratory if this is located outside of the EU.

One area that needs particular attention relates to sterile products. Within the EU, there is no difference between the standards of sterility required for commercial products or IMPs, but this is not necessarily the case in some non-EU areas where there can be an assumption that phase I studies do not require such a high standard.

Interestingly, there is a significant difference between the regulatory requirements for the manufacture of IMPs between the EU and the US. In the EU, all IMPs must be manufactured under GMP, but in the US there is a different approach taken.

The QP release for a batch of IMP is a three-stage process.

- The first stage involves issuing a QP declaration for inclusion in the sponsor's clinical trial application. This declaration will state that the site(s) of manufacture is compliant with GMP, but it does not refer to a specific batch of product.
- The second stage of the release will be that of the bulk batch of IMP following review of the manufacturing records that relate to the specific batch (there can be implications here if the manufacturing batch documents are written in the local language).
- The final part of the QP release process happens at the end of the packaging process.

Formulation

Eventually, an IMP will need to be formulated into a product that is easy and palatable for patients to take.

When considering the best formulation for a product, there are a wide range of issues that need to be taken into account. Some of the major ones include particle size distribution, crystal habit, polymorphism, dissolution rate, impurity profile, moisture content, and flow properties. In practice, the final formulation will normally be dictated by the physical and chemical characteristics of the API.

At every stage of development, full stability testing will be required in order to provide data to support a shelf-life for each different formulation.

Whilst it is true that the production process for an IMP can change during its development, it is expected that the dosage form will be fixed by phase 2B. By the time phase 3 is reached, it is vital that the trial uses the product in the planned formulation for the licensed product and is using the correct grade of excipients. The medication should ideally also be packaged in the primary materials planned for use in the commercial pack.

What is blinding?

Blinding methodologies

The majority of clinical trials are 'blinded' and this has a fundamental effect on the way in which clinical trial supplies are assembled. This section describes the concept of blinding and explains the consequences with respect to the production of clinical trial supplies.

Blinding explained

Clinical trials can be run in one of three ways (Table 17.1).

The reason for using a blinded study design is to avoid other factors potentially influencing the outcome of the trial. A couple of examples will help to explain this.

Table 17.1 Trial designs

Trial design	Description
Open-label	All medication is clearly identified.
Single-blind	Either the investigator or the patient (normally the patient) is unaware of which treatment is being taken.
Double-blind	Both the investigator and the patient are unaware of which treatment is being taken.

If the trial subject knew that he or she is taking the placebo treatment instead of an active drug, he or she would be disinclined to report that symptoms were diminishing, even if they were.

Conversely, an investigator may downplay the positive comments from a subject regarding his or her symptoms if the investigator knew that the subject in question was on the placebo arm of the trial.

For open-label trials, there are no particular considerations for manufacturing and packaging, but for single- or double-blind trials there are because it is essential that both the products and the packaging look absolutely identical in each arm of the trial. This issue is probably the most challenging of all those faced when producing clinical trial supplies.

Blinding products

The methodology used for blinding products will depend on the design of the trial. If a placebo is to be used, the challenge is to produce an inactive product which looks, tastes, and smells identical to the IMP. If a comparator is to be used, the challenge is to make a marketed commercial pharmaceutical product look like the IMP.

There are really only two ways to effectively blind products. One is to produce a matching placebo and the other is to over-encapsulate a product.

Manufacturing placebos

Manufacturers of an IMP will find arranging for the manufacture of a matching placebo (this could be tablets, vials, ointments, liquids, etc.) relatively easy, as long as the look, taste, and smell of the material is the same as the active product.

Academic institutions carrying out a trial on a commercially available product may find production of a placebo much more challenging. The manufacturer of the commercial product is not always willing to provide a placebo as it may have to stop production of the commercial product in order to manufacture the placebo. It is not as simple as subcontracting someone else to do this either; there are issues of copyright that make the manufacture of a matching placebo impossible without the express consent of the manufacturer of the active product.

The same is true for a competitor comparator as often, the comparator will need to be blinded against the trial own product which could look very different indeed. The best technique to overcome this will be dependent on the design of the trial. Sometimes, over-encapsulation is the best answer (Figure 17.1) but this only works for solid oral dose products. Another way of solving the problem is to have a 'double-dummy' study design in which

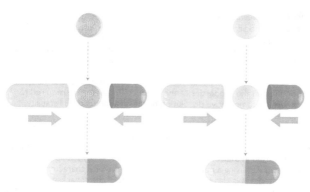

Figure 17.1 Over-encapsulation.

Table 17.2 'Double-dummy' study design

Dose group	Daily dose
Active A	Active A + Placebo B
Active B	Placebo A + Active B
Placebo	Placebo A + Placebo B

matching placebos are manufactured for each product and the subjects take an active or a placebo of each (Table 17.2).

Over-encapsulation

If you are lucky enough to be working with an oral solid dose product, the simplest way to produce a placebo and/or to blind against a comparator may well be over-encapsulation.

This relatively simple procedure results in the IMP and/or comparator being placed inside a hard gelatin capsule and it is then easy to make a matching placebo capsule (Figure 17.1).

There are a few considerations to bear in mind with this technique:
• The product must be small enough to fit inside a capsule.
• In order to ensure that the product doesn't rattle inside the capsule, it is normal to backfill the capsule with a powder such as lactose. Use the same powder to fill the placebo capsules.
• If the drug product is a large, heavy tablet, there could be a problem with a discernible weight difference. In these circumstances, the manufacturing process becomes more complex as a protocol would have to be developed which ensures that both the active and placebo capsules fall within a predefined weight range.
• Finally, the capsules could be opened by the subject and then all blinding would be in vain.

Analytical considerations

If placebo medication has been manufactured or products have been over-encapsulated, there are some significant analytical considerations.

- The placebo material is subject to the same stability testing as the active product. In addition, if the product is sterile, full sterility testing is also required.
- It is essential to ensure that the process of over-encapsulation has not affected the properties of the product. Processes are required to undertake comparative dissolution testing in addition to full stability studies.
- Active comparator testing may not be possible as it is difficult to gain access to the necessary analytical methods.
- The active comparator ideally needs the primary packaging be the same as that used in the commercial pack. This reduces any manipulation of the product having a negative impact on the physical characteristics of the material. It is also likely to limit the effect of the repackaging on the shelf-life of the product.

Blinding processes

Having managed to produce drug products that are blinded against each other using one of the methodologies described, it is important to ensure that no other processes unwittingly unblind the supplies. This section describes some of the potential pitfalls.

Packaging components

In almost all cases, bottles, cartons, labels, tamper seals, etc., will be used during the packaging process, and misuse of these could unblind the supplies as effectively as the product themselves. Manufacturers may make subtle changes to these components which, although they may make no difference to the specification, may be enough to unblind. For example, if a new mould is used for the production of a plastic bottle, the precise characteristics of the joints between the sections may be different enough for a diligent investigator to notice.

Another potentially challenging area is in the printing of labels. Each printer will have subtle variations in ink colour and 'weight' of the characters. It is therefore important that the same printer is used to print the labels for all arms of the trial.

Blinding checks should always be carried out on all packaging components before any packaging is commenced.

Packaging methodology

Having blinded the products and ensured that all packaging components are homogenous, there are still many ways in which the supplies for the trial can be unblinded during the packaging process.

The placement of labels on components and the way in which the components are assembled are critical to maintaining the blind.

In order to overcome issues such as this, it is normal to include photographs and/or dummy packs with the packaging instructions as well as to carry out detailed team briefings before any packaging is started. In addition, it is best to ensure that the same team packs the supplies for all arms of the trial if time lines and resources allow.

Distribution of blinded information

One final blinding consideration is the distribution of documentation that contains blinded information. There are three main types.

- The randomization list used to assign pack numbers to each of the treatment groups is the most sensitive information of all, and most companies have very strict policies for the management and dissemination this data.
- By default, the documentation used to record the packaging of clinical trial supplies will unblind any reviewer as the documentation will explicitly indicate which pack numbers were packed for each treatment group. Thus, it is critical that this documentation is only available to staff who have authority to view this level of detail.
- Finally, it is important to consider the documentation sent out to clinical trial sites with the supplies. For most companies, this documentation is produced automatically by their electronic inventory management system and this system will hold unblinded information. When setting up part numbers and descriptions in these systems, it is essential that consideration is given to where this information will be printed and to ensure that blinded descriptions are used where necessary.

Comparators, packaging, labelling documentation, and expiry date

This section concentrates on the issues surrounding the design of packaging and the packaging process itself.

Comparators

The blinding issues that the use of comparators raise have been discussed in detail in the preceding section, so it is assumed here that a suitable solution has been found and that the issue now is how to source and how to package the material.

Normally, a comparator that is going to be used is a product which is already marketed by a competitor and the purpose of the trial is to prove that the IMP is either more efficacious or safer than the competitor's product. It is worth remembering that the competitor therefore has a vested interest in you not being able to source this material!

In most cases, comparators are sourced through a third party so that the manufacturer does not know the final destination and the purpose for which the materials are being purchased. There are many wholesale dealers that have the necessary authorization to be able to purchase pharmaceutical products in this way. An alternative is to purchase material that is already available in the marketplace, but material is often only available from multiple sources, thus many different batches may be purchased. This can then make the packaging process very complex.

In any case, it is essential that the pedigree of the comparator is known and for this, a copy of the certificate of analysis is required. It is then possible to verify the nature of the product and the site of manufacture.

If a comparator is being used in an open-label trial for the indication for which it is approved for sale, the sole requirement is to attach a label to the existing pack which states the study number. It is important, however, that this label does not cover up any of the existing text. If a comparator is to be used in a blinded study and/or for a novel indication, the product must effectively be handled as if it was an IMP and all the labelling requirements discussed later in this section will apply.

Designing packaging

Drug administration

It is important to consider who will be administering the medication to the subjects.

In early trials, it is normal for the investigator to administer the medication in the controlled environment of a phase I unit or equivalent. In this case, the requirements for labelling in local languages (stated later in the chapter) may well be unnecessary and the issues relating to compliance become less critical.

The vast majority of medication taken during clinical trials is self-administered at home, however. It is therefore essential that consideration is given to how easy it is for the subject to understand what should be taken and when during the day the medication needs to be taken. If many subjects will need to take their medication to work, for example, it is important that the packs are as portable and discreet as possible.

Visit schedule

In most later-phase clinical trials, subjects will visit the clinic on a number of occasions for a consultation and to collect more medication. Thus, it is important that the supplies are packaged in such a way that each subject has enough medication to last between visits. It is also normal to provide a little more than subjects actually need just in case there is wastage or the next visit needs to be delayed for any reason. It might be tempting to give subjects all the medication at the first visit, but there are a couple of problems with this:

- If the trial runs over a number of years, it may not be possible to provide all the material at the start if the shelf-life of the product does not support this.
- If a subject decides to withdraw from the trial, all of the medication dispensed to him or her will be wasted.

It is good practice to package the supplies for each subject in a number of visit packs, which can be tailored to the duration of each inter-visit period (Figure 17.2).

Storage conditions

Increasingly, IMPs need specialized storage conditions and the percentage of refrigerated and frozen materials has grown significantly. If the product needs to be stored under conditions such as this, consideration needs to be given to both the packaging components and the size of the final package. For frozen supplies, for example, it is important to use labels that are

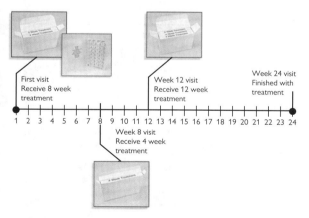

First visit
Receive 8 week
treatment

Week 12 visit
Receive 12 week
treatment

Week 24 visit
Finished with
treatment

1 2 3 4 5 6 7 8 9 10 11 12 13 14 15 16 17 18 19 20 21 22 23 24

Week 8 visit
Receive 4 week
treatment

Figure 17.2 Pack design for 24-week clinical trial.

resistant to moisture damage and that have adhesives that continue to function under these storage conditions. Many pharmacies have very limited facilities for storing refrigerated or frozen materials so bespoke storage may need to be provided or a carefully considered distribution policy adopted.

Compliance

The success of every single clinical trial hinges on the accurate consumption of medication by the subjects and the design of the clinical trial supplies can have a marked influence on this.

If the dosing schedule is very complex, providing medication in a calendar wallet may assist the subject far more than providing medication in a number of bottles (Figure 17.3).

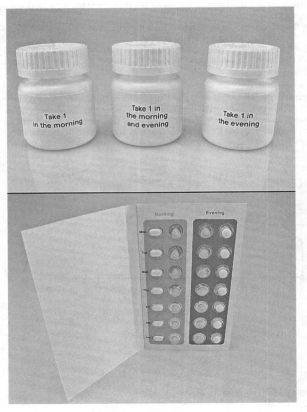

Figure 17.3 The different options of achieving compliance with a study drug.

Calendar wallets are not ideal in every situation, however. By using day names, they instantly become language-specific, but if day numbers are used instead, it is far more difficult for the subjects to determine whether or not they have taken their medication on a particular day. Finally, for long-term studies where there is a requirement to take multiple doses each day, the sheer size of the finished pack may make the use of wallets untenable.

At the end of the trial, the remaining packaging and medication is normally used to calculate compliance and to therefore validate the outcome. As mentioned earlier, it is common practice to give subjects a little more medication than they will actually use and then to base the compliance calculation on the amount that is left at the end of the dosing period. For instance, it would be logical to give a subject a bottle of 32 tablets for a four-week treatment period. Assuming that the subject returns exactly four weeks later, one would expect them to return the bottle with four tablets left in it. If there are more tablets left the inference is that the subject failed to take a tablet every day. If there are fewer, this would indicate that the subject has taken more tablets than he or she should have unless they can account for any wastage. Incidentally, the critical nature of accurate fill counts during packaging cannot be understated because of its crucial impact on the calculation of compliance.

Child resistance

In the US, it is a regulatory requirement to make all study medication child resistant and senior friendly if it is to be taken home by the trial subjects. Thus, bottles must have child-resistant caps and cartons and wallets must have specialized child-resistant features. There are many proprietary designs available so sourcing an appropriate solution is not difficult, but there are cost implications.

Overage

In almost all trials, there will be a requirement to package more material than is actually needed and, in some cases, this overage can be very significant indeed.

When calculating the required overage, a number of factors need to be taken into account.
- If the product has a relatively short shelf-life, it is likely that a proportion of the supplies will expire before they have been used.
- In any trial, a proportion of the subjects will withdraw before completion and this will lead to additional subjects being recruited to replace them.
- It is common practice to dispense a little more medication than required in order to ensure that subjects never run out of medication between visits.
- Finally and most significantly, the global distribution and the total number of trial sites will have a profound effect on the amount of overage required.

All sites will need to have a certain level of medication available whether or not they actually recruit any subjects into the trial, and there may also be a requirement to have a volume of medication available at regional depots to facilitate the timely distribution of material in some regions of the world. The necessary overage can ultimately be minimized by careful consideration of the final format of the clinical trial supplies.

The packaging process

The packaging of clinical trial supplies is a key element in any trial and one potentially fraught with peril. The risk of making mistakes is extremely high when active and placebo medication must look identical and when both need to be in the same room at the same time during the packaging process. Any mix-up of the medication can completely negate the results of the trial.

The packaging process is therefore designed to minimize risk and the two fundamental principles to ensure this are line clearance and segregation.

Before any packaging materials or products are brought into a room, it is essential to ensure that any materials left over from previous operations have been cleared away. This is particularly vital when moving between placebo and active products. This line clearance activity should be documented and then checked independently, normally by a member of the quality control team.

Once materials are received into the room, packaging components are dispensed and their storage containers closed before containers of drug product are opened in order to ensure that no drug product finds its way into boxes of components. Active and placebo drugs are never available in the same room in the same condition at the same time. For instance, if active and placebo tablets need to be dispensed into bottles before subject kits are made up containing both active and placebo supplies, the packaging would be carried in a carefully controlled manner.

1. Placebo product brought into room and dispensed into bottles.
2. Placebo bottles labelled.
3. Full reconciliation of components and line clearance carried out.
4. Active product brought into room and dispensed into bottles.
5. Active bottles labelled.
6. Full reconciliation of components and line clearance carried out.
7. Active and placebo bottles combined into subject kits.
8. Full reconciliation of components and line clearance carried out.

In some cases, post-pack ID testing is carried out to ensure that the correct materials have been packed. In this case, an independent analytical laboratory would be given sample packs from each arm of the trial in a blinded fashion and be asked to determine the nature of the contents.

Recent trends in packaging processes

There are a few recent initiatives which are starting to have a significant effect on the way in which clinical trial supplies are produced.

- The first of these is the concept of an 'adaptive trial' in which the trial design is altered as the trial runs.

For example, it may be that lower dose treatment groups are dropped if the doses in question are found not to be efficacious in the early part of the trial. These treatment groups may then be replaced with higher doses than originally planned if the drug is better tolerated than expected. In a case such as this, bespoke trial supplies would need to be packed at short notice for each new phase of the trial.

- The second initiative is 'just-in-time' labelling and this is implemented for a number of reasons. The first relates to the potential move away from multi-language booklet labels, and the second relates to minimizing

the overage of supplies that are required by only labelling once subjects have been enrolled.
- The third initiative is 'protocol pooling' where supplies destined for use in a number of different protocols are produced in one batch. The supplies are either labelled with a number of different protocol numbers and their dispatch managed through an IVRS (interactive voice-response system) system, or the 'just-in-time' labelling concept is used to add the protocol number at the point of dispatch.

The process has to be submitted and reviewed by the relevant regulatory authorities and agreement from site personnel must be sought before this process should be considered, however.

Releasing clinical trial supplies

Once the supplies have been packaged, they will need to undergo a final release before being available for dispatch. In the EU, this will be carried out by a QP, whilst in the rest of the world this will be carried out by a member of the quality assurance team. In essence, any releasing individual will be looking for the same thing: are the supplies fit for purpose?

When carrying out this release, the releasing individual will typically review the entire process and will look for the following:
- Were the supplies manufactured under GMP conditions?
- Is there stability data to support the given expiry date?
- Were the supplies packed under GMP conditions?
- Were there any deviations during either the manufacturing or the packaging operations which would shed doubt on the quality of the product?
- Do the supplies match the details specified in the IMPD (investigational medicinal product dossier), the CTA (clinical trial application), and the trial protocol?
- Does the sponsor have both regulatory and ethics approval for the trial in the country/site for which the supplies are being released?

Labelling regulations

Following the implementation of the EU Clinical Trials Directive (2001/20/EC) in 2004, the information required on clinical trial supplies labels for material to be distributed within Europe should be straightforward as the details are described in Annex 13 of the EU Guide to GMP ('Rules and Guidance for Pharmaceutical Manufacturers and Distributors', otherwise known as the Orange Guide) and referenced in the Directive (Table 17.3).

Some countries have additional requirements. For example, the EudraCT number must be included on the labels of any material destined for use in Germany, despite this requirement not being defined in the Annex.

In most circumstances, all the information detailed in Table 17.3 should be included on the labels attached to both the primary and secondary packaging.

There is also a comment in the Annex that states that some information can be omitted if its absence can be justified, for example by the use of a centralized electronic randomization system (IVRS). Indeed, there is a growing movement to omit the expiry date from clinical trial supplies in studies that are managed by an IVRS in order to avoid having to over-label

Table 17.3 Annex 13: labelling requirements

1. The name, address, and telephone number of the sponsor, CRO, or investigator.

2. The pharmaceutical dosage form, route of administration, quantity of dosage units, and, in open-label trials, the name/identifier and strength/potency.

3. The batch and/or code number.

4. The trial reference code allowing identification of the trial, site, investigator, and sponsor, if not given elsewhere.

5. The trial subject identification number or treatment number and, where relevant, the visit number.

6. The name of the investigator (if not given at 1 or 4).

7. The directions for use (but the label can reference a leaflet or other document).

8. 'For clinical trial use only' or similar wording.

9. The storage conditions.

10. The period of use (use-by date, expiry date, or retest date as applicable), in a month/year format that avoids ambiguity.

11. 'Keep out of reach of children' except when the product is for use in trials where the product is not taken home by subjects.

the supplies when the expiry date is updated. Most of the European regulatory authorities are now looking on this practice favourably, but there is still reluctance from some pharmacists to have undated material in their pharmacy.

Finally, the requirement in Europe is that the supplies should be labelled in the official language(s) of the country in which the IMP is to be used. In practice, this normally results in the use of multi-language booklet labels although this approach is currently being challenged by some regulatory authorities as they do not consider that booklet labels present the necessary data to trial subjects in a user-friendly manner.

For supplies destined for outside of Europe, the labelling requirements of Annex 13 will normally cover all contingencies. There are regional variations, however. For example, there is no requirement to put the expiry date on supplies for use in the US.

As regulatory requirements change with time and interpretations differ between organizations, best practice dictates that label text should be assessed for compliance locally in each country before any packaging commences.

Production of labels

The production of labels needs to be carried out with as much diligence as the packaging. The same issues of line clearance and segregation apply along with the wider implications of GMP.

As with packaging, labels will be produced for each arm of the trial separately. This necessitates producing 'splits' of the randomization so that each set of labels can be printed separately. This process needs careful control and checking.

Once the labels have been printed, they need to be checked for both quality and content and, on a large trial, each printing run could result in tens of thousands of labels.

At all points in the process (and during packaging), printed materials must be reconciled to 100% in order to ensure that each pack has the requisite number of labels applied. In the event of damage to a label, the reprinting process needs to be controlled in a similarly robust fashion.

Printed labels are typically stored under lock and key and are only issued to the packaging room by a member of the quality assurance department.

Packaging documentation

GMP dictates that, 'if it wasn't written down, it didn't happen'. Thus, every step of the process is recorded in precise detail and all activities signed for by the individual(s) that carried them out.

The design of the documentation should be such that the following sorts of questions can be answered easily:

- When was the packaging carried out, in which facility and by which individuals?
- Who carried out all the necessary in-process checks and what were the results of these tests?
- In which packs was IMP batch 'ABC' used?
- What were the environmental conditions during the packaging process?
- Were all the pre-printed components fully accounted for?
- Did anything unplanned happen during the packaging process (i.e. were there any deviations)?
- Which pack numbers were produced for each arm of the trial (and do these match the study randomization)?

The data contained in the packaging documentation provides essential evidence that the supplies are fit for purpose during the official release process and the documentation therefore becomes an important part of the source data for the trial. Packaging documentation should be archived under the same conditions as all source data as described in ICH GCP.

Expiry date

In Europe (though not in the US) it is a requirement to have the expiry or retest date printed on clinical trial supplies. Drugs under development have limited stability data available at the time of packaging. Thus, at the beginning of a trial there may only be enough data to support a 6-month shelf-life but, during the course of the study, further data becomes available to support an extension to a 12-month shelf-life.

In this case, the supplies will need to have their expiry date information updated and they will then need to be re-released. Expiry updating needs to be carried out under GMP conditions and documented accordingly. If supplies have already been shipped to clinical trial sites, the labels and the supporting documentation will need to be supplied to a suitably qualified individual (normally a pharmacist). This documentation will need to be completed and returned to the releasing site as evidence that the activity was carried out effectively before a new release is made available.

In Europe, there are rules as to how this activity is carried out. A label with the new expiry date and the original batch number is normally applied to the pack in such a way as to obscure the original expiry date but not the batch number, although it is also possible to apply a new label which does not obscure any of the original data. This latter approach can cause confusion however, as the old expiry date will still be visible. Typically, photographs of the updated packs would be required as proof that this requirement has been met accurately.

Dispatch of supplies

Traditionally, there has been far more emphasis on the manufacturing and packaging of clinical trial supplies than there has been on the distribution. With the advent of more and more temperature-sensitive supplies and the location of clinical trial sites in ever more exotic locations, distribution strategies need to be discussed in far greater detail earlier in the process.

Distribution strategy

This section discusses some of the issues to consider when planning the distribution strategy for the trial. Many of these issues are more relevant to later-phase trials, but some should be taken into consideration for even early-phase studies.

Nature of product

The nature of the product will have a fundamental influence on the distribution strategy that will work best. Some compounds are classified as dangerous goods and there are significant regulatory requirements which need to be considered when shipping these globally, particularly in large volumes. In addition, if a controlled drug is being used, there are also limitations on what can ship where and the mechanisms by which the shipments should be made.

By far the biggest influencing factor is the storage and therefore shipping conditions of the product, however. If a product needs to have its temperature maintained within certain limits, the entire supply chain needs to be planned extremely carefully.

The majority of products in clinical development are ambient which, in reality, normally means that their temperature should be kept between 15°C and 30°C. Traditionally, these supplies have been shipped in simple cardboard boxes with no effort made to either control or even monitor temperature, but it is not unusual for these supplies to be exposed to significant extremes of temperature. A box left on a runway in the Middle East in the summer can easily reach 50–60°C. Industry is taking a more responsible attitude and a risk assessment of the planned supply routes is a common approach now even if full temperature control and monitoring is still unusual.

For refrigerated or frozen products, fully controlled cold-chain shipments are essential and there are a number of options.

- For intra-continental shipments of relatively large volumes, the use of a temperature-controlled vehicle is advised, as temperatures will be maintained regardless of the external environmental conditions.
- For smaller shipments or for shipments over greater distances, self-contained temperature controlled and monitored modules are available that work off mains power and hold several pallets' worth of materials. This is an expensive solution however, with each unit costing several thousand pounds to hire for each shipment.
- A common solution to cold-chain shipments is the use of validated insulated shipping systems. These vary in sizes from one which could contain individual vials, to those that can handle full pallets. These systems work with the use of 'gel packs' which are packed into the

shippers. The packs need to be conditioned at specific temperatures before use, and it is important that this is done correctly in order to ensure that the temperature is maintained between the pre-determined limits.

Most systems are validated generally for a period of three to five days and, although this is long enough for many shipments, it will not allow for issues with the supply chain such as customs delays. It is therefore recommended that specialist courier companies are used for cold-chain shipments as they have the capability to replenish gel packs for shipments that have been held up at any point during transit.

Whichever system is used, it is essential that all cold-chain shipments are temperature monitored as well as temperature controlled and there are a range of devices available to do this. The device should monitor temperatures continuously and have a maximum recording period somewhat longer than the worst-case transit time. It is useful to use a device so that alarms can be set if the temperature exceeds pre-determined limits at any point.

If an excursion occurs, it may not mean the loss of the affected material. Many cold-chain products have permitted excursions to particular temperatures for a particular period of time. The QP will wish to review excursion information in order to be assured that the supplies are still fit for purpose.

Finally, clinical trial sites may have limited storage space for materials that need particular environmental conditions. This holds true for the conditions in subjects' homes. It will be possible to insist that trial sites use calibrated and monitored storage units, but all level of control over the storage conditions of the materials are lost as soon as the subject leaves the clinic.

Use of IVRS

If an IVRS is to be used to manage the randomization aspects of a trial, it will also be a very useful tool in managing the distribution of supplies. Typically, trials being run in conjunction with an IVRS require less overage of materials as supplies can be assigned to subjects centrally and re-order levels can be set relatively low. This benefit needs to be carefully weighed up against the significant costs and time that it takes to specify, configure, and validate a system however. In practical terms, it really only makes sense to use an IVRS on larger later-phase trials.

Destination countries

The shift in research to Eastern Europe, South America, Asia, and, increasingly, Africa and the Middle East, presents a range of issues. The infrastructure in many of these emerging areas is weak and there can be a naivety over what is required to supply clinical trial sites effectively. When shipping supplies to these regions, it is highly recommended that a specialist courier company is used who understands the local regulations.

These regulations will also have a significant impact on your distribution strategy. In some countries (Russia, for example) an import licence is needed every time you wish to ship supplies into the country. These take several weeks to be granted. In view of this, the alternative is to ship enough supplies to support all of the expected recruitment into the country in one go (with one import licence), and then arrange for local storage and distribution. There are a number of companies that now have depots set up in strategic locations which can support such a localized strategy.

Volume of supplies available

In a perfect world, each trial would have a significant overage of supplies available so that there is never the possibility of not being able to enrol a subject due to a lack of medication. In practice though, all trials have limited medication and, in some cases, this can be extreme. In such circumstances, the best strategy is to keep the vast majority of supplies in a central location and then ship on a subject-by-subject, visit-by-visit basis. This is time consuming and expensive, but this strategy does ensure that the majority of the available supplies are actually used by subjects as opposed to being destroyed because they have reached their expiry date before being able to be dispensed.

Site shipments

When planning site shipments, it is important to ensure that exact delivery details are known to site staff and that they understand the timelines involved. This ensures that:

• there is someone at the site to accept the delivery.
• the supplies reach the specific recipient in a timely fashion and do not sit for an extended length of time in a non-temperature-controlled reception area.

Best practice dictates that the investigator or pharmacist can confirm delivery (including an assessment of the quality of the supplies that have arrived).

• In addition to planning the timing of the shipments carefully, it is important to consider the amount of storage space that each site has available (this is particularly important for cold-chain products) and adjust the shipment strategy accordingly.
• If you are sending temperature recorders with a shipment, the site staff will need detailed instructions relating to how to manage the units and what to do in the event of a problem.

Depot shipments

If depots are to be used, it will be necessary to ship potentially large volumes of product to each one on several occasions and this can be a high-risk strategy. Losing a single subject pack during shipping due to damage or a temperature excursion is frustrating, but not critical. The same cannot be said for the loss of a substantial volume of material.

It is therefore important to plan the logistics of these shipments carefully and a higher level than normal of temperature control would typically be used. The use of a specialist courier can again help to ease the shipment through customs and any other local regulations.

For very high-value products or particularly challenging regions of the world, it is well worth considering splitting the shipment into a number of smaller ones even though this will be a more costly strategy.

Redistribution of supplies

No matter how carefully the distribution strategy is planned, there will be occasions on which supplies are in the wrong location. If redistribution between sites is to occur, it is essential to confirm that:

- the supplies have been stored appropriately at the original location (requiring temperature data to support this)
- the shipments between sites should be managed to the same degree as the initial shipments with temperature control and/or monitoring.
- any relabelling of supplies is done in a licensed facility under GMP conditions; the supplies would then need to be re-released before use.

Finally, the concept of site-to-site shipments of supplies is generally frowned upon but in general almost all sponsor companies have an SOP to address this. If the process is well controlled and documented, all will be well, but should only be considered in exceptional circumstances.

Disposal of supplies

This section describes the process for reconciling and disposing of left-over clinical trial supplies at the end of a study.

Reconciliation

As mentioned earlier, the reconciliation of the left-over medication at the end of the trial is normally used to determine compliance. Thus, this is a very important activity.

Reconciliation of drug supplies is normally a task that is carried out by the study monitors during their regular site visits. The process is to compare the site dispensing lists with the physical materials that the subjects have returned on their clinic visits. Although it is impossible to tell whether or not a subject actually ingested the medication, it is common practice to assume that any missing medication has indeed been taken as directed.

Once the supplies have been fully reconciled at site, they can either be destroyed locally or returned to the company that is managing the storage and distribution for the trial.

Return of supplies

It is not always possible to arrange for supplies to be sent back to their origins as export restrictions apply in some countries. In these cases, it will either be necessary for the sites to destroy the materials themselves or for a central facility to be found in that country to carry out this process (most regional depots will perform this service).

Returning supplies to a central location is preferable for reasons of both efficiency and control, if this option is available. Very often, the company managing the storage and distribution will arrange for the supplies to be collected and will also provide any necessary packaging materials to the site.

Assuming that the supplies are destined for destruction, it is not necessary to ship them under any temperature control. If there is a possibility that any unused kits could be re-labelled and used in the future, the same level of control used in the original shipments should be employed over the return shipments.

Once the supplies reach the central location, a further reconciliation operation is normally carried out. This generally comprises two levels of checks. Either the facility simply confirms that the correct number of outer boxes has been received from each trial site, or the outer boxes are opened and their contents (down to patient packs) are checked against the supplied packing lists.

Destruction

Destruction of supplies is normally carried out by high-temperature incineration at an appropriately licensed facility. In the case of controlled drugs, a witnessed burn is normally carried out in which a designated individual witnesses the destruction and formally signs this off.

In most cases, supplies will be retained until the final study report has been issued, just in case the results of the trial are not as expected and analysis of the returned material is required. This can of course mean that returned material needs to be retained for several years before destruction in a late-phase trial.

Once written permission is given by the sponsor, its destruction can be carried out and a certificate of destruction produced. The issuance of this certificate denotes the end of the clinical trials supplies process.

Further reading

Eudralex Volume 4 of 'The rules governing medicinal products in the European Union' contains guidance for the interpretation of the principles and guidelines of good manufacturing practices for medicinal products for human and veterinary use laid down in Commission Directives 91/356/EEC, as amended by Directive 2003/94/EC.

Eudralex Volume 4 of 'The rules governing medicinal products in the European Union' Annex 13 (referred to as the Orange Guide). ℘ http://ec.europa.eu/health/documents/eudralex/vol-4/index_en.htm

Directive 2001/20/EC of the European Parliament and of the Council of 4 April 2001 on the approximation of the laws, regulations and administrative provisions of the Member States relating to the implementation of good clinical practice in the conduct of clinical trials on medicinal products for human use.

FDA Guidance for industry 'Container Closure Systems for Packaging Human Drugs and Biologics' 1999 and Code of Federal Regulations title 16 part 1700.20. ℘ www.fda.gov

IMP accountability

Why is drug accountability needed?

Throughout the clinical trials process it is essential to be able to determine whether the protocol and GCP have been followed, that patient safety has not been put at risk, and that the integrity of the trial has been maintained. Key to achieving this are the records associated with study drug disposition, which show that the drug:

- has been labelled according to the regulations
- has been stored in conditions to keep it stable
- has been prepared and administered according to the protocol
- has been administered to the correct subjects
- has not been used outside the protocol
- has been documented and explained if used incorrectly
- has been destroyed if unused

ICH GCP 4.6.1 states that responsibility for investigational product accountability at the trial sites rests with the investigator/institution. Where allowed, the investigator (institution) may assign some or all of the duties for investigational product accountability to an appropriate pharmacist or another appropriate individual who is under the supervision of the investigator (institution).

Section 6.4.1 states that the clinical trial protocol should include in trial design, 'accountability procedures for the investigational product(s), including the placebo(s) and comparator(s), if any'.

The recommendation on the content of the trial master file and archiving describes the documentation that needs to be in place before, during, and after the clinical trial. Instructions for handling investigational products, shipping records, certificates of analysis (or in the EU, batch records released by the qualified person (QP)), unblinding procedures, and site accountability should be present at both the investigator site and sponsor. Destruction records should be held by the sponsor and also by the investigator site if the drug is destroyed at site. Sample labels and treatment allocation and decoding documentation are held only by the sponsor (Table 18.1).

The Clinical Trial Directive 2001/20/EC and the Clinical Trial Regulation 536/2014 do not refer specifically to investigational product accountability, and the only references in the GCP Directive 2005/28/EC are in Article 13b which requires IMP to be disposed of only in accordance with the legislation of the member state concerned; and Article 13f, which requires compliance with the principles and guidelines of good medical practice (GMP).

The GMP Directive, Annex 13, states: '12. Packaging Instructions. Investigational medicinal products are normally packed in an individual way for each subject included in the clinical trial. The number of units to be packaged should be specified prior to the start of the packaging operations, including units necessary for carrying out quality control and any retention samples to be kept. Sufficient reconciliations should take place to ensure the correct quantity of each product required has been accounted for at each stage of processing'.

It also states: '54. The delivered, used and recovered quantities of product should be recorded, reconciled and verified by or on behalf of the sponsor for each trial site and each trial period. Destruction of unused

Table 18.1 ICH GCP Requirements for IMP Documentation

ICH GCP reference	Title of Document	Purpose	Located in Files of: Investigator	Located in Files of: Sponsor
8.2.13	Sample of Label(s) attached to Investigational Product Container(s)	To document compliance with applicable labelling regulations and appropriateness of instructions provided to the subjects		×
8.2.14	Instructions for handling of investigational product(s) and trial-related materials (if not included in protocol or investigator's brochure)	To document instructions needed to ensure proper storage, packaging, dispensing and disposition of investigational products and trial-related materials	×	×
8.2.15	Shipping records for investigational product(s) and trial-related materials	To document shipment dates, and batch numbers and method of shipment of investigational product(s) and trial-related materials. Allows tracking of product batch, review of shipping conditions, and accountability	×	×
8.2.16	Certificate(s) of analysis of investigational product(s) shipped	To document identity, purity, and strength of investigational product(s) to be used in the trial	×	×

(continued)

Table 18.1 (Contd.)

ICH GCP reference	Title of Document	Purpose	Located in Files of:	
			Investigator	Sponsor
8.2.17	Decoding procedures for blinded trials	To document how, in case of an emergency, identity of blinded investigational product can be revealed without breaking the blind for the remaining subjects' treatment	x	x (third party if applicable)
8.2.18	Master randomization list	To document method for randomization of trial population		x (third party if applicable)
8.3.11	Relevant communications other than site visits (letters, meeting notes, notes of telephone calls)	To document any agreements or significant discussions regarding trial administration, protocol violations, trial conduct, adverse event reporting	x	x
8.3.13	Source documents	To document the existence of the subject and substantiate integrity of trial data collected. To include original documents related to the trial, to medical treatment, and history of subject	x	

8.3.23	In traditional products accountability at the site	To document that investigational product(s) have been used according to the protocol. To document the final accounting of investigational product received at the site, dispensed to subjects, returned by the subjects, and returned to sponsor.		X
8.4.2	Documentation of investigational product destruction	To document destruction of unused investigational products by sponsor or at the site	X (if destroyed at site)	X
8.4.6	Treatment allocation and decoding documentation	Returned to sponsor to document any decoding that may have occurred		X

investigational medicinal products should be carried out for a given trial site or a given trial period only after any discrepancies have been investigated and satisfactorily explained and the reconciliation has been accepted. Recording of destruction operations should be carried out in such a manner that all operations may be accounted for. The records should be kept by the Sponsor'.

Guidance on the level of accountability required for non-investigational medicinal products used in clinical trials is provided in Guidance on Investigational Medicinal Products (IMPs) and 'non investigational medicinal products' (NIMPs). This states that 'traceability of medicinal products which allows adequate reconstruction of NIMP movements and administration should be ensured taking into account the purpose of the trial and trial subjects' safety. [A trial] has at least to include a procedure to record which patients received which NIMPs during the trial with an evaluation of the compliance, where necessary.'

Note: with the implementation of the EU Regulation 536/2014 NIMPs will be referred to as auxiliary medicinal products.

What does IMP accountability involve?

Where are the records kept?

At the investigator site, the records should be kept as part of the investigator site file (ISF) (investigator trial master file, or TMF). Often the records are held by the pharmacist in a separate 'pharmacy file' or 'pharmacy manual' which is a subset of the ISF/TMF. At the end of the study the pharmacy records should be archived with the other investigator site file records.

It is important to keep the records up-to-date and well organized. This makes things easier for recording new information, checking and monitoring data, helps to prevent errors, and facilitates prompt action on an emergency or recall.

The sponsor accountability records should be kept in the sponsor TMF. If some of the records are held by the manufacturer, there should be a note in the TMF indicating where the records are held and by whom.

What needs to be accounted for?

In simplest terms, all records associated with the disposition of IMPs once they have been released for use at a trial site until the IMP is destroyed should be viewed as accountability records. This includes records for unlicensed IMP, any marketed authorized products used as IMPs, comparators, or adjuvant therapy.

If the pharmacy provides the IMP on prescription from the investigator, a full record of accountability must still be maintained at the investigator site with summary evidence also held at the sponsor site.

For NIMPs, the sponsor should determine the level of documentation required based on the study design, the nature and function of the NIMP, and the regulatory requirement to record at minimum which patients received which NIMPs, with an evaluation of compliance. In this context, where the term 'IMP' or 'drug' has been used in this chapter, the requirement might also apply to a NIMP.

Labelling records

Labelling records for the most part are classed as GMP records (please refer to Chapter 17 for details).

Records of the labelling process need to be kept with the GMP manufacturing and packaging records and batch release records. However, GCP requires a copy of the labels attached to drug to be filed in the sponsor's TMF.

Patient alert cards, distributed to patients for them to carry at all times in the event of an emergency, are classed as labels (GMP Directive, Annex 13). These may be held by the investigator for distribution to clinical trial subjects, but a copy should be retained in the investigator site file.

Delivery and transportation

When IMP is transported from one location to another, the details of transportation must be recorded, to document that what leaves one location arrives at its destination on time and intact, and that throughout the journey, the required storage conditions have been maintained. Therefore, for the purposes of accountability the shipment documents accompanying the drug should contain the following:

- Identity of each product being shipped (name, batch number)
- Exact quantity of each batch of product
- Date and time of shipping
- Required storage temperature during shipping
- Required storage temperature on receipt
- Name, signature, date, and contact details of person responsible for shipping
- Destination address, with a named recipient
- Name, signature, date (and preferably time) of person receiving the shipment

If there is any risk of a digression in the required storage conditions for the product during transportation (even if only over a short distance), that could have an impact on product stability, there should also be a temperature-recording device included with the product shipment and/or the packaging should be such that the required product storage conditions are guaranteed not to be breached. Records of any tests to validate the shipment temperature control should be filed in the sponsor's TMF.

In addition to the investigational medicinal product, GMP Annex 13 item 45 requires that for blinded studies the decoding method must be made available to the responsible personnel (i.e. the delegated person at the investigator site) before the drug is shipped to the site. In some cases, the decoding method is provided with the drug shipment (e.g. a scratch-off label attached as part of the drug labelling). In others, blind-break envelopes or access to an interactive voice response system (IVRS) with a decoding facility are provided.

If the IMP is transported over a short distance (e.g. within a site between the pharmacy and a clinic where the IMP will be administered), consideration should be given to the transportation method and conditions, IMP storage requirements, and stability data. If there is any risk that the IMP could exceed the limits of the recommended storage conditions before reaching its destination or before administration to the subject, then precautions should be taken to ensure the integrity of the product. Transportation records should be kept showing the dates and times of transport and receipt.

Receipt

Ideally, the sponsor will arrange for a receipt form to be included in the shipment, or may provide an IVRS for acknowledging safe receipt of the drug. Either way, the drug receipt records need to show the following, and this information should be kept both at the investigator site and by the sponsor:

- Identity of each product received (name, batch number)
- Exact quantity of each batch of product received
- Date and time of receipt
- Condition of receipt (intact, damaged, storage conditions complied with)
- Name, signature, date, and contact details of person receiving the shipment

There should be evidence (e.g. a receipt form) in the investigator site file that the decoding method was provided to the site before or at the time of drug receipt (unless the decoding method is incorporated into the label) (Figure 18.1).

Example Drug Receipt Form

Date received	Drug name/ description	Details (boxes, vials, etc)	Dose form	Strength	Batch No	Expiry Date	Number received	Received by (initials)	Checked by (initials)	Received intact and storage conditions correct (Yes/No)*

* If drug is not received intact or storage conditions are not correct provide details and action taken:

Details:

Action taken:

Name: Signature: Date:

          Signature: Date:

Storage location:

Figure 18.1 Example drug receipt form.

If a randomization list has been provided to the pharmacy, its receipt should also be recorded.

If the pharmacy provides the IMP on prescription from the investigator, there should be records in the investigator site file of the clinical trial related goods being received at the site.

Storage records

Storage location

It is good practice to keep a record (inventory) of where IMP is stored. If there is a problem with a storage area (e.g. refrigerator breakdown), it is then easy to tell which IMP may have been affected.

Records of quarantine

It is important to record when IMP is stored or moved into and out of quarantine. This provides evidence that quarantined IMP has been kept segregated from released products and has been unavailable for use.

Temperature monitoring

Temperature monitoring is critical to good storage and management of IMP. Each medicinal product is labelled with a required storage temperature, determined by stability testing. If the storage temperature limits are exceeded, the stability of the product could be impaired; therefore the storage temperature must be monitored and recorded throughout the study. This applies just as much to ambient storage as to refrigerated and frozen storage.

The simplest form of temperature monitoring is to use a maximum/minimum thermometer to record the temperature of the storage area, preferably at least twice a day. The record should contain the following:
- Identification of the storage area
- Date
- Minimum temperature
- Maximum temperature
- Signature or initials of person recording the temperature

A common mistake is only to record the actual temperature at the time the measurement is taken (rather than the maximum and minimum). This is insufficient as a temperature excursion could be missed at a different time of day and it will be not possible to tell how long the temperature has been out of range.

There should be calibration records of temperature monitors. In the UK, the Medicines and Healthcare products Regulatory Agency (MHRA) expects traceability in the calibration records to national standards (e.g. a 'reference thermometer' annually certified and traceable to national standards).

Some pharmacies have electronic temperature-monitoring systems that monitor ambient, refrigerator, and freezer temperatures (and sometimes humidity of ambient storage), linked to a central alarm system and often to a computer server for storage of records. The validation and maintenance records of such systems should be maintained and available for auditing and monitoring. A copy of relevant records should be filed in the investigator site file to show whether and when the IMP storage temperature has gone out of range during the course of the study.

Other environmental storage records/requirements

The most common storage requirement is temperature control. However, some products are sensitive to light or humidity, and in this case these storage conditions must also be managed, monitored, and recorded. Recording protection from light might be a simple statement as to how this is achieved, or might involve recording the time period of light exposure during IMP preparation, transport, or administration.

Practicalities if drug is self-administered by patients

If drug will be self-administered by patients, it is generally impractical to ask subjects to record the storage temperature. If temperature management is critical, consideration should be given when designing packaging as to whether a device can be included to record temperature or detect an excursion. However, it may be necessary to rely on the subject informing the investigator staff if the drug has been exposed to an extreme temperature.

Management of excursions

If the storage temperature or environmental limits have been exceeded, the sponsor should be notified immediately and their advice sought on management of the IMP. IMP that has exceeded its storage limits should not be used without direction from the sponsor, as the stability of the product may have been affected, impacting its effectiveness or safety. Records of the excursion, communication with the sponsor, action taken, and confirmation of continued stability, where applicable, should all be retained with the drug accountability records. Urgent replacement of IMP may be required.

In some cases a sponsor may provide guidance in advance about the degree of excursion that can occur (range of tolerance) without affecting the stability or safety of the product.

Inventories (drug accountability records)

The record that people most often think of as a 'drug accountability record' is basically an inventory of drug distribution at the site. The level of complexity of inventories depends on the nature of the product and the design of the study. Records for single-use vials will usually be simpler than for multiple-dose products taken over a period of time. Records should be maintained in the investigator site file and may include the following:
- Product name, batch number
- Quantity received, date
- Quantity dispensed, date
- Kit or box number (if applicable)
- Subject number
- Signatures (initials of person dispensing and checker if required)
- Quantity remaining
- Quantity returned (used/unused)
- Totals (used, unused)
- Signatures (initials of person receiving and recording returns)

Many sponsor companies have standard inventory forms for drug accountability (Figure 18.2) which are customized for different studies and products.

EXAMPLE DRUG ACCOUNTABILITY FORM

Protocol No: ....   Site No: ....   Investigator: ....

Drug Name	Batch number	Receipt date	Number received/ remaining	Dispensed to subject number	Dispensing occasion (Visit)	Date dispensed	Number dispensed	Pharmacist's initials and date	Checked initials and date	Date returned to pharmacy (if applicable)	Number used	Pharmacist's initials and date

Figure 18.2 Example accountability form.

Care should be taken when designing inventories as it is very easy to design a form that does not record enough or the appropriate information, and often this is not discovered until after the start of the trial. After designing a form, try to complete it with the drug packaging, dispensing, and returns records in mind.

All drug quantities must be accounted for. If some has gone missing or has not been returned by the subject, this must be documented and explained.

Preparation, dispensing, and administration

Dosing instructions

The protocol may provide sufficient dosing instructions. However, commonly separate instructions are provided which give more extensive details. When created, these should be quality-control checked (QC'd) to confirm the accuracy and ensure there are no instructions that conflict with the details in the protocol.

IVRS records

IVRS systems are often used for drug management, most commonly for controlling and recording shipping and receipt of IMP. However, they are also sometimes used for complex dose calculations where the investigator or pharmacist dials into the system and provides the current data on the subject and the IVRS system calculates the dose. It is critical that the system is fully validated and that the sponsor has a copy of the validation records and user-acceptance test records, as well as the calculated doses. Any changes in the programming, however small, should be re-tested to confirm that the calculations have not been affected and the system continues to work within required specifications.

Preparation records

If there are preparation steps for IMP, such as dilution or dissolution, these steps should be recorded and preferably checked and countersigned by a second person. It is not uncommon for dosing errors to occur due to the wrong vial of drug being selected or a measurement being misread. A second check at this stage can avert a potentially serious and dangerous mistake, especially for intravenous (IV) preparations.

Randomization records

If randomization is done during dispensing or dose preparation, clear records should be retained, including instructions on how the randomization has been implemented and any QC steps taken to ensure accuracy.

Dispensing records

IMP might be dispensed from the pharmacy directly to the clinical trial subject, from the investigator to the subject (if there is no pharmacy involved), or from the pharmacy to the clinic for administration to the subject by the investigational staff. In the latter case there should be a further record documenting that the dose was administered or dispensed.

Where IMP is provided on prescription from a local or community pharmacy, the batch numbers dispensed to each patient should be documented wherever possible.

Dosing records

Dosing records should document the subject number, date, and (usually) time of dosing and the dose administered. For IV drugs, the start and stop time is usually also recorded.

If subjects self-administer the drug, it is difficult to ensure accurate recording. Some sponsors ask subjects to complete diary cards or worksheets, although often these can be inaccurate or incomplete. For oral products, other sponsors invest in dispensing devices that incorporate a dispensing counter. Other options for patient-activated dosing records include Internet-based forms and phone text services. If individual dosing records are not completed, it may be necessary to rely on the dispensing and returns records to determine assumed compliance.

Compliance

In designing drug accountability records, it is essential to think about what level of compliance can and needs to be measured in order to be able to confirm whether study subjects received the correct dose, in compliance with the protocol throughout the study.

Errors and explanations in accountability

If an error is made in accountability records, that data should be corrected in accordance with ICH GCP-compliant data correction practices, striking a single line through the incorrect data, writing the correct data next to it, signing, dating, and providing a reason for the error. If accountability records have been included in an electronic CRF (eCRF), the system should prompt for an explanation of the change.

If the error is only in the documentation, there may be no further action required, but if the records have been transcribed elsewhere, changes will need to be followed through to all locations.

Management of dosing errors

A dosing error is another matter. Any dosing error presents a potential safety risk to the subject and could risk the integrity of the trial data either for the subject or the trial as a whole. The following actions are required at minimum:

- Check details of the error and confirm or manage subject safety
- Report the error immediately to the investigator and the sponsor
- Record the error in the source records with an explanation
- Establish the root cause, take corrective action, and where applicable, implement actions to prevent a recurrence

Even apparently minor errors can indicate a problem with an underlying process so it is important to investigate the cause to prevent repetition or future similar errors. In a multicentre study, practice at other sites might be implicated and changes in practice required.

A common dosing error is when a subject is dosed with IMP that has had a temperature or other environmental excursion, without receiving confirmation from the sponsor that the product is still considered to be stable or unaffected by the excursion. This poses a safety risk to the subject in terms of possible breakdown products and reduced efficacy, also with implications for the integrity of the study data.

Dosing errors should be assessed to determine if they represent a serious breach of the protocol or GCP.

Reconciliation

All IMP must be accounted for across the clinical trial. Within a clinical site IMP received, used, and unused should be reconciled, all totals should balance, and any discrepancy should be explained.

A similar reconciliation should take place at a study level (quantities distributed to sites, used, unused, returned/destroyed, and not accounted for, with explanation).

Reconciliation may be documented in paper records or through the sponsor's clinical trial management system (CTMS).

Other records

The sponsor should decide before the start of the study whether any other materials or equipment need to be accounted for and reconciled during the course of the study, such as drug delivery devices, tablet counters, etc.

Unblinding records

If the study is blinded, the investigator and sponsor must each have access to the information to be able to tell quickly in an emergency what drug a patient has taken. Traditionally this information has been provided to sites as 'code-break' or 'blind-break' envelopes, usually stored by the investigator, pharmacist or both. Before the start of the study it is important to determine who will keep these records and that there is a process in place to allow 24-hour access to the information in an emergency. It is also important that the monitor checks that the information is kept intact throughout the study and any breaking of the blind is quickly reported to the sponsor so that decisions can be made concerning the ongoing management of the subject in the trial and the management of trial data. This is because knowledge of the treatment can bias assessments and decisions by both investigator staff and the sponsor.

One way of dealing with 24-hour cover and close monitoring of blind breaking is to use an IVRS system or a 24-hour call system, which the designated investigator staff can telephone to obtain the treatment information in an emergency.

Any breaking of the blind should be documented in the subject's trial records and medical notes. However, the information should be reported and managed so that only those people who need the information to manage the subject medically are exposed to the treatment identity. This prevents further bias in managing the subject within the clinical trial and minimizes the risk of inadvertently unblinding staff to other subjects' treatment.

Where blind-break envelopes have been used, it is essential to re-secure the information in the envelope (e.g. by resealing it) to prevent other staff opening the envelope and becoming aware of the treatment information.

The sponsor must make a decision on whether the subject should be withdrawn from the study. It may not be ethical to continue treatment and assessments if the subject's data and/or further assessments have been compromised. On the other hand, it may be unethical to deny a patient further treatment (e.g. in an oncology study when no alternative treatment is available), and so the decision might be made to continue in the study, with assessments and trial management made only by investigator staff who remain blinded.

Expiry management and relabelling

The sponsor should have oversight of all drug batches and their expiry dates, where drug has been supplied by the sponsor. There should be forward planning of resupply or relabelling if drug will expire during the study, to avoid any subject receiving expired IMP or missing doses. Planning decisions need to be made well in advance of expiry so that new batch manufacturing, purchasing, and labelling can be planned or relabelling processes can be developed, individuals trained, and relabelling activities conducted before the existing batch expires.

European regulations allow expiry date relabelling to be done at the site by the clinical trial site pharmacist, other healthcare professional, or an appropriately trained clinical trial monitor. Annex 13 of the GMP Directive states:

'33. If it becomes necessary to change the use-by date, an additional label should be affixed to the investigational medicinal product. This additional label should state the new use-by date and repeat the batch number. It may be superimposed on the old use-by date, but for quality control reasons, not on the original batch number. This operation should be performed at an appropriately authorized manufacturing site. However, when justified, it may be performed at the investigational site by or under the supervision of the clinical trial site pharmacist, or other health care professional in accordance with national regulations. Where this is not possible, it may be performed by the clinical trial monitor(s) who should be appropriately trained. The operation should be performed in accordance with GMP principles, specific and standard operating procedures and under contract, if applicable, and should be checked by a second person. This additional labelling should be properly documented in both the trial documentation and in the batch records.'

Two people should be involved in the relabelling activity, one to do the relabelling, the second person to check. There should be explicit written instructions to follow, and a record of all labelling done, signed by both individuals. The old expiry date must be completely covered by the new label without obscuring any other labelling. Label quantities must be reconciled, with every label being accounted for; records and spare labels should be returned to the sponsor, although sometimes a copy of relabelling records is also filed at the site.

Local regulations vary, and in some cases IMP must be returned to a central depot for relabelling, in which case the shipment records and transportation conditions apply as already described.

For some countries outside the EU that do not require the expiry date to be included on the IMP label, extension of expiry date can be provided by a memo, to be filed in the investigator site file. If the shelf-life cannot be extended further, the drug must be replaced.

Recall and resupply

Recall can be instigated by the sponsor, by the marketing authorization holder (for licensed products) or by the regulatory authorities, and this happens when there is an issue with the IMP. How quickly the drug must be recalled depends on the seriousness of the issue. Sponsors must have a process in place to manage recall. The following need to be considered:

- assuming only a specific batch is affected, locating disposition of that batch across the entire study to enable replacement IMP to be sent
- action required for ongoing subject management (safety implications)
- contacting subjects if required to organize return or exchange of IMP
- coordination of IMP return and replacement
- continuity of subject treatment (or not)
- implementing a temporary halt (hold) on the study if required
- documentation required to ensure all IMP is returned and traceable
- substantial amendment implications (study hold and restart)
- serious breaches implications (subject safety, study integrity)

The potential urgency and implications for managing a recall show why it is essential that drug accountability (disposition) records at the site are kept up to date and accurate at all times.

Redistribution between sites

Generally the regulations do not encourage redistribution of IMP between sites. IMP is labelled specifically for a site (labelling includes the investigator name) and is shipped under controlled conditions to ensure maintenance of storage requirements throughout transportation.

If the IMP is to be redistributed after receipt at the site, it must be relabelled with the new investigator name, QP released by the sponsor's designated QP, and shipped under the same controlled conditions as the initial shipment. For a large proportion of sponsors, the cost, complexity, and risks involved in this process are considered excessive and it is easier to ship a new batch of IMP to the site. However, where redistribution is essential, this is usually done by returning the IMP to the regional distribution centre, or a regional centre with GMP facilities, for relabelling, QP release, and onward shipping. There should be full traceability and documentation at each stage.

Returns

Whether or not as a recall, periodically during the study or at the end of the study, drug returned to the sponsor must be recorded. There should be reconciliation at the site before shipping. This is usually done by the pharmacist and CRA together; one to record, the other to check, and both to sign the records.

The sponsor must determine at the start of the study what needs to be returned and what can be recorded and destroyed at the site (and when).

The returns documentation should record the IMP identity, batch numbers, quantities, dates, and signatures (Figure 18.3). If continued integrity of the product is important (e.g. PK studies where any anomaly in results might indicate a need to check the IMP), then the same care and environmental controls and records apply to the returned shipment as for the outward shipment. There should be a receipt record to reconcile the number received with the number shipped.

EXAMPLE RETURN FORM

Protocol No: . . . .   Site No: . . . .   Investigator: . . . .

DRUGS RETURNED:

Description		Number sent from site	Number received by sponsor
IMP Description	No. unused		
	No. used		
	Total returned		
NIMP Description	No. unused		
	No. used		
	Total returned		

Packing/shipping signatures:
Pharmacist: . . . .   Name: . . . . Signature : . . . . Date: . . . .
Sponsor CRA: . . . .   Name: . . . . Signature : . . . . Date: . . . .

Sponsor Receipt Signatures:
Date received: . . . .
Contents checked by: . . . . . .   Name: . . . . . .   Signature : . . . . Date: . . . .
Comments:

Figure 18.3 Example drug return form.

Where a separate decode mechanism has been provided (e.g. blind-break envelopes), its return must also be documented.

Destruction

It should be determined at the start of the study when and by whom each type of study drug will be destroyed. The sponsor may require all IMP to be returned to a central storage location for storage under controlled conditions until after the data have been analysed. In some cases it may be impractical or unnecessary to return IMP to the sponsor, who will agree to destruction by the site.

In both cases all drugs should be accounted for and there should be:
- a policy or written procedures for destruction
- a detailed record of what has been sent for destruction (identity, batch numbers, quantities, date, signature)
- a certificate or confirmatory record of the destruction

Considerations for non-commercial studies

In cases where the IMP is manufactured and/or labelled and released at the same location as the investigator site (e.g. healthcare institute-sponsored single-site studies), some of the records described here may be combined or may not be required, such as shipping and returns records. However, receipt, inventories, dispensing, dosing, and returns records are still required between the pharmacy, investigator, and subject, and there may be environmental transportation considerations for movement across the site.

Local GMP activities

UK phase I clinics and sites with an MIA (IMP) Licence

In the UK, the MHRA has applied the strictest interpretation of the regulations for manipulation of IMP at site. Where there are GMP activities conducted by the site, such as end-stage manufacturing and packaging and labelling at phase I clinics, an MIA(IMP) licence is required and all applicable records must be generated according to GMP requirements, in addition to the investigator's GCP records. In this case, there will be two stages of QP release. Bulk product may be QP released and shipped from the sponsor to the site, to be received under quarantine. All transportation and receipt records which have already been described apply here. Further manufacturing steps are then undertaken according to GMP and the product is QP released by the site's QP and moved out of quarantine storage. At this final QP release stage, the QP must also confirm that the required regulatory documentation is in place, such as the clinical trial application (CTA) approval and ethics committee (EC) approval. The move from quarantine to released storage locations should be recorded.

Exemption 37 to the UK Medicines for Human Use (Clinical Trials) Regulations 2004 allows hospitals and health centres in the UK to perform assembly activities for IMPs, without the need to hold an MIA(IMP) licence. The assembly activities are defined in the regulations as:

- 'enclosing the IMP in a container which is labelled, before the IMP is supplied or used in a clinical trial'
- 'where the IMP is already contained in the container in which it is to be supplied or used in a clinical trial, labelling the container, before it is supplied or used in a clinical trial, in that container'

This exemption only applies for hospitals or health centres performing the assembly and by hospitals or health centres actively involved as a clinical site for that trial.

Documents and forms

It is good practice to QC all forms designed for drug accountability to ensure that they collect or present the correct information. This is essential for dosing instructions and documents that provide calculation methods. The following is a list of documents and forms relating to IMP accountability and management that should be considered when setting up the clinical trial. Not all forms will be required, depending on the design of the study. Some forms may be combined if the records are simple.

- Shipment request
- Shipment record (drugs, devices, materials, decode records)
- Shipment receipt
- Internal site shipment/transportation record
- Temperature monitoring record
- Temperature excursion record
- Equipment calibration records
- Accountability (inventory) record
- Dispensing record
- Preparation record
- Prescription/request for dispensing
- Dosing record
- Returns record (inventory)
- Subject compliance record (e.g. diary)
- Relabelling record
- Recall record
- Returns shipment documentation
- Returns acknowledgement
- Destruction records
- Reconciliation at site
- Final reconciliation for the study (sponsor only)
- Sterile preparation instructions
- Dose calculation worksheets
- Dose preparation worksheets
- Instructions for using IVRS system
- Expiry/extension memos (where applicable for sites outside of the EU)
- Randomization list (if applicable)
- Patient alert cards (part of IMP labelling)
- Disposition records for NIMPS not supplied by sponsor
- Instructions for handling IMP (reconstitution, dilution, freeze–thaw instructions, considerations for blinded studies, etc.)
- Instructions for handling temperature excursions

Further reading

ICH E6 Guidelines for Good Clinical Practice.

Directive 2001/20/EC OF the European Parliament and of the Council of 4 April 2001 on the approximation of the laws, regulations and administrative provisions of the Member States relating to the implementation of good clinical practice in the conduct of clinical trials on medicinal products for human use.

Commission Directive 2005/28/EC of 8 April 2005 laying down principles and detailed guidelines for good clinical practice as regards investigational medicinal products for human use, as well as the requirements for authorisation of the manufacturing or importation of such products.

Commission Directive 2003/94/EC of 8 October 2003 laying down the principles and guidelines of good manufacturing practice in respect of medicinal products for human use and investigational medicinal products for human use, Annex 13.

Eudralex Volume 10 Guidance on Investigational Medicinal Products (IMPs) and 'non investigational medicinal products' (NIMPs), rev. 1, March 2011.

Medicines for Human Use (Clinical Trials) Regulations 2004 (Statutory Instrument 2004 No 1031) and related amendments.

Clinical Trial Regulation. ℘ http://eur-lex.europa.eu/legal-content/EN/TXT/?uri=uriserv:O J.L_.2014.158.01.0001.01.ENG

Safety reporting

Introduction

One of the reasons for good clinical practice (GCP) is to protect the subjects in a research trial. In all research the subjects' well-being should be paramount.

Safety checks, procedures, and reporting are fundamental to any research study involving human subjects. This includes the timely detection and management in line with duty of care of side effects related to (or unrelated and occurring in parallel with) a research study, adverse events (AE), serious adverse events (SAE), adverse reactions (AR), and suspected unexpected serious adverse reactions (SUSAR). In addition, excellent record keeping, follow-up, and reporting are essential so that appropriate decisions can be taken relating to study participants as well as those which help steer the course of the study, based on emerging safety information.

In commercial organizations conducting clinical trials in investigational medicinal products (CTIMPs) there are entire departments whose role it is to deal with safety information received from investigator sites. Staff have to decide, based on the information, if the event is an SUSAR as there are very strict reporting requirements that must be followed if this is the case. These will be discussed in this chapter.

Adverse events

During a research study or clinical trial, any medical event that may happen to the participant must be recorded, even if it appears to be unrelated to the study. The classification of these events is fairly complex and it is important that they are reported in the correct way and the appropriate people notified.

Figure 19.1 and Figure 19.2 illustrate flow diagrams showing how to report adverse events and these can be adapted to a range of healthcare settings.

The clinical trial regulation defines an adverse event (AE) as 'any untoward medical occurrence in a subject administered a medicinal product and which does not necessarily have a causal relationship with this treatment.' This definition includes any incident that happens to an individual; for example, falls, headaches, nausea, intercurrent events, worsening of pre-existing

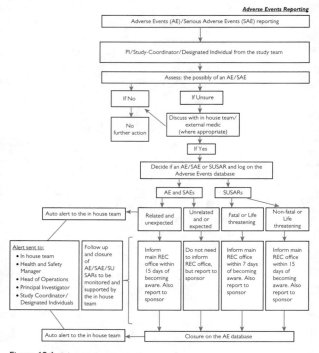

Figure 19.1 Adverse events reporting procedure.

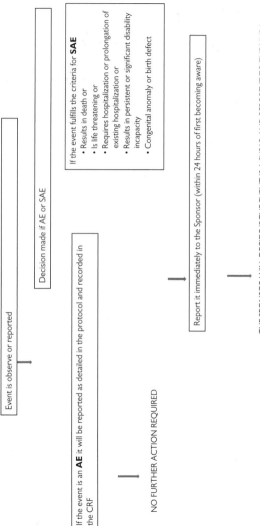

In a CTIMP study sponsored by a commercial organization the reporting requirements are simple.

Event is observe or reported

Decision made if AE or SAE

If the event is an **AE** it will be reported as detailed in the protocol and recorded in the CRF

NO FURTHER ACTION REQUIRED

If the event fulfills the criteria for **SAE**
 • Results in death or
 • Is life threatening or
 • Requires hospitalization or prolongation of existing hospitalization or
 • Results in persistent or significant disability incapacity
 • Congenital anomaly or birth defect

Report it immediately to the Sponsor (within 24 hours of first becoming aware)

THE SPONSOR WILL DECIDE IF THE EVENT IS A SUSAR AND REPORT IT TO THE MHRA

Figure 19.2 Adverse events reporting procedure in CTIMP studies.

conditions, aggravation of the condition being treated, and clinically significant abnormal laboratory values or vital signs.

An adverse event does **not** include:
- procedures such as pre-planned or elective surgery
- hospitalization for procedures for pre-existing condition (not aggravated during the study)
- hospitalization for social reasons

A participant must be given information regarding potential AE for any study procedures. This should be provided via the participant information sheet and the consent process and should be offered verbally prior to a procedure being carried out.

Types of adverse events

Adverse event

An adverse event is 'any untoward medical occurrence in a subject admin-istered a medicinal product and which does not necessarily have a causal relationship with this treatment'.

Serious adverse events

An SAE is any untoward medical occurrence that at any dose:
- results in death, or
- is life threatening, or
- requires hospitalization or prolongation of existing hospitalization, or
- results in persistent or significant disability or incapacity
- results in a congenital anomaly or birth defect,

or
- is otherwise considered medically significant by the investigator
  (Note: this is not an ICH E6 GCP definition)

With either an AE or SAE there are levels of relatedness which must be taken into account when reporting these events. The definitions of causality include:
- Definite—*clearly* related to the research
- Probable—*likely* to be related to the research
- Possible—*may be* related to the research
- Unlikely—*doubtful* that it is related to the research
- Unrelated—*clearly* not related to the research

In order to determine relatedness or causality to the treatment being given, various forms of evidence must be reviewed. It is vital that this judgement is made by a medically qualified person.

What kind of evidence may point to a causal relationship?
- That the participant has taken the drug
- Whether or not the participant experienced this event previously
- Timelines; for example, does the event occur when there is the maximum concentration of the treatment in the body (Cmax)
- Class effect: some treatments have well-known effects (e.g. ACE inhibitors may result in a cough so a similar treatment that produces a cough can be attributed to the treatment)
- The event stops when the treatment is withdrawn
- 'De-challenge, re-challenge' is the best proof of causality

'De-challenge'—where the treatment is stopped the event disappears; the treatment is then reintroduced (re-challenge) to see if the event recurs. This is the best proof of causality but not many investigators will expose the patient to this process to prove the point.

The causality of an event is attributed by the investigator. If the sponsor does not agree with the investigator, then both opinions (the investigator's and the sponsor's) must be documented in the clinical study report.

In addition, the investigator needs to take into account whether the AE or SAE is expected or unexpected. For example, an expected AE could be the participant fainting during venepuncture, while an unexpected AE would be a participant having a cardiac event during venepuncture.

The severity of the event must also be assessed. There are a number of definitions for mild, moderate, or severe events. The definition must be clearly recorded in the protocol. Examples are:

• Mild—transient symptoms, no interference with subject's daily activities, acceptable
• Moderate—marked symptoms, moderate interference with the subject's daily activities, but still acceptable
• Severe—considerable interference with the subject's daily activities, unacceptable

Adverse reactions

An adverse reaction (AR) is any untoward and unintended response in a subject to an investigational medicinal product or a medicinal product taken as part of a trial which is related to any dose administered to that subject. This is the definition contained in the Medicine for Human Use (Clinical Trials) Regulations (2004) as amended.

Suspected unexpected serious adverse reaction

A suspected unexpected serious adverse reaction (SUSAR) mainly refers to a drug trial when undergoing a CTIMP.

> *The definition of SUSAR as written in the Clinical Trial Regulation*
> 'Unexpected serious adverse reaction': a serious adverse reaction the nature, severity, or outcome of which is not consistent with the reference safety information. The information regarding the treatment can be found in the investigator brochure or, if the drug is marketed, in the summary of product characteristics (SmPC). If there event is not recorded in the IB or SmPC, it is unexpected.

SUSARs are defined by regulations 2(1) of the Medicine for Human Use (Clinical Trials) Regulations 2004. A reaction is considered to be:

• **suspected**—because they are in a clinical study environment.
• **unexpected**—the nature, severity, or outcome of which is not consistent with the reference safety information.
• **serious**—if it results in death, is life threatening, requires hospitalization, or prolongs existing hospitalization, results in persistent or significant disability or incapacity, or consists of a congenital abnormality or birth defect.
• **adverse reaction**—any untoward and unintended response in a subject to an investigational medicinal product which is related to any dose administered to that subject.

Reporting adverse events

Investigator responsibility

If an SAE does occur during the study, it should be reported to the sponsor immediately and certainly within 24 hours of staff first becoming aware of the event. With the implementation of the EU Regulation it will become a legal requirement to report SAEs within 24 hours of first knowledge.

Sponsor's responsibility

The sponsor has to review the SAE and decide whether or not it is a SUSAR. The questions to ask are:

• Is it related? That is, it resulted from administration of any of the research procedures, and

• Unexpected? That is, it is a type of event that is not listed in the investigator brochure as an expected occurrence.

If the SAE is an SUSAR, the sponsor has to report the event to the competent authority, which in the UK is the MHRA.

If it is a fatal or life-threatening SUSAR, the sponsor has to report within *seven calendar days* and then send a follow-up report within 8 further days.

A non-fatal or non-life threatening SUSAR must be reported to the MHRA within *15 days* of first knowledge.

The sponsor reports SUSARs via the EudraVigilance database (EVDB). Step-by-step information can be found at: ॐ https://eudravigilance.ema. europa.eu/human/evdbms01.asp

Sponsors are required to submit complete data on all SUSARs occurring in EU member states to EVCTM (EudraVigilance clinical trial module). This enables the relevant competent authorities, in collaboration where necessary, to maintain an effective overview of the safety issues in a clinical trial.

In the UK regulatory context, the MHRA will actively monitor the safety of clinical trials through its access to the European databases. Where the MHRA raises safety concerns with the sponsor, it will directly inform the main research ethics committee (REC) so that any implications for the ethics of the trial can be considered in parallel.

If appropriate, the information has to be communicated to the ethics committees and participating investigators.

In addition to the expedited reports sponsors must submit annual developmental safety update reports (DSURs). DSURs update the status of the clinical trial, summarize the sponsor's understanding, and manage identified and potential risks, describe new safety concerns that could affect the protection of trial subjects, and examine whether the information collected in the previous year accords with current knowledge of the product's safety. They standardize the way in which yearly reports are submitted.

The guideline instructs sponsors to focus on data from interventional trials. However, it also recommends the inclusion of other findings that may have a bearing on the safety of trial subjects. Such information could include findings of non-clinical trials, as well as clinical trials conducted by the sponsor's development partners and non-interventional or compassionate-use studies.

The primary responsibility for monitoring the safety of research partici-pants lies with the trial sponsor. The sponsor has a duty to take action which may include taking urgent safety measures, making amendments to the pro-tocol, or even suspending or terminating a trial where the safety profile or the risk/benefit analysis changes significantly.

It is also important to collect safety information even when a treatment is on the market. In fact many marketing authorization procedures require PASS studies be performed (post-authorization safety studies) in order to collect additional safety information. PSURs (periodic safety update reports) are required for post-marketed drugs and companies have an obligation to collect any safety information for the lifetime of the product.

Medical care

Medical care must be provided to the participant throughout the study. This fits in with the principles of good clinical practice. ICH GCP 4.3.2 states that 'during and following a subject's participation in a trial, the investigator ensures that adequate medical care is provided to the subject for any adverse events, including clinically significant laboratory values related to the clinical trial. In addition, the investigator would inform a subject when medical care is needed for any other illness of which the investigator becomes aware'.

Furthermore, the AE must be followed up until it has either stabilized or is resolved. The participant's GP must also be informed by the investigator (e.g. through a GP's letter).

The rules outlined in this chapter do not state where the investigator's responsibilities for an AE end. Here again, the study protocol will provide direction to the investigator. For example, the protocol may state the following requirement: all AE/SAEs will be followed through to resolution or until the investigator attributes the AE/SAEs to a cause other than the study intervention/procedure or assesses them as chronic or stable.

If the protocol is more stringent than this guidance, the investigator should follow the protocol or vice versa. The patient information sheet and informed consent form should state how medical care decisions will be made and who will provide the medical care.

Protocol deviation

A protocol deviation is a planned departure from the requirements of a study protocol in order to deal with unforeseen circumstances. Such deviations should be agreed with the sponsor and, in the case of an urgent safety measure (USM), as soon as possible after the event. Minor protocol deviations may be considered minor (or 'non-substantial') amendments and do not need to be routinely notified to the ethics committee or the competent authority. However, if the deviation meets the criteria for a 'substantial amendment' it should be notified to the EC and/or the MHRA and an opinion sought. In particular, where the deviation is made to protect a subject from an immediate hazard to his or her health or safety, this should be notified to the EC as an urgent safety measure and reviewed accordingly.

The sponsor or the local principal investigator may implement a deviation from, or a change in, the protocol to protect subjects against any immediate hazard(s) to their health or safety without prior EC/MHRA/sponsor approval/favourable opinion. As soon as possible, the implemented deviation or change, the reasons for it, and, if appropriate, the proposed protocol amendment(s) should be submitted:

• to the REC for review and approval/favourable opinion;
• to the sponsor for agreement, and, if required;
• to the regulatory authorities, that is the MHRA and main REC (CTIMPs only)

In the UK, the initial notification to the EC should be made immediately by telephone. Notification in writing should be sent to the main REC (and MHRA) within three days that such measures have been taken, the reasons why, and the plan for further action.

In the UK, the responsibilities of the EC are inevitably more limited. RECs do not have to review the SUSARs as they do not have access to comprehensive safety data (in particular, SUSARs outside the UK), nor do they generally have the resources and expertise required to carry out in-depth analysis of the available data. The REC should, however, be ready to act on safety concerns that are brought to its attention by the sponsor or the MHRA. In particular, the REC is responsible for ensuring that the consent of participants continues to be based on accurate and up-to-date information about risks and benefits.

Breaches

It is relevant to consider breaches alongside safety reporting because an inappropriate protocol deviation or breach can result in compromise to participant safety.

Breaches are:
• Deviations to a pre-agreed change to protocol, or
• Violation of protocol or GCP.

Serious breaches include:
• A breach of the protocol or GCP that is likely to affect to a significant degree:
  • the safety or physical or mental integrity of the trial subjects; or
  • the scientific value of the trial.

Reporting breaches

Breaches need to be reported to the EC and/or the MHRA. Some breaches may need expedited reporting, depending on the degree of severity. Breaches (non-serious violation/deviations) need to be taken into account when the data are analysed.

When a serious breach does occur, the investigator must report the event to the sponsor. The sponsor then reports the event to the EC and must report to the MRHA within seven days of becoming aware of such a breach.

Further reading

EudraVigilance database. ℘ www.eudravigilance.org/human/evDbms01.asp

The Commission Directive 2001/20/EC of the European Parliament and of the council of 4 April 2001.

The Commission Directive 2005/28/EC of 8 April 2005. ℘ http://eur-lex.europa.eu/LexUriServ/ LexUriServ.do?uri=OJ:L:2005:091:0013:0019:en:PDF

The Commission Regulation 536/2014.

Data management

Ensuring confidentiality of data

Confidential information is any information imparted on the understanding that it will not be disclosed to others. Whenever people give personal information to researchers, it is confidential as long as it remains personally unidentifiable.

Personal data is subject to the Data Protection Act 1998 in the UK and similar law throughout Europe and many other parts of the world. The Data Protection Act sets out requirements to protect people's fundamental rights and freedoms and in particular their right to privacy with respect to the processing of personal data. The Act covers the collection, processing, and disclosure of personal data.

Unless due to specific circumstances, research participants should be required to provide informed consent. In practice this means that potential study participants are given adequate information about the study in a way that is easily understandable and they should be invited to ask any questions they may have. Consent must be given freely and the participant should be told that consent can be withdrawn at any time. It is useful to provide a volunteer information sheet giving an overview of the research along with contact details for a member of the research team. The data collected should be adequate, relevant, and not excessive for the requirements of the study.

All medical research using identifiable personal information, or using anonymized data from the NHS that is not already in the public domain, must be approved by a research ethics committee.

Anonymization

Anonymization is a vital tool in the protection of personal data. Personal information should be anonymized as much and as soon as possible after collection. Although the anonymization process may cause delays and increase the risk of error, even a simple anonymizing system provides a safeguard against accidental or deliberate release of confidential information. There are two main methods of anonymizing data:

- Linked anonymized data separates personally identifiable information from research and published data. It is possible to re-link if needed using a unique identifier, (subject ID) which is allocated at the beginning of the participant's involvement in the study. Access to the identifying data should be limited to only those people who need it for the care of study participants or the running of the study (e.g. to provide blood results or send appointment letters). Access to the personal identifying data should be controlled by the principal investigator or by the custodian of the research database. Linked anonymized data must be handled in accordance with the Data Protection Act.
- Unlinked anonymized data contains no data or links to other information that could potentially be used to identify individuals.

Ensure that anonymized data cannot be reconstructed to become personal data. It is conceivable that a combination of data in a particular dataset, perhaps in conjunction with data in the public domain, may be unique to an individual or family who could therefore be identifiable from that information.

Transfer of confidential data

All research data should be kept on secure network servers. The folders containing the data should be set up to allow groups of users to have appropriate access permissions. There might be separate groups for users who are allowed to update data and for those who may only view data (editing rights). It is wise to take advice from the IT section and abide by the rules of the research institution. Avoid keeping data on PCs, laptops, mobile phones, and removable media. When this is not possible, consider methods of encrypting the devices and the use of passwords.

Transferring data from one organization or site to another introduces risk to the security of data. It is strongly advised not to use e-mail to transfer unencrypted data or to convey any personal data. There are several secure ways to transfer data. Secure free transfer protocol (FTP) sites and virtual private networks (VPN) are the most secure. If neither is available, personal data could be transferred in an encrypted, password-protected zip file, which can be written to a disk or sent via secure e-mail. Ensure the password is complex (more than 10 characters, containing a mix of upper- and lower-case letters, numbers, and special characters). Do not send the password in the same e-mail as the attachment or enclose it with the disk. Organizations should have robust policy or procedures in this respect.

Research organizations will have policies and guidance regarding data confidentiality and security. Abide by the requirements and, if in doubt, seek advice; there will be people who can help.

Planning the trial and the database

A well-designed database is a great asset to a study. The degree to which it will help will depend on a number of factors including the complexity of the data, the number of fields collected, 'external' data, and the number of cases.

It is possible to develop and run a study using anything from a spreadsheet to a database that is very robust. An Excel spreadsheet is quick and easy to set up; setting up a database may take a very long time.

A robust system is preferable so if possible try to avoid using a spreadsheet, even for the simplest study. A little time spent learning the basics of a simple database (e.g. Microsoft Access or FileMaker) is well worthwhile. On the other hand, a complex database might represent something of an overkill. A balance must be struck; the prime objective is to create clean, usable data using a robust and validated system.

Benefits of using a database

There are many benefits of using a database. It will generally ensure:

- clean data—due to the validation, checking, automated routines, and other aspects of the database design. This goes a long way towards preventing data errors.
- all data is in one place—this is a benefit in time and accuracy that cannot be overstated. If all the study data is in a well-structured database, it is very quick and easy to relate the various data and to produce reports and data extracts to a range of requirements. The queries or views created to do this can be documented, saved, and run repeatedly. If reporting data, for example, from a spreadsheet of blood results, a separate spreadsheet containing physical measurements, and a further one containing demographic data, the time spent linking, merging or, worse still, copying and pasting the data could be quite considerable. In a database, a query could be created in minutes.
- database tables and the fields they contain can be documented. Metadata is easy to document.
- archiving—the data can be archived as a single entity (supporting documents and files should also be stored).
- publishing data—if the data are to be made available to other researchers (e.g. on the Essex Archive), the data can be extracted and easily documented.
- future use—the database, being well-structured and documented, will enable future users of the data to make full use of the data.
- future studies—when developing or designing a database for another study it is highly likely that future users will be able to utilize aspects of previously developed databases (Figure 20.1).

When the decision is made to develop a database, it is wise to discuss requirements with developers as early as possible. If the trial is not using experienced developers then speak to people who may be able to help with design. The developer should gain a thorough understanding of the study protocol and how the data will be captured, manipulated, and reported. Early discussions may allow for changes in protocol to facilitate

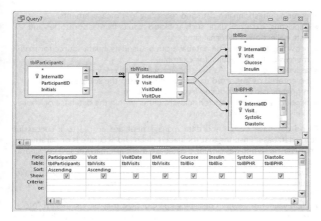

Figure 20.1 An example (Microsoft Access) query reporting data from four different, but related datasets.

a more effective study. Understanding the protocol will almost certainly allow the developer to suggest database features and functionality that had not previously been considered. Once the requirements of the database are fully understood the developer will be able to design the general structure, ensure data integrity, validate data, and produce accurate results. The developer will need to consider deployment, security, and ongoing support issues. The database will probably pass through several iterations of development, testing, demonstration, and change before acceptance by the researcher.

What is the database used for?

A database may be used in several ways throughout the life of the study. It can be used for:

- screening. By testing the input against inclusion and exclusion criteria, manual checking can be avoided. Not everyone wants to record screening data but it can be very useful. For example, a study protocol says that BMI must be in the range 25–28 and that recruitment is proving difficult. The screening data might show that a significant number of people with a BMI in the range 28–30 have been excluded. It might be too late to amend the protocol for the study in progress, but this data could be very useful when designing the next study.
- managing visits. The database could be used to generate lists of participants who have appointments during a given period, which could be used to generate reminders, perhaps as text messages. It could also be used to identify participants who have failed to attend an appointment.

- entering questionnaire data and recording visit measurements.
- importing 'external' data, such as blood results from laboratories and data collection at external sites.
- providing feedback. The database can be used as a data source for mail merges of blood results, for example.
- as a data repository. As the study proceeds, all relevant data can be entered or imported to the database. Keep the source data. All reporting can be produced from the database.
- producing final datasets for analysis, either within the database or, more likely, using statistical software.

Good database design and data management are crucial to a successful study database. Ensuring that the data is clean and accurate is of paramount importance. When developing a database there are many design considerations; for example:

- Data types—if a particular field expects a number as a result, then make sure the field type is numeric; if a field is a date then make sure it is in date format.
- Field validation—when designing an input field that allows 'Yes' or 'No', make sure these are the only options available (although it might be wise to want to code missing values). If a field has a valid range between 100 and 200, validate against values outside that range. Date of birth should not be in the future. However, consideration must be given to how data, shown on a form, that is outside the valid range should be handled. One option is to record the data in a notes field, another is to allow the value to be recorded and to report it in an exceptions report. Messages and conditional formatting can be used to bring the out-of-range value to the attention of the person entering the data in case there was a genuine typing error. At some point, before the data is analysed or reported, a decision will have to be made regarding any invalid data.
- Form design—when designing an input form, it is quicker and more accurate to enter data if it is looks similar to the paper version. Also important is the need to enter the data as it appears on the form; if the form has 'Yes/No' responses to questions, then make the input 'Yes/No' and not 1/0. The final data may require 1s and 0s but this can be achieved in a number of ways without recourse to requiring data-entry staff to interpret when inputting. If the database and study have been planned in parallel, relevant documents can be adapted to mirror the database form. An experienced data-entry administrator is a valuable asset to the design and development of data-entry screens. Ask for feedback of issues, such as tabbing order, swapping from keyboard to mouse, look-up options, and other design issues that affect the speed and/or accuracy of data entry. Data-entry staff should always be encouraged to talk to database developers to ensure the most efficient system possible is developed.

- Missing data—checks will often be made for missing data so ensure that any data that is genuinely missing is marked as such. Consider and design the original form in a way to minimize valid non-responses. A (real) example:

  Question 3. If you experienced the following symptoms how would you describe the severity? (Select one for each symptom)

  - Nausea   Mild/Moderate/Severe
  - Heartburn   Mild/Moderate/Severe
  - Abdominal Pain Mild/Moderate/Severe

  In this example, if the study participant did not experience the symptom there would be no response. Ideally the form would be changed to include the option 'Not applicable', but if designing the database retrospectively, add a field to indicate there was no response.

- Double entry—although entering the same data twice has an obvious cost, it is a very useful tool to improve data quality. An exception report should also be used to report discrepancies. It may not be practical or desirable to apply double entry to all fields. Comments and notes fields are more prone to discrepancies due to rewording, abbreviating, changing of spelling mistakes, etc. They are also less likely to be critical research data.

- Cross validation—if there are data on a form (e.g. date of birth) that is held elsewhere in the database, then compare the two. Exceptions reports will help pinpoint problems and guide the way to correct inscription.

- Exceptions reports can be used to compare the same data from different sources, doubly entered data, and to report missing values (e.g. blood results).

As well as entered data, there are likely to be electronic data generated by laboratory or clinic instruments. This is invaluable data and so it should be imported into the database. If the import process needs to happen on a regular basis then consider automating the import routine and subsequent data reconciliation checks. It is a fact of life that data from laboratories is not always 100% clean. Mistakes can happen with IDs at more or less any stage during the process, from sticking the barcode on a tube to manipulating a spreadsheet file of results. For this reason it is strongly advisable to have at least three identifiers on samples (e.g. date of birth, gender, initials, and barcode) that can be validated and reported in the results data.

Data entry

Data entry is a skilled discipline. It requires attention to detail and a great deal of patience. The source data can be missing, handwritten answers from subjects can be illegible or unclear, and the data can be incomplete; the list of possible scenarios is almost endless.

Include data-entry staff in discussions or presentations about the study throughout its life course. Staff like to understand the importance of the work they are doing, how it fits into the study, and the impact the study will have when published. Presentations early in the study, most of which can be produced from the protocol, can give an overview of the study, its relevance, and anticipated impact. Include some interesting facts such as number of subjects, uniqueness and details of the experiments or intervention. At the end of the study it is useful to present the results and findings to the whole team and, hopefully, announce details of where the study will be published. Developing and delivering presentations helps engage the entire team, lets everyone see the study from a different angle, and polishes presentation skills.

Including data-entry staff in the preparatory and subsequent work means they may be more likely to:
- be able to suggest changes to forms or to the database.
- identify 'strange' data and know when to raise queries.
- provide some insight as to the volume of work, which could be very useful when applying for grants or funding.
- understand the study, the deadlines, relevance, and importance of the data, which motivates staff to produce the best possible results. Knowing deadlines allows them to prioritize their workload.

Data-entry work requires careful planning to meet deadlines: when does the work need to be finished? At what stage does it need to be checked? Are there multiple deadlines, like monthly provision of blood results, that need to be met? Deadlines should be established at the beginning of the study and reviewed on a regular basis.

The day-to-day planning will depend on other work commitments and the individual entering the data. It will not always be possible to employ the use of dedicated data-entry staff. Data entry might have to be undertaken by multi-skilled administrators, a student, or maybe even the principal investigator.

If there is a large volume of work data entry might well comprise a full-time job. If not, consider how to organize the work. Data entry is often best done in batches as this allows a rhythm to develop. Some people may find it best to spend a day at a time on one type of form; others may find half a day the most they can manage before their attention wanders.

The database will ideally have been designed to make the data entry as error-proof as possible. The design may incorporate double-entry of data; if so it is recommended to use two different people to enter the data or to enter the data on different days. Differences between the double-entered data may be identified by messages or by highlighting fields on the second entry screen that do not contain the same data as the first. The data-entry staff should act on messages and notice highlighted data. When discrepancies are found both entries may need to be checked.

Data that is not double entered may need to be checked for accuracy. Data to be checked should be defined by the study principal investigator. Ideally, checking is conducted by two people; one reading the database (or an output from it), the other the form. The checks completed should be documented. This could be a note of the number of forms checked or by recording the IDs of the checked records. The database will need updating to show the checks have been done to avoid double-checking later. Data-entry work completed by inexperienced staff should be thoroughly checked.

In large commercial sponsor companies vast amounts of money are spent on sophisticated computer systems. The same rules apply; data management and IT support teams need to be fully aware of database requirements. Double data entry is always done if paper CRFs are employed, but many companies now use eCRFs or electronic data capture (EDC) systems where data may go directly into the database. However simple or complex the system may be, validation is a vital step.

Validation of data systems

Throughout the course of the study, the systems to manage the data are critical. In the UK, for example, there is a requirement for a data management plan to be submitted when applying for a grant from the Medical Research Council and other research funding organizations.

Whether or not there is a requirement to submit a data management plan, it is important to take all reasonable steps to ensure data quality, security, and confidentiality. Furthermore, consideration should be given to requirements, or desires, to share the study data, possibly on a research data archive.

The level of testing undertaken will depend on the complexity, nature, and scale of the systems used and the risk the study poses. A simple diary or calendar will need moderate testing to ensure it meets requirements, whereas a database with multiple input fields, especially where the result of one field can be validated against another, will require more vigorous testing. A database developer should ensure as far as possible that the database works as expected before handing over full acceptance testing to the research team. With a complex database there will often be the need for several records, not only to test the input forms and import routines but also to ensure the data can be reported as required.

During the course of the study there are often changes and new requirements. Changes have to be handled with extreme care to ensure integrity of existing data, and these will need to be tested accordingly.

In addition to the testing of the 'mechanics' of the systems, it is important to recognize that the content of the data may require validation. Validation of data entered by data-entry staff should be handled by the design of the relevant paper and database forms, double-entry and checking processes. Imported data must undergo an appropriate checking process as well. Always run as much validation as possible to ensure imported data is accurate.

Important points to consider
- Ensure results are for the correct people and time point. Possible checks include that:
  - there is a valid participant ID for the result.
  - there is a result expected (e.g. that the participant gave blood). Cross-check any other data available in the results data against data already in the database. Where discrepancies are found, these related data may be used to identify the cause of the discrepancy and to assign the result to the correct participant.
  - there is the correct number of results for the participant. This check will identify results that have either been reported twice, perhaps from two separate aliquots, or where an ID has been entered incorrectly.

- Ensure results are within a reasonable range. Checking that data is within a reasonable range is problematic. For example, a height of two metres might be acceptable; a height of three metres is not. Where is the line of acceptability? Continuing this example, if age and gender were to be taken into account, the acceptable height might vary. Acceptance of the data will also vary depending on the source of the data. Results from an accredited laboratory are far more likely to be accurate than those from a study participant who recorded weight using bathroom scales.
- Ensure missing values are coded or explained.

Once a significant amount of data has been collected it may be possible to check the data in relation to itself. The timing of these final checks will depend on the study protocol; at a minimum the results should be checked before they are published. Possible checks include:

- Reasonableness checks or peer review; both very useful tools for checking data for outliers. Consult relevant experts who will advise how the data should be broken down; some results may need to be subdivided by age and/or gender, for example. Graphs, box plots, and scatter diagrams can be used to compare results.
- Batch checking. Consider comparing the average mean of batches of results. The batches could be a batch or run number provided in the results data by a laboratory, a nurse, a time point, geographic location, or any other variable that might have an impact on the result. Such comparisons could, for example, detect a significant difference between heights measured by one nurse to those measured by another. Take advice from experts to decide whether there is likely to be a real difference; for example, vitamin D in blood is likely to vary throughout the course of the year. Statisticians will advise whether the difference is significant. Subsequent follow-up action would depend on the nature of the difference and the opportunity to re-measure or re-analyse.
- Results below level of detection. Some results (e.g. C-reactive protein) may be reported by a laboratory as below the level of detection. A decision has to be made as to how to use these 'results' in analysis and published data. One solution is to remove results below the lower detection limit, but this reduces the value of the data. An alternative is to create a notional value. For example, C-reactive protein in the National Health and Nutrition Examination Survey (NHANES) calculated this notional value as the lower detection limit divided by the square root of two. It is important to document any decisions made regarding the reporting of notional values.

When trial data are to be included in submissions to regulatory authorities for a drug licence, all the software used to collect, transfer, edit, and archive the data must comply with ICH GCP sections 5.5.3 and 21 CFR (Code of Federal Regulations) Part 11—system validation. Both these regulations specify similar expectations, in that all clinical computerized systems will be developed in a structured manner by qualified developers, tested methodically and used, as specified in documented procedures, by users who have been formally trained. The programs used to cross-check data must also be validated in the same way as the computerized systems and, where systems include the functionality to change data if necessary, the details of the changes, including original values, details of who and when changes were made, must be captured in a secure audit trail.

Further reading

National Health and Nutrition Examination Survey: 2009–2010 Data Documentation, Codebook, and Frequencies ℘ www.cdc.gov/nchs/nhanes/nhanes2009-2010/CRP_F.htm
Gillespie BW, et al. Estimating population distributions when some data are below a limit of detection by using a reverse Kaplan-Meier estimator. *Epidemiology* 2010 Jul;21 Suppl 4:S64–70.

Research project management

What is a project?

A project is a temporary piece of work which typically has defined resources (people or budget) and a set time frame to achieve a clear objective or outcome.

A clinical research trial is a good example of a project. This involves a group of people (a clinical project team) working together to try to answer a specific medical question (e.g. does this compound work in a specified group of patients with a certain disease?), aiming to obtain the answer within a set time frame and budget.

What is project management?

Clinical project teams are made up of a variety of people with different skills and backgrounds (e.g. investigators, nurses, scientists, pharmacists, clinical research associates, data managers, and statisticians). The leader of this team is the project manager who acts like the conductor of an orchestra ensuring all the members of the project team work together harmoniously towards the same goal which is the delivery of a successful project.

Stages of a project

All projects go through four different stages:
- Stage 1. Definition—defining and agreeing the subject and aims of the project.
- Stage 2. Planning —planning how the project will be conducted.
- Stage 3. Implementation and control—running the project.
- Stage 4. Close-out—delivery and the end of the project.

Stage 1: Definition: defining and agreeing what the project is about

Before a project starts it is important to identify key stakeholders that have a significant interest in the outcome of the project and to determine their requirements and expectations.

What is a stakeholder?

A stakeholder is anyone with an interest in, or is affected by, the outcome of a project. This can include the people funding the project, members of a research team, heads of department, data safety review boards, data monitoring committees, patients (including patient groups), ethics committees, and regulatory authorities.

Examples of clinical research project stakeholders are:

- Project funders—grant authorities (the Medical Research Council, Wellcome Trust), medical charities (Cancer Research UK), and commercial sponsors (e.g. pharmaceutical company).
- Project performers—investigators, nurses, laboratory staff, pharmacies, patients, drug supply teams, clinical research organizations, site management organizations, NHS clinical research networks, and clinical research associates.
- Project design—investigators, scientists, statisticians, medical writers, regulatory managers.
- Project approval—ethics committees, NHS trusts, NHS R&D departments, regulatory agencies (e.g. Medicines and Healthcare products Regulatory Agency, US Food and Drug Administration, and European Medicines Agency).

What is a successful project?

A successful project is one where the needs of the stakeholders are either met or exceeded. Ensuring the success of a project depends on having a good understanding of the aim of the project, the needs of the key stakeholders and their respective success criteria. This is known as the project scope. Time spent defining, and agreeing the scope of a project before it starts will save a lot of wasted time and heartache later on.

Defining the scope of a project

Ideally, a meeting (or teleconference) should be held attended by key people with an interest in the project (especially anyone funding the project) to discuss, decide, and agree:

- what **exactly** is being attempted (e.g. what question or hypothesis will be investigated?)
- what form the investigation will take (e.g. clinical trial, patient audit, market research). This should be a 'top line' agreement; the fine detail (e.g. actual study design) can come later.
- what are the different options for conducting the investigation in a practical way? Choose the best with an agreed rationale.
- what timescales are involved? Are there any important deadlines (e.g. conference submission dates, PhD research grant funding end date, planned registration submission date for a commercial project)?

- what is the intended output or outputs (e.g. clinical study report, academic research thesis, manuscript, abstract, presentation)?
- what costs will it involve (e.g. study budget)?
- are there any risks that can be identified, and how will these be handled? (e.g. for a clinical trial this may be the expiry date of the investigational medicinal product (study drugs)).

Write down and circulate the answers to these questions after the meeting with a deadline for comments. This provides people a chance to consider what was agreed, and will help to ensure everyone has the same understanding. Once agreement has been reached, finalize this in a project scope document and ask all the major stakeholders to sign to confirm their agreement. The more detail and precision that can be achieved at this stage, the less likely it wil be that difficulties will arise later.

The project scope should be continually referred to as the project progresses. If any changes are requested during its course, the project scope document can be used as a basis to consider the implications, especially in terms of the following:

- Aim—is this still realistic and achievable?
- Timelines—will changes affect the timelines?
- Output—how would the envisaged changes affect the proposed output?
- Cost—what is the cost implication?

The impact can then be discussed, agreed, and documented, and an amendment to the project scope signed off again by the key stakeholders. This ensures that everyone is kept up to date with the progress of the project, understands and agrees the reason for any changes, and accepts their impact as they arise. Defining and agreeing a process for making scope changes at the beginning of a project can save a lot of time during the project, which will help to achieve the timelines.

Stage 2: Planning: planning how the project will be conducted

Once the project scope has been defined and agreed, a good project plan is essential for the successful delivery of the project. Although it is tempting to rush into actually doing the project, any time spent planning is extremely valuable and helps achieve a successful outcome. This planning can be done in parallel with the development of the study design or protocol and should take into account the results of any feasibility studies conducted.

Feasibility studies

Checking the feasibility of the proposed project can provide valuable information to be used in the project scope and plan. For a clinical trial, this can involve circulating a proposed study outline, a suggested patient population (using the draft study entry and exclusion criteria), the patient numbers required, any important non-routine equipment/patient assessments/laboratory tests required, and timelines circulated to the wider stakeholders (especially any clinical teams who will be involved in enrolling the patients, and any teams involved in providing investigational product/drugs or laboratory supplies). Obtaining this feedback will provide valuable information about potential challenges in the proposed project and allow these to be taken into account at the planning stage.

If the proposed study design changes significantly (e.g. major change to the patient exclusion criteria), it may be wise to repeat the feasibility to assess the impact and take this into account in the project plan.

Contents of a project plan

A good project plan will contain the following:
- The aim and required output of the project (taken from the approved project scope). This should match the final study protocol.
- Details, outcome, and the impact of any feasibility studies performed.

How the project will be achieved
- Study design and required statistical power. This will directly affect the amount of investigational product and study supplies required (i.e. the study budget).
- Study end points—specific patient assessments required.
- Total number of patients required, and how they will be enrolled including:
  - The sort of sites/clinics that are required (e.g. primary or secondary care).
  - Numbers of investigational sites used to recruit these patients.
  - Location of these sites.
  - Number of hospitals/clinics.
  - Areas located (e.g. number of hospitals under one NHS Trust).
  - Countries (e.g. UK only, or multiple countries).
  - Number of regions (e.g. Europe only or US, Asia Pacific, etc.).

Study timelines
These should take into account the number of patients required and the geographical area where the study will be conducted. Regulatory and ethics approvals will probably be quicker to achieve for a single hospital in one

country than for multiple hospitals in different countries in a variety of geo-graphical regions (e.g. Europe, US, Asia Pacific etc.).

Study budget

Cost of study, including all supporting resources (e.g. supplies, personnel, any required approvals, printing, transport).

Team roles and responsibilities

These are linked to timelines and are extremely important, especially if different organizations are involved in the project (e.g. use of contract company to pack blinded study drugs/investigational medicinal products). They should be used as a reference point when producing any contracts with external organizations.

Assumptions and risks

Including a risk management plan and predefined 'triggers' that will activate this plan.

For example, for a clinical trial:
* the risk may be that not enough patients enrolled.
* the plan may be to open more centres/sites.
* the trigger for this plan could be enrolment being 80% or less of the planned target after 25% of the enrolment period has passed.

The project plan should include how the success of the risk management plan will be measured and what other actions will be taken if the project risk continues.

Patient safety management

Actions to take if unexpected adverse events/serious adverse events are seen in the study participants.

Patient confidentiality

How data will be handled to ensure patient confidentiality is maintained.

The project plan should be a 'living document' and be referred throughout the life of the project when tracking its progress. The original plan can be considered the 'baseline' plan as it contains the original scope of the project.

Project management tools

The aim of project management tools is to help plan and track the scheduling and timing of the tasks required to complete the project.
This can be done using:
* work breakdown structure—listing all the tasks that need to be done (each task has a single deliverable).
* project network—tasks are put in the correct order, indicating any which have to be completed before another task can be started (e.g. for a clinical trial, ethics and regulatory approval has to be obtained before patient recruitment can start).
* project timings—estimate the duration of each task, then add target start and end dates.

Costs can be set against individual tasks to allow planning and tracking of budget expenditure.

Consider running a simple sub-project to submit a clinical study to an ethics committee:

Step 1: Identify the work breakdown structure

For example, a list of individual tasks that need to be done for the ethics submission.

A task list might include:
- Complete the ethics submission application
- Finalize the study design
- Complete and finalize the study specific patient information leaflet (PIL) and consent form (PIL/consent)
- Sign off the submission form
- Produce any recruitment aids (e.g. patient letters, posters, flyers, advertisements)
- Book a slot with the chosen ethics committee
- Submit the clinical trial application

Step 2: Produce a project network using these tasks

This puts tasks in the correct order, identifying any which can occur at the same time (termed 'in parallel'), and which tasks have to be completed before the next task can start ('in series').

Working in parallel is a good way to save time, but it is important to ensure that the relevant tasks can actually be done in parallel (Figure 21.1), that the start of one doesn't require the output of another, and that there is sufficient resource to run a number of tasks simultaneously.

Identification of the critical path

As Figure 21.1 shows, there are a number of key tasks that link together and have to be performed in the correct order to achieve the submission. For example, the design of the study has to be finalized before the ethics submission is completed (in case it changes), and the submission form has to be completed before it can be signed. Sign-off has to happen and a slot booked before the form can be sent to the ethics committee. This set of tasks is known as the 'critical path' (dark blue in the diagram) and defines the shortest feasible time in which the project can be performed. A delay in any single aspect will cause the delay of the whole project.

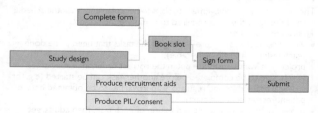

Figure 21.1 Project network production.

The timing of other 'non-critical tasks' is more flexible (i.e. these tasks can move without affecting the duration or final end date of the project). Care should be taken as a non-critical path task (e.g. completion of the patient information leaflet and consent form) can become critical and hold up the whole process (termed a 'rate limiting step') if undertaking this task is delayed.

Adding durations and timing (project milestones)

If you know how long a task should take (e.g. six weeks to write a protocol), this information can be added to the task network, along with target dates (called 'project milestones'), which help to plan how to deliver the project within the agreed time frame. This information can be expressed as a table, or as a series of bars, known as a Gantt chart (Figure 21.2).

Identification of key project milestones

The milestone dates on the critical path are known as the key project milestones. Tracking achieved dates against the planned date of these milestones helps the project manager know if the project is on track to achieve all its key deliverables by the relevant deadlines.

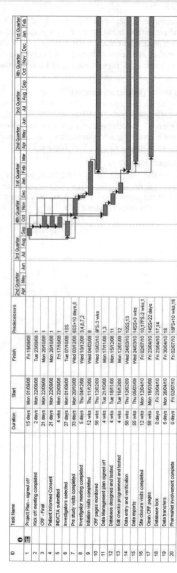

ID		Task Name	Duration	Start	Finish	Predecessors
1		Project Plan - signed off	15 days	Mon 01/09/08	Fri 19/09/08	
2		Kick off meeting completed	2 days	Mon 22/09/08	Tue 23/09/08	1
3		CRF - Final	21 days	Mon 22/09/08	Mon 20/10/08	1
4		Patient Informed Consent	21 days	Mon 22/09/08	Mon 20/10/08	1
5		IND/CTA submitted	4 wks	Mon 22/09/08	Fri 17/10/08	1
6		Investigators selected	27 days	Mon 01/09/08	Tue 07/10/08	1SS
7		Pre study visits completed	33 days	Mon 20/10/08	Wed 03/12/08	6SS+10 days,5
8		Investigator meeting completed	5 days	Thu 04/12/08	Wed 10/12/08	3,4,6,7,2
9		Initiation visits completed	12 wks	Thu 11/12/08	Wed 04/03/09	8
10		CRF pages monitored	56 wks	Thu 12/02/09	Wed 10/03/10	9FS-3 wks
11		Data Management plan signed off	4 wks	Tue 21/10/08	Mon 17/11/08	1,3
12		Database designed and tested	4 wks	Tue 18/11/08	Mon 15/12/08	11
13		Edit checks programmed and tested	4 wks	Tue 16/12/08	Mon 12/01/09	12
14		Data entry and verification	58 wks	Thu 12/02/09	Wed 24/03/10	10SS,13
15		Data imports	55 wks	Thu 05/03/09	Wed 24/03/10	14SS+3 wks
16		Site closure visits completed	12 wks	Mon 12/04/10	Fri 02/07/10	10,17FS-2 wks,1
17		Clean CRF pages	58 wks	Mon 16/03/09	Fri 23/04/10	14SS+22 days
18		Database lock	0 days	Fri 23/04/10	Fri 23/04/10	17,14
19		Data transfers	5 days	Mon 26/04/10	Fri 30/04/10	18
20		Premarket involvement complete	0 days	Fri 02/07/10	Fri 02/07/10	16FS+10 wks,16

Figure 21.2 Example of a Gantt chart for a clinical trial.
Reproduced with kind permission of the Institute of Clinical Research.

Stage 3: Implementation and control: running the project

Monitoring and reporting

Once the project has started it is important to monitor its progress against the plan regularly to ensure it is kept on track. This can be done by actively checking as each of the project milestones is achieved to see how this fits with the project plan. If it looks like a milestone is going to be missed, the appropriate risk management plans can be triggered, or project constraints considered to allow the project to be delivered to the stakeholders in line with the plan.

Some of the project stakeholders, especially those providing funding, may require regular reports on progress against the plan. This is very important where funding is linked to achieving project milestones.

Project constraints: cost, time, quality

Projects have three main components:
- Cost/resource
- Time
- Quality/scope

Changing one of these components can have a direct effect on the other two. Project progress can be speeded up by adding in more resource (which for a clinical trial could mean opening more centres so increasing the cost), or reducing the quality (this may be achieved by a reduction in the study statistical power to require less enrolled patients).

Similarly, constrained costs might require the project to take longer due to a scarcity of resource, or might call for a reduction in the project scope.

It is important to discuss any such proposals and obtain the agreement of the key project stakeholders. Referring to the original project scope will help decide which changes can be made whilst ensuring the project will still meet the needs of these stakeholders.

Managing the project team

Projects involve a team of people. Often, these people:
- have different backgrounds/individual skills (e.g. statistician, medics, nurses, scientists, and data managers).
- are located in different places. This may be different organizations (hospitals, laboratories, or companies) or countries (possibly involving different time zones).
- are not directly managed by the project manager.
- work on a number of different projects/roles at the same time (e.g. investigators may have to run clinics and wards in addition to conducting the project).

To ensure project success, the project manager needs to:
- encourage the team to have high levels of collaboration and solidarity. A face-to-face meeting at the start of the project can help the team get to know each other, develop project ownership, and promote successful working relationships.

- provide clear objectives and responsibilities; these need to be specific, measurable, achievable, realistic, and time-bound (also known as SMART). Objectives should be based on the key milestones in the project plan. The team should be encouraged to notify the project manager immediately of anything that may stop them achieving their project objectives. The project manager can then plan to minimize the effect on the project.
- be flexible and willing to initiate the 'risk management plan' and other required changes to bring a project back on track.
- provide good information and feedback on the progress of the project to the team. Congratulating the team on achieving key milestones on an ongoing basis increases team motivation and encourages success.
- listen and value feedback from team members and be willing to act upon this, especially if problems are being identified.
- support team members in finding solutions to any challenges. As a clinical trial project team is multidisciplinary, the project manager does not have to be the expert in all the disciplines, and will not have all the answers to problems that arise during the project. The project manager should seek the advice of the relevant team experts on an ongoing basis.

For projects involving multidisciplinary teams, often located in different places and not directly managed by the project manager, good communication is essential. Time should be spent at the start of the project devising a communication plan (implemented by whom, circulated to whom, when, and how).

Communication can be achieved in many ways including:
- face-to-face meetings
- e-mails
- teleconferences/web conferences

Meeting agendas circulated (ideally one week) in advance of project meetings allow the team to:
- add the meeting to busy diaries, ensuring staff can attend.
- prepare for the meeting—especially important if staff are expected to provide information or updates.

Brief minutes detailing decisions reached and actions agreed (including deadlines) should be circulated to all team members (especially those who could not attend the meeting). Starting each meeting with a progress review of the previous meeting's agreed actions is important for successfully monitoring the project and identification of any issues.

The frequency of this communication will change during the project, with communication more frequent at the planning and start-up phase, reduced during implementation before becoming more frequent again towards the end when the deliverable (e.g. study report, abstract, or manuscript) is being produced. Different team members will be involved at varying levels at different stages of the project.

Stage 4: Close out: delivery and the end of the project

The end of the project is when the deliverable (e.g. study report, abstract, or manuscript) has been produced and given to the stakeholders.

It is really important to make time to conduct a close-out meeting, or series of meetings, with all the project participants. The actual agenda will vary depending on the participants. Items to include are:
- Results/outcome of the project, plus any impact they might have
- Feedback or lessons learnt
- Acknowledgement and thanking the participants

Further reading

Schwalbe K. Healthcare Project Management, 2013, Schwalbe Publishing, Minneapolis, Minnesota.

꩜ http://www.nextscientist.com/manage-a-large-research-project/

꩜ http://www.mrc.ac.uk/research/research-policy-ethics/good-research-practice/

Essential documents

Introduction

The trial master file (TMF) is the collection of essential documents, historically in hardcopy, but increasingly in electronic format, generated during the conduct of the clinical trial. The regulations and the increased importance given by regulatory inspectors to the content and maintenance of the trial master file have greatly increased its significance. The EU Directive and Regulation states that the TMF 'shall consist of essential documents, which enable both the conduct of a clinical trial and the quality of the data produced to be evaluated.' It is a legal requirement that a TMF is established before the start of the clinical trial.

There are three basic components to a TMF:
- Sponsor's generic documents applicable across the whole study and all sites
- Investigator site file collected and maintained at site (belongs and remains with the investigator)
- Central investigator file: a 'mirror' set of the site file with a few important exceptions, that the sponsor or contract research organization (CRO) maintains.

The sponsor should not have documents that reveal the subjects' names; the subjects must remain anonymous to the sponsor. For phase 1 trials, normally based in a specialist unit with no additional sites, there is often no individual investigator file held centrally by the sponsor/CRO.

It is the TMF that forms the basis of both independent audits and regulatory inspections. The GCP E6 Guidelines define an essential document as 'Documents which individually and collectively permit the evaluation of the conduct of a study and the quality of the data produced'. The essential documents should be filed in an organized way that will facilitate management of the clinical trial, audit, and inspection (Rules Governing Medicinal Products in the European Union, Volume 10, Clinical Trials). It should be remembered that essential documents may come in a variety of formats including: written, electronic, magnetic and optical records and scans, X-rays and electrocardiograms. Anything that describes or records the methods, conduct, and/or results of a trial, the factors affecting the trial, and the actions taken is an essential document and so must be filed and retained. These documents may also be held in a separate location from the main TMF during the trial, such as the drug-dispensing records held in the pharmacy department.

The documents may be held in paper format, electronically, or in a combination of both formats provided that the documents can be made available to inspectors on request. Many documents are held electronically during the conduct of the trial and only printed out at the end of the trial. Inspectors want to review the documents that have actually been used and referred to during the trial, so may request access to electronic documents if these are the documents that the clinical research associates (CRA) and clinical trial administrators (CTA) have been using regularly.

Any institution conducting clinical research should have a standard operating procedure (SOP) or work instruction (WI) covering the establishment and maintenance of the TMF. This should include responsibilities, security, storage, filing, and quality control of the TMF. The filing structure should be added as an associated document, along with templates for file labels, table of contents, and notes to file.

The ICH/GCP E6 Guidelines contain a helpful list of essential documents listed in section 8, with guidance as to whether they are applicable to the sponsor/CRO only, the investigator only, or to both parties. However, it is worth noting that this list is regarded by regulatory agencies as a minimum requirement and so should not be considered comprehensive (this is discussed in detail later in this chapter). The TMF provides transparency of conduct and an audit trail to facilitate the full reconstruction of the trial at a later date.

Documentation required before the trial starts

It is a legal requirement to maintain a TMF which should be established by the sponsor and the investigator *before* the start of the trial, (Rules Governing Medicinal Products in the European Union, Volume 10, Clinical Trials). This is the period of high activity when the majority of documents have to be filed. The GCP E6 Guidelines list the essential documents in section 8 according to the different phases of the clinical trial: before the trial begins (section 8.2), during the conduct of the trial (section 8.3), and at the completion of the trial (section 8.4).

Investigator brochure (IB)

The latest version of this document or the summary of medicinal product characteristics (SmPC) must be on file to ensure that the participating investigators are fully aware of all the current information about the drug being researched. The IB contains a summary of all the known information and research for the compound being tested. The IB must be regularly updated so it is essential that editions are clearly identified with a version number and date. It is strongly recommended that the issue of the IB is tracked to ensure that all sites have the current version of the IB. If the drug is already a licensed product, then the SmPC should be on file.

Protocol

The protocol is the 'bible' of the clinical trial. It includes all aspects of the design and methodology, number of subjects to be recruited, tests and visits, and publication of the results at the end of the trial. The sponsor/CRO approval and review process for the protocol must be fully documented. A protocol fully approved, by the regulatory authorities and independent ethics committee (IEC), must be available before the start of the trial. Any subsequent amendments must be clearly identified with version and date, must go through the internal approval process, and be submitted to the regulatory authorities and IEC for approval.

Informed consent form (ICF) and patient information sheet (PIS)

It is a fundamental principle of GCP that all participants in a clinical trial give their informed consent to participate in the trial. Documentation of this consent must be approved prior to the start of the trial and versions of the consent must be clearly controlled. If there have been local requirements to amend the ICF/PIS, then the version control of the documents becomes vital. It is usual practice within the UK for the ICF/PIS to be issued to subjects on institution-headed paper but this practice is not widespread throughout the rest of Europe. If there are subjects in the trial whose first language is not English then these documents must be translated. Best industry practice dictates that the local language documents given to a patient, such as ICF/PIS, are 'back translated' into English.

Financial aspects of the trial

There must be a signed agreement in place clearly stating the payments to be made to investigators/institutions for conducting the trial, before any trial activities take place at site. Financial disclosure documentation, usually associated with trials conducted under US Federal Drug Agency (FDA) regulations, requires the investigator to confirm that he or she has no financial interest in the study results or any proprietary interest in the product being tested. This demonstration of due diligence helps show that there is no bias from investigators while conducting the trial. Sometimes there is a separate financial agreement, in addition to the contract. This is also covered in the signed agreements section.

Insurance statement

The safety and well-being of subjects taking part is a fundamental principle of GCP. The provision of insurance to compensate subjects for any trial-related injury suffered during the conduct of the trial is confirmed by an insurance certificate.

Signed agreements

Before the start of the trial, contracts must be in place between the sponsor and CRO, if applicable, and between the sponsor/CRO and the institutions/investigators. Any other vendors, such as laboratories, translators, data management staff, or medical writers, who will provide specific services during the course of the trial, must also have a contract. The contracts should clearly state what payments will be made, when, and what are the individual responsibilities under the contract. While not an essential document, a vendor selection document is advisable. Inspectors often expect to see evidence of vendor selection and a breakdown of vendor responsibilities available within the TMF.

Ethics committee approvals

It is a GCP requirement that an independent ethics committee (IEC) gives its approval prior to the start of the trial. The approval letter from the IEC must be on file prior to the release of any study drug to site and prior to any subject screening. The TMF should include, in addition to the approvals, the completed submission forms with lists of submitted documents and their versions. The composition of the IEC and a statement confirming that the IEC operates in accordance with the GCP guidelines should also be on file. In the UK, if the research is to be conducted in a National Health Service (NHS) institution, it is also required to have research and development (R&D) committee permission.

Regulatory authority approval

All clinical trials conducted in Europe must be registered on the EudraCT database. A EudraCT number will be issued for a trial when it is registered and this number must be quoted in all correspondence with the competent authority (CA) and the IEC. In the UK, clinical trial authorization (CTA) from the MHRA must be in place prior to the start of any trial activities. Also in the UK, if the research is to be conducted in an NHS institution, it is required to have R&D approval, as mentioned above.

Curricula vitae

It is necessary for the trial team to demonstrate that all members are suitably qualified by education, training, and experience to participate in the trial. CVs should be recent, usually recommended to be not more than two-years old, and should include information such as Medical Council registration numbers and evidence of GCP training. It is generally accepted that the CVs of all site team members should be kept on file and a delegation log should be maintained specifying which tasks may be performed by which individual team members.

Laboratories

The laboratory used for analysing the subject samples must be part of an accreditation programme, and a current certificate of accreditation must be on file. The laboratory's standard reference ranges and any instructional manual should be on file.

Investigational medicinal product

Includes certificates of analysis, investigational medicinal product dossier (IMPD), qualified person (QP) signed release, import licence (if applicable; this may be considered part of the regulatory approval process), templates for shipping receipts and drug accountability, and labelling for the drug. Instructions for the handling and/or reconstitution of drug at site and also for the storage of drug and temperature logs if required.

Decoding procedures and randomization

The decoding procedures document how the treatment of a single subject in an emergency may be identified without 'unblinding' all subjects in the trial. This can be achieved by individual random code envelopes. The randomization list specifies which treatment has been allocated to each subject. The list is either generated by the statistics department or by third-party vendors that specialize in interactive voice-recognition systems (IVRS) or interactive web systems (IWS). The master randomization list will be opened by the statisticians after the database has been locked and analysis of the trial performed. At this point it becomes apparent if the trial has successfully demonstrated efficacy and safety or not.

Pre-trial monitoring and trial initiation monitoring reports

The investigators taking part in the study must have been assessed as suitable, so there may be feasibility questionnaires and a pre-study site selection visit. These must be reported and included in the TMF. Before a site can start screening subjects there must be a site initiation visit or visits which cover all aspects of the trial including some protocol specific training and frequently some GCP training. This visit must be reported and note taken of all site staff who attended the training. Any presentations or training materials used at the visit must be retained in the TMF.

The following documents are not specified in section 8.2 of the GCP guidelines but they are normally produced prior to the start of a trial.

Case report form

The document, either hardcopy or electronic data capture (EDC), in which the subject data is collected and associated documents such as patient diaries, diet sheets, or quality of life questionnaires. These must be approved by the IEC.

Safety

A serious adverse event (SAE) plan, a document to explain the process for the handling of SAEs and the procedure for processing SAEs, is required.

Documentation during the trial

While the trial is underway, the documents updating versions and amendments, monitoring, and data collection are the types of documents that need to be collected. These are specified in the GCP guidelines and comprise the following.

IBs and protocol amendments

The IB must be revised regularly, particularly to incorporate safety information, any revision or changes to the protocol, ICF/PIS, CRF must be approved internally by the sponsor/CRO. The new versions must be clearly identified as such.

Approvals and updates

New versions of IBs, protocol amendments, ICF/PIS, and CRF must be submitted to CA/IEC and R&D departments, and the approval letters filed in the TMF.

Curricula vitae

For new staff members, and updated ones for existing staff must be collected.

Laboratories and IMP

Any revision of reference ranges, manuals, and procedures must be filed. Also, new certificates of authorization must be filed.

Monitoring visit reports and monitoring log

A log should be maintained recording each time the monitor, clinical research associate (CRA), or other sponsor/CRO staff visit the site, including the date of the visit and the reason for the visit. Routine monitoring visits, including the checking of source data, discussion of any issues or difficulties with the site team, and review of completed CRF pages, must be written up and reviewed, as detailed in the monitoring plan.

Relevant communication

Throughout the trial communication with IEC or CA, sites or vendors must be documented. The communication may be in the form of telephone conversations, faxes, letters, e-mails, or meeting minutes. Much of this communication may be held electronically. This can be a difficult area to control simply because there is a great deal of documentation generated. This is discussed further later in the chapter.

Signed consent forms and source documents

The subject must sign a consent form prior to participation in the trial. The form also permits access to the subject's medical records by CRAs, auditors, and inspectors. Within the EU, permission is usually included for the export of personal data outside the European Economic Area (EEA). The source data includes the subject's medical history and documents the subject's existence. These documents are not part of the sponsor/CRO's TMF; they remain at site.

Data collection

CRFs, subject diaries, and questionnaires record information about the subject's participation in the trial. Data clarification forms (DCFs) document the changes or corrections raised by the data management team, after the initial completion of the CRF.

Serious adverse event (SAE) reports

Any SAE must be reported by the investigator 'immediately' (within 24 hours of becoming aware) to the sponsor/CRO, including follow-up reports and related correspondence. Information about SAEs must be sent to all other investigators involved in the trial.

Notifications to IEC and CA

During the trial SAE reports, IB updates, and interim reports must be submitted to IEC and the CA (and the R&D department if in the UK).

Screening and enrolment logs

A log should be maintained to record all subjects screened for potential inclusion in the trial. The enrolment log and study identification code list records all subjects taking part in the trial. These documents remain at site.

Signature sheet

GCP guidelines identify this document as recording signatures and initials of site team authorized to make corrections to the CRF. It is more common now to use a delegation sheet. This incorporates the signatures and initials of site staff, along with the duties they may perform. The delegation sheet must include new members of the site team as the trial progresses and the dates that team members leave the project.

Record of retained body fluids/tissue samples

The identification and location of samples must be documented in the TMF, and these must be retained during the conduct of the trial.

Documentation requirements after the trial

After the completion of the trial the following documents need to be added to those already collected to complete the TMF. These documents are listed in section 8.4 of the guidelines.

IMP and drug destruction

A full accountability of all drug dispatched to site, dispensed to subjects, and drug to be returned at trial completion. After close-out of the sites and full drug accountability, all unused drug is destroyed either at site or centrally. A certificate of drug destruction must be issued.

Samples destruction

On completion of the trial, all samples and tissues collected during the trial must be destroyed and a certificate of destruction issued (unless arrangements have been made to retain for 'future research' projects).

Audit certificate

Certificates, not the reports, of any audits conducted during the trial either at site, of the TMF or of third-party vendors must be filed in the TMF if required by applicable law or regulations (e.g. Japan).

Close-out visit

All sites must be formally closed out at the end of the trial and any outstanding documents collected from site, even if the site did not recruit any patients into the trial. A summary trial report must be sent to all investigators.

Notification to IEC and CA

IEC and the CA (and R&D departments) must be informed when the trial is complete and a copy of the summary report must be submitted. If part of a multinational trial then the authorities should be informed on completion of the trial at the site and also when the trial is completed worldwide, as these times may be different.

Clinical study report (CSR)

A report must be produced for all trials. This may either be a comprehensive trial report including all the statistical report, with the tables, listings, and figures (TLFs), or the latter may be issued separately. Even if the trial is terminated prematurely, as a minimum a safety report must be produced.

Additional documents

The GCP E6 guidelines list approximately 87 documents required for inclusion in the TMF. This is widely considered to be an inadequate list, with regulatory inspectors frequently requesting additional records. The GCP guidelines do not include data management documents as part of the required list and makes no mention of e-mails. Inspectors frequently request to see documents that support the clinical trial process, such as evidence of vendor selection and a breakdown of vendor responsibilities. These documents are now generally accepted as part of the TMF, but they are usually filed separately from the clinical operations documents. Their location should be known so that they may be made available, along with reports on computer validation and other supporting documents, if required by the inspectors.

Figure 22.1 illustrates these additional documents.

To address this gap in guidance about the content of the TMF, the Drug Information Agency (DIA) has produced a fully inclusive list of documents that should, depending on the type of trial, be included in the TMF. It is known as the TMF reference model: ✆ http://tmfrefmodel.com. The model is based on phase 2/3 studies, but the group is currently working on guidance for phase 1 studies and for investigator site files. The reference model indicates those documents that are core (i.e. mandatory) for inclusion in the TMF and also those that are recommended for inclusion in the TMF. It also highlights alternative names for some documents.

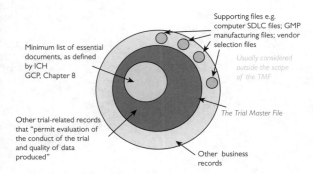

Figure 22.1 The trial master file.
© 2009 Rammell Consulting Ltd. Reprinted by permission of Rammell Consulting Ltd.

Correspondence and e-mails

One of the most difficult sections of a TMF is the correspondence. The GCP guidelines require that 'relevant communications other than site visits—letters; meeting notes; notes of telephone calls' that 'document any agreement or significant discussions regarding trial administration, protocol violations, trial conduct, adverse event reporting' must be included in the TMF. Where things become difficult is when deciding just what is relevant and what is not. The danger is always that rather than make a decision, every single piece of communication is included. The GCP guidelines, as they were finalized in 1996 when e-mails were virtually unknown, makes no reference to e-mails at all. The handling of e-mails continues to be a problem. Should they be printed out? Ought they be preserved in electronic format? This is recommended, as they were originally available only electronically, but they must be available on demand if required. The e-mails must be saved and organized in a manner that allows for searching and easy retrieval and also can be preserved throughout the time required for the retention of the clinical trial documents.

All communication should be regularly reviewed throughout the conduct of the trial to confirm that it is still relevant and required to be on file. The GCP-RMA have produced a useful guidance paper on handling clinical trial communication. ✍ www.gcp-rma.org

Notes to file

If there are issues during the conduct of the trial, such as missing or damaged documents, these are frequently recorded in notes to file. This practice is being discouraged by the FDA and CAs as issues regarding TMF documents should be treated in accordance with the corrective and preventative actions procedures of the relevant company/institution. However, if a note to file is added to the TMF, it should explain the problem and what steps have been taken to rectify it, and any preventative measures that have been put in place to ensure it does not occur again. For consistency there should be a template for these notes and they should always be signed and dated. If notes to file are being used, they should be numbered, tracked, and generated as soon as the team becomes aware of the issue, not on completion of the trial prior to archive. Notes to file highlight problems, so they should be avoided if possible. Inspectors can have findings about excessive use of notes to file.

Organization of TMFs

Although the GCP Guidelines and Volume 10 give some assistance with the documents that are considered to be essential for the conduct of the trial and therefore must be included in the TMF, it does not give any assistance in how the TMF should be filed, other than 'in an organized' manner. Given that the same basic information has to be collected for the TMF, it is somewhat surprising how very different approaches are taken by companies and institutions to their TMF. For investigators and institutions participating in a large commercial trial sponsored by a pharmaceutical company, this will be decided for the trial team, as the company will have its own filing structure, the site file will be established for the team, and the company's CRA will maintain this file.

If the study is sponsored by a non-commercial institution or is investigator-led, this assistance is generally not provided, although many do now have SOPs to support creation of these structures. To create a useful and practical filing structure for a clinical trial is quite challenging. Any filing structure needs to ensure completeness and ease of use both to the study team and to any auditor or inspector who needs to refer to the TMF. The most common approach to the TMF is to use a numeric system, with appropriate subsections. For example, a basic filing structure could follow a simple listing as shown in Table 22.1.

Annotating the file structure with the documents to be filed in a particular section and reminders about signatures will assist the teams in filing documents and provide assistance for new team members, in both filing and retrieving documents. One of the most important aspects of the TMF is the consistency of filing. The policy on filing of documents should be included in the SOP, to cover date order and date format and how regularly documents will be filed. A backlog of documents sitting in a filing tray are neither 'readily available' nor secure. The files should be clearly identified with protocol number, sponsor name (if applicable), and sections of the TMF included in that file. At the front of the file there should be a list of the sections contained in that file. This information should remain current, so if an additional file is needed, the information on the old files should be amended to reflect the inclusion of an additional file.

TMF training should always be given to the team at the start of the study. If the TMF is being held by a CRO and the filing structure and SOPs to be followed belong to the sponsor, then the sponsor should arrange for training to be given to the CRO team. When a CRO is maintaining the TMF, the filing structure, document format, and return to the sponsor on trial completion should all be agreed in the service level agreement.

A simple spreadsheet can be very helpful in tracking documents, giving a central list for number and dates of protocol amendments, approvals by authorities, and current versions of other approved documents such as ICF/PIS. A hyperlink can be set up from an Excel spreadsheet to a Word document, for quick reference. It is particularly useful if there is more than one investigator site to record the status of documents from a particular site (e.g. principal investigator's CV is out of date).

Table 22.1 Table of Contents: Trial Master File

Section	Document type	Purpose/comments
Section 1	Trial personnel	
1.1	Sponsor team	Include contact details, CVs signed and dated, training records
1.2	CRO	Include contact details, CVs signed and dated, training records
1.3	Vendor teams	Include contact details, CVs signed and dated, training records
Section 2	Protocol	
2.1	Final protocol and approval form	Original signature page, signed and dated Protocol must be version controlled Internal approval form signed and dated
2.2	Protocol amendments and approval forms	Original signature pages, signed and dated for all amendments Amendments must be version controlled Internal approval forms signed and dated
2.3	Protocol translations	Original signature page, signed and dated Protocol must be version controlled Internal approval form signed and dated If translated into several languages arrange by language or by country
2.4	Protocol synopsis	If applicable
2.5	Protocol deviations and Notes to file	Filed by sequential number or chronologically
2.6	Correspondence	File in reverse chronological order
Section 3	Independent ethics committee (IEC)	
3.1	Approvals	Approval for trial protocol and amendments
3.2	Submissions	Initial application for approval to conduct trial, must include list of all documents and versions of documents submitted
3.3	Notifications and acknowledgements	SAE reports, interim reports, updated IBs, etc., notified to IEC
3.4	Membership	Members approving the protocol and amendments
3.5	Constitution and/or SOPs	Approved authorized copies
3.6	Statement of GCP compliance	If included on approval letter, add note to file
3.7	Correspondence	File in reverse chronological order

Translations

It is a GCP requirement that all documents given to subjects are in their own language. This is not just for large multinational trials; in trials where recruitment will come from a local ethnic population, there may well be a need to translate documents from the generic English. The documents given to the subject include ICF/PIS, quality of life questionnaires, recruitment adverts, and also the labels on the IMP, so these must be translated. There should be a formal certificate of translation, signed and dated to verify the accuracy of the translation, filed along with the original English and foreign language version. There should be a CV or confirmation of the translator's qualification to perform the translations. Many companies also require a 'back' translation of the foreign version into English (performed by a different translator), and then a comparison with the original English version against the version translated from the foreign language. This is not mandated, but is considered to be best practice. In addition, if trials are being conducted in a number of countries, it is a GCP requirement that essential documents are in English, so regulatory and ethics committee approvals, contracts, and insurance, for example, are translated into English from the local language.

Version control

An area of weakness often highlighted by MHRA inspectors is the version control of documents. It is essential that the study and site teams are always working to the latest version of a document. So IBs, protocol amendments, ICF/PIS, CRFs, and any study monitoring or data management plans, must be clearly identified with a version number and date. Ideally, a list of previous versions should also be included. While previous versions must be retained on file, steps should be taken to ensure the latest version is being followed by all the study and site teams.

Storage of TMFs

It is a GCP requirement that the TMFs are securely stored in a manner which prevents their premature destruction and maintains subject confidentiality. Increasingly, inspectors have come to expect dedicated document rooms, with security and environmental controls. However, this is not mandated within the legislation. It is perfectly acceptable for smaller companies or academia, investigator-led and charity-funded research institutions to store their TMFs in a more basic manner. The TMFs should be secured, in lockable metal cupboards, not wooden because of the fire risk. However, the cupboards must be locked while not in use and there has to be a secure system for the safe storage of the keys, such as a locked key cupboard. Where records are not being stored for long periods of time (i.e. active filing areas), there is no requirement for any special environmental controls other than protecting records from extremes of temperature and humidity to avoid immediate damage.

Non-commercial and academic trials

The EU Directives do not distinguish between commercially sponsored trials and those conducted by non-commercial or academic organizations. All subjects taking part in clinical research are entitled to the same levels of protection. Some trials, including epidemiological and registry studies, are not included in the scope of the EU Directives, but researchers are expected to adhere to the principles of GCP. The definition of non-interventional trials under the EU Directive is quite narrow. Basically, the IMP must be used in accordance with its licence, must be following 'standard treatment', and no additional tests or procedures are being performed. One of the aspects of the EU Regulation is the definition of non–interventional trials. The additional administrative burdens imposed by the EU Directives have adversely affected these types of trials, greatly reducing the number of academic trials conducted in the UK. The definition of a 'non-interventional' trial is widened in the EU Regulation, while at the same time ensuring harmonization across the EU member states.

When establishing a TMF for all of these types of trials, the GCP essential document list should be assessed as to the applicability of each document type to the trial, and it should be made very clear exactly who is the sponsor of the trial. For example, at the very minimum there will be a basic protocol, proposal or feasibility, consent will have to be obtained from participants, information given to subjects about the trial, data will need to be collected and analysed, and a report produced. Permissions will be required, possibly from the IEC and definitely from R&D, if the study is being conducted on an NHS site. If the ethics committee confirms that the trial does not need ethics approval, this written confirmation should be included in the TMF. There may or may not be documents about IMP, randomization, laboratories or third-party service providers. Having decided which documents will be applicable to the trial and a basic filing structure produced, then the TMF should be set up prior to recruitment of subjects. The filing should be completed regularly with sections within the TMF clearly indicated and files labelled with trial number or name. The documents should be filed in reverse chronological order and at the beginning of the file there should be a contents list. If the files become too full then additional files must be made up and contents sheets and labels amended.

Quality control (QC) of the TMF

It is strongly recommended that some QC reviews are specified in the TMF SOP and that these are routinely followed during the active phase of the trial. It is very much easier to locate a missing document, obtain a signature for a CV or document an issue, while the trial is still active. The QC should cover completeness of the TMF, appropriate to the phase of the trial, quality of documents, and accuracy of filing. These routine checks will encourage staff to keep filing up to date and make end of study checks very much easier. The QC checks that have been performed should be documented.

Electronic trial master files (eTMFs)

Traditionally the TMF has been in paper format. This has been changing, with most of the large pharmaceutical companies and the large CROs now using and declaring the electronic TMF as the master for inspection. In many ways this is a logical step; the majority of the essential documents in the TMF are generated electronically by the sponsor or CRO. There are some documents that will not be available electronically, such as ethics approval letters, which must therefore be scanned for inclusion in the eTMF. Also 'wet-ink' signature pages must also be scanned, although the increasing acceptance of 'electronic signatures' means in reality that there are very few documents that cannot be generated electronically.

The advantages of an eTMF include the visibility of documents, regardless of time or location, electronic back-up, and the granting of different levels of access according to need to all team members. So far, the eTMF has mainly been adopted by the large sponsor companies and CROs. Just as EDC has become the standard format for collecting data from the CRF, eventually there will be eISFs. This will solve one of the perennial problems of lack of space and storage at sites.

Retention requirements

Under the GCP guidelines, all essential documents must be retained for a period of two years after the last marketing approval in any of the ICH/GCP countries, or for two years after the formal end of research on that compound. The EU Directive 2001/20/EC requires compliance with the principles of GCP, so confirms this retention period. The patient identification codes, CRFs, patient files, and source data, along with other specified essential documents, must be retained for at least 15 years under EU Directive 2003/63/EC, or for as long as the product is authorized. This reference to patient records means it is often considered to be mainly applicable to investigator sites. The EU Directive 2005/28/EC requires essential documents to be retained for five years after completion of the trial or longer if so required by national law or institutional policy. These requirements are primarily aimed at the commercial IMP research trials and interventional trials, so are not necessarily helpful for non-interventional, non-IMP, or devices research. As there is less guidance for these types of trials, many researchers use the five-year minimum retention time, as laid out in the 'GCP Directive'. All R&D departments (in the UK) and academic institutions should have a retention schedule in place for the guidance of their research staff. On its implementation, the Clinical Trial Regulation 536/2014 requires that essential documentation is retained for 25 years.

Conclusion

The maintenance of the TMF is an essential part of demonstrating the transparency of conduct of the clinical trial. A well-ordered, accurately filed, and complete TMF is evidence that the principles of GCP and the legal requirements of the EU Directives, UK statutory instruments and EU Regulation have been followed.

Further reading

International Conference on Harmonisation of Technical Requirements for Registration of Pharmaceuticals for Human Use. Guideline for Good Clinical Practice (ICH E6), April 1996. ℘ www.ich.org

Directive 2001/20/EC of the European Parliament and of the Council of 4 April 2001, on the approximation of the laws, regulations and administrative provisions of the Member States relating to the implementation of good clinical practice in the conduct of clinical trials on medicinal products for human use. Official Journal L 121, 1 May 2001: 34–44.

Commission Directive 2005/28/EC of 8 April 2005, laying down principles and detailed guidelines for good clinical practice as regards investigational medicinal products for human use, as well as the requirements for authorisation of the manufacturing or importation of such products. Official Journal L91, 9 April 2005: 13–19.

The EU Clinical Trial Directive.

DIA reference model 2012. ℘ www.diahome.org/

Eudralex volume 10. The rules governing medicinal products in the European Union, *Chapter IV* Guidance for the conduct of GCP inspections—Sponsor and CRO, Annex IV. ℘ http://ec.europa.eu/health/documents/eudralex/vol-10/>2009-06-30 GCP-RMA Relevant Communication Policy v1.0.doc Policy gcprma.files.wordpress.com/.../2009-06-30-gcp-rma

Archiving

Introduction

Unfortunately, archiving of the clinical trial documents is rarely considered at the beginning of the trial and consequently this causes many difficulties and problems when the trial is completed. From the very start of the project, thought must be given to where and when the documents will be archived, who will perform the archiving, and who will continue to manage them throughout the retention period. There is little guidance about archiving except regarding retention periods, which in themselves can be confusing, although the inspectors invariably do look at archiving procedures and usually make time to interview the archivist. It is a legal requirement to archive the clinical trial documents.

The GCP Directive 2005/28/EC Article 17 and the EU Regulation article 54 states that 'Essential documents shall be archived in a way that ensures that they are readily available, upon request, to the competent authorities'. This clause means that a procedure must be in place to control and track the clinical trial documents on completion of the trial and throughout their retention period.

The GCP E6 guidelines give no help with guidance for archiving, only stating the period of retention for documents. There is no definition of an archive, minimum building and storage conditions for security and long-term preservation of the documents. However, there is guidance available from the related discipline of good laboratory practice (GLP), which can be helpful when establishing an archive for GCP records.

The GLP—Guidance on Archiving published by the Medicines and Healthcare products Regulatory Agency (MHRA) provides a definition of an archive, 'Archives: The facilities and supporting resources necessary for the secure retention and maintenance of materials accumulated by an organization in the conduct of regulatory studies'.

There should be a standard operating procedure (SOP) in place for archiving the clinical documents. It should include the preparation for the trial master file (TMF), the transfer to the archive, the security and management of TMFs at archive, and the eventual destruction of the clinical documents. There should be similar procedures for the investigator site file (ISF).

The archive

The most useful guidance for the requirements for an archive is found in the quality standard ISO11799—Information and Documentation—Document Storage requirements for Libraries and Archives.

Location

Very few people have the opportunity to oversee the provision of a purpose-built archive; the majority either inherit an archive or are allocated a space within the company's building or site that will become the archive. When considering the location of the archive, some factors should immediately cause alarm, such as an archive sited on a flood plain or in close vicinity to a river or canal. If the site is part of a manufacturing/business park, the type of companies based there need to be assessed. Do the factories emit excessive smoke, dust, or harmful gases? Also, does any installation or depot create a risk of fire or explosion? As an example, the Hertfordshire Oil Depot in Hemel Hempstead in the UK, which caught fire after a series of explosions in December 2005. This was a major incident and it took several days before the area to be declared safe, and during this period even buildings not damaged by the fire were not accessible. Consider the nature of the companies close to the proposed archive. Could they be a target for terrorists, political activists, travellers?

If the archive is to be located on the pharmaceutical company's site, it should be located away from any manufacturing activity or distribution/storage warehouses that might increase the risk of fire or explosion.

Archive building

The physical structure of the building must be weatherproof and provide some degree of fire resistance. The walls and roof should be constructed from a material with a high thermal capacity, such as brick, which is a good insulating material. The building must be large enough to house not only the current archive contents but allow for future deposits to the archive, preferably with at least room for the next five years. Doors must be waterproof, secure, and have excluders fitted to ensure that rodents cannot slip in under the doors. The archive should not have windows, for both security and environmental reasons, excluding harmful light and assisting in reducing temperature fluctuations. Ideally, there should be a covered area for the delivery and collection of archive boxes.

If the archive is to be an assigned space within an existing building, for security reasons it should be a self-contained unit. If possible, siting an archive in a basement should be avoided because of the risk of flooding and the presence of water and heating pipes. The water and heating pipes must not be run through the archive because of the danger of leakage from them. The ground floor is the best location for the archive for convenience of deliveries and also because of the weight of the storage of archive boxes. If located on an upper floor, then a survey will be needed to check the load-bearing capacity of the floor, and construction work may be needed to reinforce the floor.

The internal structure of the archive, walls, floors, and doors should all be fire-resistant as should other materials used, such as paints. The material used should not attract or retain dust. Electrical installations should be kept to a minimum. It is recommended that computers are located outside of the archive in a separate working area. Any electrical installations should be checked annually. Lighting should be low-level, only illuminating in sections in a large archive, sufficient to allow deposits and retrievals. The lights should be situated over the aisles between the racking and shelving. If there are any windows, these should be boarded up both for security and to reduce sunlight. There should be no naked light bulbs within the facility.

Suitable racking (i.e. metal not wooden shelving), fixed to accommodate the standard size of archive boxes used, will allow for the most economic use of space. There should be a clearance of at least 10 cm from the ground to the first shelf, which allows the air to circulate and in the case of a flood, the boxes would be clear of any standing water.

Archive staff should have a working area separate from the archive because access to the archive should be limited to the process of depositing and retrieving boxes. The environmental conditions most suited to the preservation of paper are not ideal for people.

Security

Whether the archive is within the company offices, a separate building on the site, or an off-site unit, security of the archive is of the highest priority. Ideally, the archive site should have secure perimeter fencing, closed circuit television, and overnight, if not full-time, security guards. There should only be one door into the archive and this should have an intruder alarm fitted. If there are windows these must also be fitted with intruder alarms. The alarm system should be part of a 24/7 monitoring service and the system should automatically alert the nearest police station to an intrusion.

Access to the archive should be controlled by means of an entry key code or magnetic swipe card; the latter is preferable as it will produce a record of all access to the archive. All visitors and contractors must sign a log recording the time and purpose of their visit and they must be accompanied by archive staff at all times. This applies equally to workmen employed for building work or general maintenance. Companies used for this work must be carefully selected and their staff should have been fully vetted.

When storing large volumes of paper records, the other major security risk is fire. There have been incidents of fires at off-site storage facilities, most notably at the Iron Mountain Bromley-by-Bow depot in July 2006. The company's annual report of 2007 attributed the cause of the fire to arson, which is an extreme event and very difficult to detect. Even though this modern building had both fire-detection and sprinkler systems, the building was completely destroyed, with the loss of many pharmaceutical records stored at the site. Rather than detecting a fire quickly it is much better to prevent the fire starting in the first place. Obviously smoking must be absolutely forbidden in the archive or around the archive. The construction and furnishings of the archive with fire-resistant material, the use of metal rather than wooden fittings, and minimal electrical installations all contribute to the fire prevention. Regular maintenance of any electrical installations and wiring, and good housekeeping to keep the archive neat and tidy will help with this.

There must be a fire-detection system in the archive which alerts both the staff and the local fire brigade. Consideration should be given to installation of a water or gas suppression system in the archive as this can be activated automatically. If a system is installed, it should allow for activation in sections rather than the whole system at once. Also the system and archive boxes immediately below the sprinklers and water pipes need frequent routine checks to ensure there are no leaks from the system. A gas suppression system does not have the same risks as a sprinkler system; however, these are very expensive to install and to be effective the archive must be completely air-tight. There should also be hand-held water and electrical fire extinguishers within the archive. Staff must be trained in archive evacuation procedures if a gas suppression system is in place. There should also be routine fire drills for the staff, all of whom should be trained in the use of hand-held fire extinguishers, which may well contain the fire until the fire brigade arrives.

Environmental controls

It is widely accepted that lowering the temperature and humidity will lengthen the storage life of paper. With humidity, there is a risk of microbiological activity above 60%, while if the relative humidity is too low then there is a risk that the paper will become brittle. With temperature, the biggest problem is large fluctuations either between different seasons or even day- to night-time temperatures. The generally accepted temperature ranges are 14–18°C + /– 1°C, assuming that staff are regularly accessing the archive. For humidity, the recommended ranges are 30% to 50% +/– 3%. If the archive is storing other media, such as magnetic tapes which require a cooler temperature, consideration should be given to perhaps dedicating a specific area of the archive for their storage.

An air-conditioning unit is the simplest way of controlling temperature/humidity in the archive. When environmental conditions are included in the storage quality manual or SOP then there has to be regular monitoring and recording of the conditions. If the temperature or humidity goes out of the specified range then remedial action must be taken and this action must be documented. An air-filter and smoke-extraction system should also be considered for the archive.

Potentially rodents such as rats, mice, and squirrels can do much damage, an archive box and its contents providing both home, bedding, and food all at the same time. Doors to the archive should never be unattended and they should be fitted with excluders so no creature, however small, can slide under the door. Regular maintenance checks should be made of the building to ensure there are no holes or gaps in brickwork or around windows, etc. A pest control company should be contracted to monitor the archive and its surroundings. It should have a schedule for regular visits which must be increased if they find evidence of rodent activity, or in the autumn when there is a natural increase in rodent activity.

Insects can also cause problems in the archive. If there is an infestation, a commercial company can be employed to fumigate the archive. The regular circulation and filtering of air will help control dust within the archive. The dust should be removed as it carries fungi spores, mould, and bacteria harmful to paper. Archive staff should make sure the archive is always clean and tidy.

The ideal storage conditions for paper (cool and dry) are not really suitable for people, therefore it is better to limit staff activity in the archive to adding archive boxes to the shelves or retrieving the boxes. All other staff activities such as preparing files for archive, cataloguing of box contents, maintenance of databases, are best performed in a separate, dedicated area adjacent to the archive. This also has the advantage that computers, photocopiers, and other electronic equipment are not required within the archive.

Management of the archive

The management of the archive and the archived documents should be the responsibility of an archivist. The 2005 GCP Directive requires that all sponsors (and CROs) appoint an archivist to be responsible for the control and long-term preservation of the clinical trial documents. In a small organization, it is perfectly acceptable for this role to be combined with other duties such as clinical trial assistant (CTA). It is also a legal requirement to restrict access to the archive. An access log must be maintained recording all non-archive staff who visit the archive, for whatever reason, and all visitors should be escorted in the archive.

Preparation for archive

Prior to archive, the TMF should be reviewed for completeness and accuracy of filing. Any omissions or issues requiring explanation should be documented in a note to file. It is the responsibility of the study manager to sign off the TMF as ready for archive. There should be timelines for this quality review of the TMF and transfer to archive included in the SOP. Materials that may perish or cause the paper to deteriorate must be removed; rubber bands will perish, bulldog clips will rust, and most significantly of all, plastic wallets that sweat, potentially causing mould and mildew to develop. In addition, after time in plastic wallets, the print can stick to the plastic, literally pulling the ink from the paper. It is also recommended that the documents are removed from the lever-arch files, a cover sheet containing the information from the spine label be added, and the documents secured by a plastic archive or 'e' clip. This offers the most effective use of space within the archive box, while keeping the documents securely filed, and allowing for the re-use of the lever-arch files. A contents list of the archive box should be produced. All these tasks may either be completed by the archive staff or by members of the clinical operations teams.

Transfer to the archive

There must a documented procedure for the receipt of the TMF into the archive. If the preparation for archive is not performed by the archive staff, then the contents lists provided by the clinical operations team must be verified and any discrepancies resolved before the archive team takes responsibility for the TMF.

Indexing and cataloguing

If the boxing up and the cataloguing of the TMF and possibly other related clinical trial documents is performed by the archive staff, then a second person should check contents lists for accuracy. It is essential, even in the smallest of archives, to ensure accurate cataloguing and indexing of the archived TMFs to ensure that they really are readily available on request by the authorities. As a minimum, the following information should be captured in the index: compound name and/or number, trial name and/or number and date. Other information to be captured includes investigator names and site numbers, study manager name, and possibly therapeutic area. The cataloguing, or listing, of the box contents should be on a standard form to assist in the capture of all of the relevant information required for the indexing. It is strongly recommended that these contents are not hand-written. They must include sufficient information to enable the identification of specific pieces of information (e.g. ethics approvals, individual CRFs by number). A copy of the contents list should be included in the archive box and a copy of this, either paper or electronic form, held centrally for use by the archivist.

'Chain of custody' and tracking

The change from active TMF, while the trial is still ongoing and the responsibility of the study manager, to the inactive archived TMF when the TMF becomes the responsibility of the archivist, is known as the 'chain of custody'. This transfer of responsibility must be clearly defined and documented. It is much more apparent when an off-site storage facility is being used, but it is equally important to establish the transfer of responsibility for small on-site archives. A master archive log must be maintained for the archive. It is most practical to hold the archived TMFs in archive boxes. These should be issued with a unique sequential number or barcode. The shelving within the archive must have individual location identification (e.g., row number, column number, and shelf number or a barcode). Then each archive box is assigned to a location and the location recorded. Here, a spreadsheet is quite adequate for a small archive. As long as everything is well documented there is no requirement to keep the whole TMF together (e.g. the CRFs may well be ready for archive ahead of the rest of the TMF). A spreadsheet can also be used to demonstrate how much unallocated space is available in the archive and warn management when the archive is likely to run out of space.

Information about exactly who is allowed access to the archive and who is allowed to authorize retrievals from it must be held by the archivist. Routinely, a check should be made to ensure that these access rights are being followed. It is also useful to track the use of the archive, the number and frequency of requests for retrievals, and the number and size of TMFs being deposited.

Retrievals from the archive

Any request for a retrieval of an archive box or a complete TMF from the archive must be authorized by management as stipulated in the relevant SOP. The retrieval must be documented, with the reason for the retrieval given, and signed by the appropriate manager. If possible, the information required could be accessed by the archive staff and either a scanned copy or photocopy sent to the requestor. This is preferable as it allows the TMF or archive box to remain in the safety of the archive. If a complete TMF is required or a large number of boxes required, this may not be possible. Any retrievals from the archive must be tracked. While on loan from the archive, the boxes/TMF become the responsibility of the person requesting the retrieval. The boxes/TMF should be kept securely, ideally in a locked cupboard or room and returned as soon as possible to the archive. Loans should always be for a limited period, as specified in the SOP, and the archivist must actively follow up retrievals as they approach the end of the loan period. There must be a valid reason for extending the loan period.

When the archive boxes are returned to the archive, the person who has had the responsibility for them must inform the archivist if there have been any changes to the contents of the box. The archivist must check the contents of the archive boxes against the contents lists before the boxes are returned to the archive, and the retrievals tracking sheet completed with the date of return.

Audits and inspections

During regulatory inspections it is usual both for the archivist to be interviewed by the inspectors and also for the facility tour to include a visit to the archive. The inspector must sign the access log and be escorted at all times when visiting the archive. The inspectors will review the archiving SOPs and other records held in the archive such as any recording of environmental conditions, pest control, and security monitoring contracts. They will look for the clear breakdown of responsibility for the TMF between the clinical operations staff and the archive, and for the documented process of transfer of TMFs into the archive and control of any retrievals from the archive. During an inspection, many documents that are not traditionally defined as part of the TMF are routinely requested by the inspectors. These documents may not have been included with the TMF when the trial was closed and sent to archive, but staff training records, computer validation reports, and contracts are frequently looked at during an inspection. If these documents are not included within the archive, it is recommended that someone, not necessarily the archivist, knows exactly where these documents are located.

Retention times

The most commonly asked archiving question is 'how long do I have to keep my documents?' This should be a relatively simple question to answer but it is complicated by conflicting timelines included within the GCP guidelines and the regulatory requirements of the EU Directive. The EU Regulation when fully implemented (expected to be 2016) will clarify the retention period as 25 years but in the meantime the debate about this continues. When establishing a retention period for clinical research documents, other factors such as business or legal requirements may have to be considered. As the GCP Guidelines were produced primarily for use in clinical trials that would result in licensing applications for the compound, they may not be very helpful for non-commercial, academic, or non-drug research. Before the introduction of the GCP Guidelines it was common practice to retain clinical trial documents for 15 years.

The GCP Guidelines state that essential documents should be retained for two years after the last approval of the marketing application in any ICH GCP area or there are no contemplated marketing applications in any ICH GCP area. If research on the compound is discontinued, then the essential documents need only be retained for two years after completion of the trial. The retention times are the same for sponsor and investigators. It is the sponsor's responsibility to inform the investigator when he or she may destroy the documents. However, the essential documents may be retained for a longer period if so required by the regulatory authority or the sponsor. The EU Directive 2001/20/EC does not specifically mention retention times for clinical documents but confirms that documents should be retained in accordance with the principles of ICH/GCP.

It would be much simpler to write a retention schedule if there was a fixed period of archiving for essential trial documents, which is the basis for the archiving requirements under the GCP Directive. The 2005 Directive, incorporated into UK law under SI 2006/1928, states a period of only five years after completion of the trial for the retention of essential documents. If the institution where the trial was conducted or national laws require a longer retention period, then the TMF must be retained for this increased period of time. The UK does not specify any additional retention period over the five years minimum.

There is a further EU Directive 2003/63/EC which is applicable to licensed products and marketing authorization holders. In the 2003/63 Annex 1 the requirement is: 'The sponsor or other owner of the data shall retain all other documentation pertaining to the trial as long as the product is authorised.'

It specifies that essential clinical trial documents, including case report forms (CRFs), other than a subject's medical files, must be retained for 15 years after the completion or discontinuation of the trial. It also requires that the subject's medical files should be retained in accordance with the applicable legislation and in accordance with the maximum time permitted by the hospital, institution, or private practice. This reference to both the CRFs and the subject's medical files implies that this particular retention period applies to the investigator site files, thus these files should be retained for a minimum of 15 years. The Clinical Trial Regulation, when implemented, will remove the ambiguity as it clearly states that essential documents be kept for 25 years.

As litigation in all areas has increased within the UK, there are examples of court cases involving clinical research and pharmaceutical products. If a compound is subject to a court case, then an order for a 'litigation hold' will be applied to the clinical research documents. In these circumstances, none of the clinical documents are allowed to be destroyed, even if they have reached the stipulated retention period. A 'litigation hold' on a compound or product overrides any retention schedule or standard company procedure.

Investigator site file archiving

As previous stated, currently the investigator or institution is required to retain documents for a minimum of 15 years, with the implementation of the EU Regulation this will be extended to 25 years. Even with the introduction of electronic data capture (EDC), thus replacing the large paper CRFs with an electronic format, many investigators and institutions find it very difficult to archive the clinical trial documents for the required periods of time in suitable environmental or secure conditions. It has become quite a common practice for sponsors of commercial trials to assist their investigators with this long-term storage. This assistance may be included in the financial arrangements for the conduct of the clinical trial, or it may be in the form of a one-off financial payment to cover the archiving for 15 years (25 years in the future), or the sponsor may have an arrangement to provide off-site storage for the investigator's archiving. If the latter is the case, then the process must be established in a manner which allows the investigator to retain control of and access to his or her archiving. The investigator archiving should not go the sponsor offices or be under the control of the sponsor. At no time should the sponsor access the investigator archiving boxes.

Off-site storage

The sheer volume of clinical trial documents generated during a research programme and the length of time documents must be retained have resulted in the utilization of specialist off-site storage facilities. These facilities must provide the security, environmental controls, and administration already discussed. In fact, many of them are able to offer a far higher level of security and control than would be available in small company offices. They normally have their own dedicated transport and can offer additional services such as 'image on-demand'. This service offers the contents of an archive box or file to be scanned and sent electronically to the client, so avoiding the need to recall and transport the box from archive to client.

As when selecting any third-party service provider, a documented selection procedure must be followed. Ideally, a minimum of three companies should be approached and asked to tender for the contract. All the companies should be asked to submit a proposal and all the potential facilities should be visited. It is essential, if the storage has more than one location, that the location visited is the one where the trial's boxes will be archived. Factors to be considered when selecting an off-site storage facility include distance from the trial site, levels of security, fire prevention and suppression, transport services, a client working area, scanning facilities, and awareness of pharmaceutical regulations. An auditor, experienced in the assessment of archive facilities, should audit the site prior to signing a contract.

The contract should include the service level agreement (SLA), which specifies the standards of service required. This includes how quickly archive boxes can be returned, normally the next working day with a provision (usually at a premium) to have 'emergency' same-day retrievals if required. 'Deep storage' facilities are something to consider (the storage of documents unlikely to be recalled). How much notice of a collection of new or returned boxes will the facility need? Can the account be set up with different access levels for various personnel? Can individual department accounts be established under the one contract? Are there any circumstances when a courier rather than the facility's own transport may be used? If a box is damaged or deteriorates through old age, should the box be returned or can the facility's staff re-box? Are there any special instructions to bear in mind (e.g. when an archive box must only be returned to the investigator depositing archive box)? All such questions should be considered when compiling the service level agreement.

It is important to demonstrate ongoing oversight of the storage facility other than just routine contact maintained in order to collect new archive boxes for inclusion in the archive. This can take the form of a request for a report on the archive boxes on deposit to be verified against the archive log held by the archivist. After the initial audit, prior to signing the contract, regular audits should be conducted, and a two-yearly programme is recommended. However, if there any issues—such as non-compliance with the SLA—between the scheduled audits, the storage facility should be visited and the issue resolved immediately.

eArchiving

The problems associated with guaranteeing the long-term preservation of electronic documents has largely meant that while electronic documents are used widely during the clinical trial, when it comes to archiving, many companies and institutions rely on the paper copies. The increasing acceptance of eTMFs, the use of EDC for CRFs, and the analysis of samples and specimens by computers, have all led to progress in electronic archiving standards. The use of electronic signatures has now been widely accepted by the regulators, so the pressure to retain original wet-ink signatures has been removed. If the original raw data are in electronic format, then ideally it should be preserved in that format.

In the US, the FDA has issued guidance for the use of electronic signatures and electronic documents in Rule 21, CFR Part 11. This is the FDA ruling for electronic GxP-compliant records created after 19 August 1997. One of the objectives of this ruling is to preserve and protect electronic GxP records and prevent fraud. This guidance is widely followed within the EU, and the standard is frequently referred to by the regulatory inspectors.

Both hardware and software can create problems when archiving electronic documents. Will the current format be compatible as new devices and technology emerge (e.g. can today's portable devices read yesterday's floppy disks)? In addition, there are issues surrounding early versions of software packages, many of which cannot be opened by current versions. Also, the responsibility for archiving electronic documents normally belongs to the IT department and is not under the control of the GCP archivist. The use of pdf files to ensure that the electronic document is not edited or altered does not guarantee that the document can be opened many years later. The pdf/a standard has been introduced to preserve the accessibility of electronic documents in the long term.

When establishing an electronic archiving process, first the format and media must be selected, and a full back-up of the data included in the system. The meta-data should be set down to allow for quick searching for and identification of individual documents. The data must be held in a format that prevents the accidental or deliberate overwriting, alteration, or deletion of these records. Only authorized personnel should be able to access these records and any requests for access to the archived electronic records should follow a similar documented procedure to the access to paper records. If the company/institution is using magnetic tape to create weekly/monthly/quarterly back-up copies, these should be held at a separate and secure location. Many of the contract archive companies offer this type of specialist storage in addition to the more traditional storage of paper.

When preparing to archive electronic data it must be remembered that this data may be in various different locations, held on memory sticks, on CD/DVD, held in the laboratory, or even on personal laptops. If the data are to be transferred to an alternative media, then a fully documented and validated process must be in place, with suitable quality control checks to verify that all the data have been transferred and all the electronic documents are complete. This is particularly important if there are software/hardware developments that necessitate the transfer of all the clinical trial data to an alternative media. Electronic records should be read periodically to confirm that they can still be read and that they have not started to deteriorate. There must be an SOP to cover this.

In addition to the pdf/a standard and 21CFR Part 11, the British Standards Institution (BSI) has produced a code of practice regarding the legal admissibility of information stored on electronic document management systems.

Conclusion

The GCP Directive 2005/28/EC has made it a legal requirement for an archivist to take responsibility for the archiving and long-term retention of clinical trial documents. The attention that regulatory inspectors, particularly those from the MHRA, pay to the archiving process has increased the focus on the archiving process within companies and institutions. Standards within archives have improved and QA departments now regularly conduct audits of their own or contracted archiving services. There is still limited guidance around the archiving process and for many archivists archiving is only part of their role. The Scientific Archivists group provides the opportunity to meet and share knowledge and discuss issues and problems with other members, along with presentations and workshops by industry experts. ℛ www.sagroup.org.uk

Further reading

ISO 11799:2003: Information and Documentation—Document Storage requirements for Libraries and Archives.

International Conference on Harmonisation of Technical Requirements for Registration of Pharmaceuticals for Human Use. Guideline for Good Clinical Practice (ICH E6), April 1996. ℛ www.ich.org

Directive 2001/20/EC of the European Parliament and of the Council of 4 April 2001, on the approximation of the laws, regulations and administrative provisions of the Member States relating to the implementation of good clinical practice in the conduct of clinical trials on medicinal products for human use. Official Journal L 121, 1 May 2001: 34–44.

Commission Directive 2005/28/EC of 8 April 2005, laying down principles and detailed guidelines for good clinical practice as regards investigational medicinal products for human use, as well as the requirements for authorisation of the manufacturing or importation of such products. Official Journal L91, 9 April 2005: 13–19.

The EU Clinical Trial Directive Regulation 536/2014.

Legally admissible standards PD0008/1996.

ISO 19005:2005 Document management: Electronic Document File Format for long-term preservation Part 1 Use of PDF2005.

Audits and inspections

Introduction

The requirement for quality data is recognized by everyone who works in clinical research. The ability to maintain accuracy and quality throughout a clinical trial is a dynamic process which involves both ongoing quality control steps and systematic and independent quality assurance. Good quality entails a system or process that is fit for purpose and that meets the required standards to ensure accuracy, reliability, and conduct. Synonymous with this is the quality management system.

With the introduction of the first European Good Clinical Practice (GCP) Directive (91/507/EEC) nearly 20 years ago, sponsors have been responsible for introducing a system of quality assurance (QA), audits, and quality control (QC). Recently, these processes have greatly developed and increased in complexity, especially with the introduction of other significant documents such as ICH GCP Guidelines 1996,[1] the Data Protection Directive (95/46/EC),[2] the Clinical Trials Directive (2001/20/EC),[3] the GCP Directive (2005/28/EC),[4] and the Clinical Trials Regulation (536/2014)[5].

The Clinical Trials Regulations regulate the clinical trials of investigational medicinal products (CTIMPs). NHS organizations that sponsor and host CTIMPs must ensure that systems are in place so that CTIMPs can be managed and conducted in accordance with the Clinical Trials Regulations as defined previously and the Research Governance Framework. Under the Research Governance Framework (2005), research organizations are required to audit compliance with legislative and governance requirements. NHS organizations must conduct formal audits on a selection of their research projects or the activities they perform. The minimum standard as defined by the Department of Health for research governance states that at least 10% of projects should be routinely audited. Additionally, audits should be conducted if there is any suspicion of reduced research governance standards in a project.[6]

This chapter outlines the comparison between QC and QA and how these important processes form part of a quality management system for an organization. Audit strategy and methodology, site and sponsor audits, and regulatory authority inspections are also discussed.

Why do we have QA and QC?

Any discussion about aspects of quality in clinical research must start with consideration of good clinical practice (GCP). GCP applies to both commercial studies as well as non-commercial studies that may be conducted within the NHS. It defines a set of ethical and scientific quality standards for the design, conduct, recording, and reporting of clinical trials. The purpose of GCP is to ensure that the rights, safety, and well-being of trial subjects are protected and that the data generated are credible.

It is a GCP requirement to implement both QC and QA within an organization or at a trial site. ICH GCP 5.2.1 states that the sponsor or the CRO should implement quality assurance and quality control, and that 'systems with procedures that assure the quality of every aspect of the trial should be implemented' (ICH GCP 2.13).

The quality management system is a term encompassing audits (QA), standard operating procedures (SOPs), the how, what, and when of trial implementation, quality control, training, etc. Together, these activities contribute to the quality of the output or deliverable.

Quality control

Quality control (QC) refers to the operational techniques and activities undertaken within the quality management system to verify that 'the requirements for quality of the trial-related activities have been fulfilled' (ICH GCP 1.47). These are processes that are implemented to improve the accuracy, to meet established standards, or to improve the timeliness of the outputs.

QC verifies that the requirements for quality of the trial-related activities have been fulfilled, which should be reflected in SOPs. QC is conducted 'in process', day to day as the trial is underway, and should be applied to each stage of data handling to ensure that all data are reliable and have been processed correctly. QC review is typically on a large sample or may even comprise a complete review of the deliverable/output.

Another aspect of quality control is training, which is a key component for clinical research success. This can include investigator training programmes covering GCP, protocol training, and other study-specific training. Today, training is often web-based, which is particularly useful for 'just in time' training on routine topics like SOPs.

Table 24.1 illustrates examples of quality control activities seen in clinical trials.

Table 24.1 Example of quality control reviews

Investigator selection	Feasibility and review of investigator selection criteria are one of the first QC steps in a clinical trial
Document reviews	Such as informed consent form, protocol, statistical analysis plan, data management plan, clinical study report. 100% QC by at least the same department that produces the output (plus additional appropriate cross-functional review)
REC/CA submission documents	100% review of all documents prior to submission to the research ethics committee(s)/competent authority(ies)
Regulatory document package	Review prior to release of investigational medicinal product (IMP) to site (100%). This is often called the 'green light' review, one of the most important QC checks prior to IMP release and subjects recruitment
Vendors/sub-contractors	Selection and ongoing maintenance is another QC process
Site monitoring	Source data verification (SDV) (100% or sampling), drug accountability (100% or sampling) are part of the QC of site activities conducted by the monitor/CRA
Co-monitoring	Review of monitoring process (not 100% of all CRA activities, but theoretically 100% of monitors would undergo/be involved in a co-monitoring visit at some point).
Training	University courses, workshops, GCP/Statutory Instrument (SI) training, investigator/site staff training
Review of TMF	Ongoing reviews and final review prior to return to sponsor (100%)/archiving

Quality assurance

Quality Assurance (QA) refers to all those planned and systematic actions that are established to ensure that a trial is performed and the data generated, documented (recorded), and reported in compliance with GCP and the applicable regulatory requirements (ICH GCP section 1.46). The processes that are established by this independent group are conducted in order to validate that the operational activities and controls (as defined by QC steps) are employed.

Under ICH GCP guidelines, the sponsor organization (this can include a contract research organization (CRO) or an NHS Trust) is responsible for implementing and maintaining both QA and QC systems described earlier, with written SOPs to ensure that trials are conducted and data are generated, documented, recorded, and reported in compliance with the protocol, GCP, and the applicable regulatory requirements. QA also looks for evidence that appropriate QC activities have been undertaken and it will assess the reliability and integrity of the quality control systems. Audit usually involves a small sample of the output/deliverable with a focus on the review of the process and ensuing documentation. QA will identify errors that lead to one-off corrections; however, the aim of QA is to improve processes (Table 24.2).

Table 24.2 Example of quality assurance audits

Site audit	Approximately 10–20% of sites audited are generally audited. Includes audit of the deliverable (investigator site file and case report forms (CRFs)) and site processes (conduct of the trial and evidence of QC (monitoring activities))
TMF audit	The main TMF and small % (normally 10–20%) of in-house investigator site files are audited. Includes audit of the deliverable (appropriate documentation in the TMF and site files), and audit of the clinical/biometric processes, and evidence of QC of the files (by clinical personnel)
Database audit	Small % (usually up to 10 CRFs) of CRFs vs deliverable (database) audited and data management processes, and evidence of QC of database (including review of data management error-rate determination)
Clinical study report audit	Audit of a sample (perhaps a small % of table of contents, % tables, figures, and listings, 100% text) of deliverable (CSR) and audit of biostatistics and medical writing (possibly medical affairs) processes; and evidence of QC of CSR

The role of the QA unit

Establishing a QA unit, especially in the healthcare environment, can be daunting. There always seems to be so many priorities and there are often pressures from within the organization or from other teams for help and support. It is important to allocate resources carefully to ensure the QA unit is effective. In order to establish basic QA activities, a certain critical mass of staff is required. Smaller units should focus on auditing activities rather than processes which can be covered by other groups.[7]

The role of QA is to provide an effective auditing programme for internal and external audits to verify GCP compliance and effectiveness of systems and processes. Some units also perform contractual audits. Resources do need to be carefully allocated to ensure both internal and external stakeholders are satisfied. Typically, the QA team provides advice, support, training, and consultancy; the team provides feedback to management regarding quality issues, and also conducts vendor/subcontractor audits. The overall aim of the group is to assist the organization in process improvement. QA may also be involved in due diligence auditing before acquisition. For smaller QA units, there tends to be a higher proportion of document audits and a lower proportion of system and vendor audits. Larger QA units conduct more system audits (but still only approximately 6%) and more vendor audits (but still only approximately 6%).[8]

QA is also involved in SOP reviews, SOP coordination, and change requests. SOP deviations need to be recorded and tracked. SOP training matrices may also be coordinated by QA.

Once audit reports have been written, corrective and preventive actions (CAPAs) are requested from auditees. Review and follow-up and elevation of significant findings to senior management are performed by the QA group. Most QA units maintain a database in order to track responses and record action plans and timelines. A CAPA database is usually maintained for internal audits/findings and for sponsor audits or regulatory inspections. The tracking and follow-up of inspection findings is particularly significant.

QA staff are frequently involved in training related to their area of specialty, most specifically GCP (or other GxPs), regulations, ISO, risk assessment, etc.

Quality assurance metrics

A variety of metrics are measured and assessed by a QA unit. Measurements include internal performance evaluation, for example, the time it takes to send out an audit report to the auditees, timelines on responses from the organization, and timelines on the CAPAs. The number and type of various audits/inspections are also recorded as well as information on numbers of 'critical' findings, numbers of 'major' findings, and number of 'other' findings/recommendations which could be identified during an inspection, a sponsor audit, or during an internal audit. The percentage of audits with 'critical' findings, % of audits with 'major' findings, etc., could also be measured over each year to review how the organization is improving. Most QA groups regularly update the organization on CAPAs and provide trend analysis on audit findings.

A risk-based audit approach

In order to anticipate, prevent, and address protocol, regulatory, and/or GCP non-compliance issues, organizations use a best practice risk-management framework that considers all parts of the process, which controls are in place, and then tests the strength of these controls. Each potential risk is then prioritized to enable the QA team to focus its efforts on a particular process or clinical trial. Quality management staff conduct the planning and prioritize the process. Management is often aware of the risks and formal assessment may not be conducted when scheduling all audits.

A simple way to calculate risk integrates recognition of potential/actual risks to quality and/or business continuity (threats), the risk assessment/analysis (functions are prioritized according to risk levels), developing strategies to manage and mitigate risk using relevant resources and assuring the traceability of decisions.

The guidelines for assessing risk can be based on the three criteria as listed in Table 24.3.

Frequency of use
- Used often = 3
- Used sometimes = 2
- Used seldom = 1

Regulatory risk
- High risk = 3
- Medium risk = 2
- Low risk = 1

Business risk
- High risk = 3
- Medium risk = 2
- Low risk = 1

Table 24.3 An example of a simple risk assessment that can be performed by a QA Unit

System / Vendor	Frequency of use	Regulatory risk	Business risk	Total
System A (e.g. clinical monitoring)	3 = Used often	3 = High risk	3 = High risk	9 = High risk
Vendor A (e.g. CRF Printer)	3 = Used often	1 = Low risk	1 = Low risk	5 = Low risk

The risk analysis can then be determined as high risk (with a value of 8 or 9), medium risk (with a value of 6 or 7), and low risk (with a value of 3, 4, or 5). All high risk assessments need to be audited. Medium-risk systems/processes are usually scheduled as a routine audit, occurring perhaps every two years. Low-risk systems/processes may not be audited. When vendors are assessed, it may be relevant to schedule a remote assessment rather than conducting an on-site audit.

Site audits can be assessed in a similar way. Patient safety, data integrity, medical ethics, and/or regulatory risk need to be considered.

Audit strategy and methodology

By having an effective quality management system and a QA programme of effective audits means that a range of possible risks may be prevented. To ensure that quality is inherent in every aspect of the process, the Shewhart model is often considered the best guide. This was popularized by the father of quality control, Edward Deming. The model defines the essential steps for QA in all clinical studies: Plan, Do, Check, Act.

Most organizations audit according to risk. This is often due to resource constraints. Projects or programmes of work are chosen that are required to meet strict legislative requirements, or where there is suspicion of reduced research governance standards. The NHS R&D Forum has produced excellent guidance on monitoring and audit.[9]

Some Trusts have developed specific research governance auditing tools or checklists for use either for completing by researchers themselves or for external auditing by, for example, a peer NHS organization or the R&D office. Trusts have different levels of auditing for the different classes of research; some Trusts do not actively review commercial projects to the same level as other research. Internal audit programmes in Trusts need to be built to cover the Research Governance Framework and clinical trial regulations.

Study-specific audits are used to assure the quality of the individual activity/service or product; for example, an audit of a site will focus on the quality at that site and the actions that may follow the audit are mainly study-specific. Sometimes findings/actions may also be applied to other sites taking part in the study.

A systems-based approach is far more common in larger QA units, but the importance of site/study-specific types of audits must be borne in mind. Systems/process audit focuses on the delivery of a particular system/process. There can be several interfaces that need to be considered. Systems/process audits look across programmes of studies and can target particular areas of concern. By looking at several studies, the findings can have more impact on the organization as they can be seen as evidence of some kind of systematic failure, rather than merely an isolated incident.

Internal audit of clinical trials within a Trust is conducted in accordance with the Research Governance Framework (2005), the Medicines for Human Use (Clinical Trials) Regulations 2004, and according to the quality steps defined in GCP. The R&D department is responsible for organizing internal quality audits; often an annually published audit timetable is available. The R&D manager assigns audits to a person or a team, with the lead auditor being independent of the area being audited and appropriately trained/qualified staff undertaking the audit.

In the pharmaceutical industry, the QA auditor is responsible for the planning, execution, and reporting of independent audits, including follow-up and close-out activities, with input and support from the head of QA or designee as required. The head of QA (or designee) is responsible for collaborating with the QA auditor, as required, to provide support during the audit planning phase, for review and approval of the audit report, and the escalation of issues, as appropriate, to senior management.

The audit process

The audit process can be broken down into five main areas. These are audit planning, preparation, conduct of the audit, reporting, and follow up/close-out of the audit (Figure 24.1).

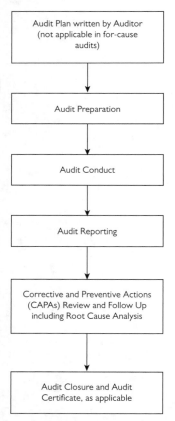

Figure 24.1 Audit process flow diagram.

An audit plan is written by an auditor prior to the commencement of the audit, involving the auditees and any other relevant staff. Audit plans are not generally written prior to 'for cause' audits, as these audits can change direction during the course of the audit. Audit preparation involves review of applicable standards, regulations, guidelines, SOPs, project documentation, etc., prior to the audit. Standard audit checklist(s) may be customized during this phase. Letters/e-mails are used to notify auditees that an audit will be taking place, and usually two to three weeks' notice is provided.

An opening meeting usually takes place prior to the commencement of the audit, and a close-out meeting conducted at the end of the audit. Both meetings should ideally involve the same staff. The close-out meeting is when findings are summarized and discussed with the auditees. Following an audit, a report is generated based on the findings presented in the close-out meeting. It is good to avoid surprising auditees with new findings, if at all possible. The recipients of the audit report are asked to complete the corrective action and preventive action (CAPA) sections of the audit report and respond within a specific timeline. A root cause analysis should be performed to determine all causes and influences that have led or may lead to a quality problem. Effective root cause analysis is essential to addressing quality problems and leads to continuous improvement. Audits can be closed when CAPAs have been satisfactorily addressed (although perhaps not resolved). Audit certificates, if produced, are circulated at this stage.

In a Trust, the R&D department is responsible for ensuring that corrective or preventive actions are closed out in a timely fashion, in conjunction with the representative of the area being audited (Table 24.4). Completed audit activity is reported back to the chief investigator and the research governance committee.

Table 24.4 Examples of corrective and preventive actions

Corrective action	Preventive action
• To eliminate the cause	• To eliminate the cause and/or reduce the probability of the issue (re) occurring.
• Identify/define the problem	• Identify/define the problem/potential problem
• Identify and understand the cause of the problem	• Identify and understand the cause of the problem
• Identify actions to correct the problem	• Identify and develop a plan to prevent occurrence/recurrence
• Implement the action plan	• Implement the plan
• Evaluate effectiveness of the correction	• Evaluating effectiveness in preventing occurrence/recurrence of the problem

Investigator site audits

If only a single audit is to be performed, this is routinely performed early in the study process. If more than one audit per study is to be performed, they should take place when appropriate (e.g. early or later in the clinical phase, prior to interim analyses, etc.). Sites chosen for audit are selected by the auditor, in consultation with the relevant staff (project director/manager and/or sponsor) and are based on, for example, high enrollers, rapid enrollers, geographical location, high number of protocol violations/deviations, high number of SAEs, etc. For contracted audits, the sites may also be selected by the sponsor.

An audit notification letter should be sent to the principal investigator and include who will be present, and their titles, the dates and the scope of the audit (e.g. opening meeting and interviews), review of TMF, review of informed consent forms, drug accountability, and review of CRFs/source data, etc. If there is a pharmacy involved, the pharmacy visit should be very clearly documented in the audit notification letter and the pharmacist be copied in, or a separate letter to the pharmacist should be written and a copy sent to the principal investigator. Ensure the letter to the principal investigator states very clearly that his/her presence is expected and give an approximation of the amount of time expected of the site personnel during the audit.

At the commencement of a site audit, an opening meeting is held with the principal investigator and site staff responsible for trial activities. Interviews with the investigator and site staff are conducted in order to obtain information about site set-up, study conduct, source documentation used and its location, etc. A tour of the facilities to include all areas relevant to the conduct of the study (e.g. investigational product storage, record storage, clinics, study-specific equipment, etc.) will also take place during a routine audit.

Documentation reviews include a full (100%) review of the investigator site file, (usually, but this may vary for larger studies) and informed consent forms (ICFs) for all subjects. Source data and CRFs/eCRFs are reviewed to ensure that records are available for all subjects in the study (including screening failures), all record types are available (paper and electronic), records are located in a secure environment, and that electronic records are compliant with regulations or paper copies are printed, signed, and dated.

Source data verification (SDV) is performed on an appropriate sample of subjects (e.g. subjects with SAEs, early terminations, protocol deviations, etc.). The routine sample size is $\sqrt{n} + 1$. The sample size may be adjusted due to size and complexity of study. Review of monitoring documentation (monitoring visit reports, log, and notes) may be conducted at the site (or as part of the preparation), and investigational medicinal product (IMP) management may include a visit to pharmacy, as appropriate. It is very important to review all safety reporting documentation.

At the end of the site audit, a close-out meeting is conducted with the investigator and site staff, as appropriate. The close-out procedure follows the route defined in the section on audit process.

Sponsor audits

When arranging a sponsor company audit at a research site or at a CRO, many of the issues remain the same. Most sponsors wish to audit within two weeks, so there is always the question of making sure QA or a similar representative is available to host the audit. CROs often need to consider if they have a policy for when a competing CRO is required to audit them. If this is an audit at the pre-contractual stage, then it is unlikely that the offer of an audit by another CRO is refused.

As with any audit, preparation is important. The operational teams need to make sure they have routinely reviewed documents ready for the audit. If a previous audit has been conducted, a record of the outcomes and the actions (CAPAs) that were promised need to be re-reviewed. Typically, documents are requested by the auditor prior to arriving at the site. The type of documents that may be requested are listed in Table 24.5. Before any documents are released to an external organization, a confidentiality agreement needs to exist.

Staff availability needs to be considered. Not all staff members are required to be present throughout an audit. It is usual for the study team to be present at the opening and closing meeting. The principal investigator and any co-investigators also need to make themselves available at pre-agreed times. Relevant SOPs or working guidelines must be accessible and consider how this ought to be achieved if these are stored electronically—access rights may need to be arranged with IT departments in advance. QA will work closely with all staff/groups to make sure documents are ready for the audit. QA do not routinely audit these documents in advance, but operational staff should QC these to make sure they are complete and up to date. QA may also wish to remind staff how to conduct themselves during an audit and what is routinely expected of them.

The actual conduct of the audit and any follow-up is similar to what has been described previously in this chapter.

Table 24.5 Type of documents requested by auditor

Typical documents requested/ reviewed for a pre-contractual audit	Typical documents requested/ reviewed whilst a clinical trial is ongoing
• SOP index/relevant SOPs	• As per the pre-contractual audit
• Organograms	
• Training files, CVs, and training records	• TMF (all documents as defined in ICH E6, section 8 and EudraLex Volume 10)
• Validation documents for IT/systems proposed for the clinical trial/21 CFR Part 11	• Pharmacy file (if separate from the TMF)
• Regulatory authority inspection list	• CRFs and source data (subject notes, laboratory test, X-rays, etc.)
• Disaster recovery/business continuity plans	

Inspections

When comparing NHS Trusts with a large pharmaceutical company, there are significant differences in how each operates. However, there is just as much risk for subjects in studies being run in academia as there are for pharmaceutical or biotechnology company studies, and therefore all need to be inspected.

In the UK, the Medicines and Healthcare products Regulatory Agency (MHRA) may conduct a routine inspection at a site. Sometimes they come to sites because they are aware of issues occurring and this type of inspection is called a 'triggered' inspection. Where an organization is named as the 'sponsor' or co/joint sponsor of the CTIMP, the MHRA may conduct a 'sponsor' inspection. An MHRA inspection in the NHS will include review of Trust-wide systems to confirm the organization has fulfilled its sponsor responsibilities. When the NHS is hosting a clinical trial for an external sponsor, an investigator site inspection may be conducted. Other bodies such as the Human Tissue Authority (HTA) and the Human Fertilisation and Embryology Authority (HFEA) also have statutory authority and perform inspections of relevant licensed establishments in the UK. Other European competent authorities may inspect, as can the EMA, the FDA, and other authorities. It is more likely that other authorities will inspect if the IMP has been submitted under a marketing authorization application (MAA) in the EU, or a new drug application (NDA) or biologics licence applications (BLAs) in the US.

Inspection preparation

It is useful to have an SOP to follow when preparing for an inspection (and it is just as useful to have something similar when preparing for a sponsor audit). Just as with sponsor audits, QA staff need to be available, but this is even more important for inspections as they will help the process run more smoothly.

Following an MHRA announcement of an inspection, usually two to three months in advance, they expect to be provided with a pre-inspection dossier within 28 days. The information that needs to be provided in the dossier includes organization details, contact name of the person who will manage the logistics, details of clinical trials of medicinal products being run, and an index of SOPs and any other processes. The inspector reviews the dossier and then agrees inspection dates and the agenda. Each inspectorate has a slightly different approach when it prepares for an inspection.

If a previous inspection has occurred, it is very important to spend a significant amount of time reviewing the previous CAPAs and the action plans proposed. When a site is re-inspected, these will be very carefully reviewed from a process improvement perspective. Any actions that have not been completed will need to be investigated prior to inspection and staff will need to address the reasons for failure to comply and will need to be prepared to answer questions on this during the inspection.

It is also vital that the QA unit staff spend time preparing themselves for an inspection. They need to consider making sure that all inspection history documents are ready, and that QA files and any tracking management systems are up to date. CAPA follow-up and close-out timelines are particularly important. The number and type of audits conducted by the QA unit may be reviewed. Audit reports are not generally reviewed (unless a 'triggered' inspection is being conducted); however, they are sometimes requested. Audit plans, audit schedules, and the like may also be reviewed. QA staff CVs, job descriptions, and training records will also need to be up to date, which is not usually a problem for this group.

General points to consider

QA will assist with the planning process, will check for availability of relevant staff, will ensure all relevant SOPs and processes are ready. Senior management will need to be notified. Mock inspections looking at specific studies may be conducted and this will help prepare the team and promote efficient and effective interactions with the inspectors. They also help in establishing and confirming roles and responsibilities during the inspection. Preparation is very important to ensure that systems and processes for conducting the clinical trial are adequate. It is important to be inspection-ready, so do not wait for inspection notification before you start to prepare. The necessary systems and processes should already be in place and should be reviewed regularly. Investigator site files and trial master files should always be up to date. Preparation in inspection response techniques, GCP training, and Statutory Instrument (SI) training may also need to be conducted with staff. For inspections that are being hosted for external sponsors, it is important to make sure these sponsors have been notified. Data that have been archived may need to be retrieved. Appointing an inspection lead is useful, as is definition of the core team who will be hosting the inspection.

The MHRA works to a fixed list of questions for routine inspections. Its questioning style is 'open', so staff cannot provide a 'yes' or 'no' answer. A full response is required. If the inspector feels too brief a response is being offered, he or she will ask the question again until a complete answer is provided. For every answer provided, written evidence must be to hand, and it may be requested for presentation within a reasonable time frame. Remind staff that it is important to remain calm and listen carefully to what is being asked. It is perfectly acceptable to ask for the question to be repeated.

During the inspection, inspectors will wish to see the processes in action. Just remember, if you are opening an electronic TMF and other documents are visible, the inspector may also wish to take a look at these.

MHRA inspections—what to expect

Introductory meeting

At the start of the inspection a brief introduction of all attendees will need to be conducted. The inspectors will introduce themselves and they will confirm the purpose of the inspection, the agenda will be reviewed, and staff or facility availability are discussed. Usually there is a top-level description about the type of services offered/number of trials conducted and staff involvement.

The inspection process

The inspection is a detailed examination of documents along with a discussion with team members as to the processes that were conducted to ensure they are adequate and applicable to the clinical trials that have been selected for inspection. The type of documents that are reviewed are the TMF/investigator site file, pharmacy file, and drug accountability records, source data versus CRFs (usually two to three subjects are selected, depending on trial complexity and number of inspectors), and subject information sheets and informed consents and CVs and training records of the staff involved in the clinical trial.

A tour of the facilities is usually conducted at some stage during the inspection. If this is a repeat inspection and the facility has not re-located, then this step may not be a priority and may not be conducted. In a hospital, the research unit, ward(s), X-ray or other test facility, and pharmacy are visited. Additionally, TMF or archive facilities, IT server rooms, and laboratories may also be visited.

A significant part of the inspection process involves discussion and interviews with the staff who were involved in the clinical trial(s) being reviewed. All key staff are interviewed. See Table 24.6 for the type of questions that may be asked. However, do also consider other staff who play a significant part in the study as they may also be questioned (e.g. R&D managers, pharmacovigilance staff, regulatory affairs, quality assurance, training managers, biostatisticians, and medical writers).

Inspection closing meeting and post-inspection follow-up

A closing meeting is conducted usually with the personnel who attended the opening meeting; this is usually the decision of the site or organization as to who should attend. A summary of the findings and grading of these will be given by the inspectors. Findings are usually defined as 'critical', 'major', or 'other' or similar findings depending on the inspectorate involved. Additionally, recommendations may be given and positive observations may also be presented. It is important to remember that inspectors are not willing to discuss the findings when they are presented at the close-out meeting. Inspection reports can take several months to arrive, but most inspectorates do intend to issue a report within 30 days of the end of the inspection. A response is usually expected within 30 days from the auditees, so it is important to prepare an internal summary of the verbal findings and to start any work that is necessary prior to receiving the report. A copy of all the documents provided to the inspectors during the inspection process should also be retained.

Table 24.6 Type of questions asked in an MHRA inspection

Function/ responsibility	Example of the type of questions asked
Common generic questions	• Can you describe your roles and responsibilities? • When was your last GCP/SI training? How is training recorded and maintained? • How is SOP training conducted and recorded? • What is the SOP creation and review process? • How do you maintain an up-to-date knowledge of regulations? • What is the agreement/contracts process? • What access levels do you have to IT systems, TMF, etc?
Principal investigator/ co-investigator	• What is the patient recruitment process? • How would you ensure a study has the necessary approvals? • Who deputizes? • How often did you meet the Monitor? • Define an SAE?
Co-investigator	• How many trials are you involved with? • What are your roles and responsibilities? • What was your training on the study? • What is the randomization process? • What are you interactions with Pharmacy? • How do you report an AE/SAE?
Project manager/study coordinator	• What is the process for the PM to find out about a new study? • How are staff members assigned to studies? • What is the consent review process? • Do you check the contents of documents provided by the sponsor for a clinical trial authorization (CTA) application? Do you need to? • What is the IMP process used for: sourcing, release, transfer, qualified person certification, shelf-life extension, label checks? • Amendments to the protocol—how is the insurance policy checked? • What is the process used to update an investigator's brochure? • What is the process for protocol waivers? • Do you document handover of trial responsibilities following a change in project team member? • Do you maintain documentation of quality control reviews? • How do you check sponsor insurance? • How are exemptions to insurance taken into account (e.g. HIV studies)? • How do you ensure UK patients are adequately covered by the insurance/indemnification? • Are ABPI guidelines being followed?

(continued)

Table 24.6 (Contd.)

Function/ responsibility	Example of the type of questions asked
Pharmacist	• When was GCP, GMP, and SI training conducted? • How are studies set up in the pharmacy? • How do you know all agreements and ethics/regulatory approval are in place? • How are you notified about trial progress? • What is the 'out of hours' process? • What happens if the temperature deviates where IMP is being stored? • How is IMP prescribed? • Were dispensing procedures reviewed by the CRO? • What is the accountability process? • What is the recall procedure for IMP? • How often did the monitor go to the pharmacy?
Monitor/ clinical research associate	• What is the process when a monitor changes to another study? • How often do monitors go to pharmacy, labs, X-ray (GCP, confidentiality issues)? • Sponsor SOPs: how does a CRO/site know when they are updated? What training was given on sponsor SOPs? • What tests are performed to test the SAE fax/phone lines?
Data manager	• What contracts do you have with third parties, e.g. CRF printers? • What is the change control process in data management? • What is the database lock/unlock process? • How do DM staff deal with personal data if they should receive it?

What regulations do GCP inspectors inspect against? A comparison between the MHRA, EMA, and FDA

Table 24.7 summarizes the regulations that are used by Inspectors when they audit in the UK, EU, and the US.[10]

Table 24.7 Summary of regulations

MHRA	EMA	FDA
ICH Guideline E6: Good Clinical Practice	ICH Guideline E6: Good Clinical Practice	ICH Guideline E6: Good Clinical Practice
Declaration of Helsinki 1996 version	Declaration of Helsinki 1996 version (some country variations)	
Clinical Trials Regulation 536/2014	Clinical Trials Regulation 536/2014	
Clinical Trials Directive 2001/20/EC	Clinical Trials Directive 2001/20/EC	
GCP Directive 2005/28/EC	GCP Directive 2005/28/EC	
2001/83/EC amended by 2003/63/EC, as applicable	2001/83/EC amended by 2003/63/EC, as applicable	
Associated Guidance Documents	Associated Guidance Documents	
Volume 10: The Rules Governing Medical Products in the European Union	Volume 10: The Rules Governing Medical Products in the European Union	
Additionally local UK laws, Statutory Instruments (SIs):	Local member state laws, as applicable	Compliance program 7348.810: Bioresearch Monitoring for Sponsors, CROs and Monitors
S.I. 2008 No.941: The Medicines for Human Use (Clinical Trials) and Blood Safety and Quality (Amendment) Regulations 2008		Compliance program 7384.811: Inspection of Clinical Investigators
S.I 2006 No.2984: The Medicines for Human Use (Clinical Trials) Amendment (No.2) Regulations 2006		21 CFR Part 11 (Electronic Records, Electronic Signatures) 21 CFR Part 50 (Protection of Human Subjects)
S.I. 2006 No.1928: The Medicines for Human Use (Clinical Trials) Amendment Regulations 2006		21 CFR Part 54 (Financial Disclosure by Clinical Investigators)
S.I 2004 No.1031: The Medicines for Human Use (Clinical Trials) Regulations 2004		21 CRF Part 56 (Institutional Review Boards) 21 CFR 312 (IND Applications) 21 CFR 812 (IDE) 21 CFR Part 11 Local/State laws, if applicable

☐ = common requirements

Summary

Having a good quality management system in place with ongoing periodic operational checks within each function, as well as conducting more systematic and independent audits, will ensure that clinical trials are being carefully managed and controlled to guarantee data integrity and accuracy, as well as ensuing that clinical trials are being run to applicable standards. Inspection is the final step in the process to make certain that the ongoing challenge of managing the quality of clinical data is being achieved in order to ensure that subjects are being protected when they take part in clinical research.

References

1. International Conference on Harmonisation of Technical Requirements for Registration of Pharmaceuticals for Human Use. Guideline for Good Clinical Practice (ICH E6), April 1996. ℘ www.ich.org
2. Directive 95/46/EC of the European Parliament and of the Council of 24 October 1995 on the protection of individuals with regard to the processing of personal data and on the free movement of such data. Official Journal L 281, 23 November 1995: 31–50.
3. Directive 2001/20/EC of the European Parliament and of the Council of 4 April 2001, on the approximation of the laws, regulations and administrative provisions of the Member States relating to the implementation of good clinical practice in the conduct of clinical trials on medicinal products for human use. Official Journal L 121, 1 May 2001: 34–44.
4. Commission Directive 2005/28/EC of 8 April 2005, laying down principles and detailed guidelines for good clinical practice as regards investigational medicinal products for human use, as well as the requirements for authorisation of the manufacturing or importation of such products. Official Journal L91, 9 April 2005: 13-19.
5. Commission Regulation 536/2014 of the European Parliament and of the council April 16th 2014. Official journal L158 27 May 2014.
6. Study Initiation and Management: Audit and Inspection. ℘ www.dt-toolkit.ac.uk/routemaps/station
7. The Role of the Quality Assurance Unit, European Forum for Good Clinical Practice, Audit Working Party, 2008.
8. Clinical Quality Assurance Benchmarking, Heiner Gertzen, Applied Clinical Trials, June 1, 2004 ℘ www.appliedclinicaltrialsonline.com/node/243034?rel=canonical
9. Research Governance Monitoring and Auditing. NDS R&D Forum, Research Governance Working Group, Examples of Good Practice, August 2003.
10. Hubby S and Dodsworth N. A Comparative Review of Inspectional Techniques and Regulatory Considerations between the EMA, MHRA, and FDA for Clinical Research Trials, Professional Poster at 23rd DIA Annual Euro Meeting, Geneva, Switzerland, March 2011.

Fraud and misconduct

Introduction

When it comes to determining the meaning of fraud and misconduct, it is important that some background information is presented on what constitutes good data quality and data integrity.

One universal standard that can be applied among regulators for evaluating data quality is defined as per the ALCOA principles (Box 25.1).

Box 25.1 ALCOA principles

A stands for Attributable to its source
L stands for Legible = fit for use (readable data such as those recorded using pen and ink)
C stands for Contemporaneous = timing/recording of data in real time
O stands for Original = the first recording of data (raw or source data)
A stands for Accurate = error free, exact recording of source data

Note: ALCOA term coined by Stan Woolen in 1990 while serving in the Office of Enforcement at the FDA (principles based on various FDA regulations, GMP, GLP).

Data integrity is important to consider as well when evaluating data quality. When discussing data integrity, the measurement of data contributing to dependability, reliability, and credibility pertaining to the systems and processes must also be scrutinized. Typically, this focuses on surrounding the capture of data, how data are corrected and maintained, as well as the transmission and retention of data. Regulators place their focus on significant end point data that supports safety and efficacy determinations when evaluating the quality of data submitted for research applications.

Regulators also define high-quality data as data 'fit for purpose'. This means data that sufficiently support conclusions and interpretations equivalent to those derived from error-free data (i.e. data to support regulatory decisions, sponsor claims about a product and labelling). Therefore:

Data Quality + Data Integrity = Data 'Fit for Purpose'

It is important to keep in mind that the consequences of falsification of data affect the overall clinical trial results and subject safety. If falsification takes place in a clinical trial, it places all subjects in that trial under possible risk for their safety. Finally, falsification of data jeopardizes the reliability of submitted and/or published data and undermines the regulatory agency's mission to protect and promote the public health.

The basis for reaching a conclusion that an individual is responsible for misconduct in research relies on the judgement that there was an *intention* to commit the misconduct and/or recklessness in the conduct of any aspect of a research project.

Definition of fraud and misconduct

There is no single accepted standard definition of fraud or scientific misconduct. The problem with this lack of a standard definition is exacerbated in countries in which multiple bodies have been involved in responding to the problem. For example, in the UK, the Association of the British Pharmaceutical Industry defines 'research fraud' as the generation of false data with intent to deceive, and the Royal College of Physicians defines 'scientific misconduct' as piracy, plagiarism, and fraud. In contrast, the Medical Research Council Policy defines scientific misconduct as 'fabrication, falsification, plagiarism, or deception in proposing, carrying out, or reporting results of research and deliberate, dangerous, or negligent deviations from accepted practice in carrying out research'. It includes failure to follow established protocols if this results in unreasonable risk or harm to human beings, other vertebrates, or the environment, and also the facilitating of misconduct by collusion in, or concealment of, such actions by others. Misconduct does not include honest error or honest differences in the design, execution, interpretation, or judgement in evaluating research methods or results of misconduct (including gross misconduct) unrelated to the research process.

The UK Research Integrity Office (UKRIO) lists the commonly accepted types of misconduct and makes it clear that interpretation is open to individual determination in each case. Interpretation of the terms will involve judgements, which should be guided by previous experience and decisions made on matters of misconduct in research. The UKRIO describes misconduct in research as:
- fabrication;
- falsification;
- misrepresentation of data and/or interests and/or involvement;
- plagiarism; and
- failure to follow established procedures or to exercise due care in carrying out responsibilities for:
  - avoiding unreasonable risk or harm to humans, animals used in research, and the environment.
  - the proper handling of privileged or private information on individuals collected during the research.

For the avoidance of doubt, misconduct in research involves acts of omission as well as commission. In addition, the standards by which allegations of misconduct in research should be judged should be those prevailing in the country in question and at the date that the behaviour under investigation took place.

Another definition of fraud and misconduct in medical research as defined by Wells and Farthing[1] as 'under-reporting of research is another form of misconduct, given that this can lead to seriously misleading recommendations for clinical practice and for new research.'

The US Commission on Research Integrity (1996) states the following regarding research misconduct: 'Research misconduct is significant misbehaviour that improperly appropriates the intellectual property or contributions of others, that intentionally impedes the progress of research, or that risks corrupting the scientific record or compromising the integrity of scientific practices. Such behaviours are unethical and unacceptable in proposing, conducting, or reporting research, or in reviewing the proposals or research reports of others'.

Some regulators, such as the FDA, have further defined fraud and misconduct in an application integrity policy (AIP) aimed at the review of applications that may be affected by wrongful acts that raise significant questions regarding data reliability. This policy contains several definitions which are applicable to evaluating fraud and misconduct and include additional definitions for regulators to consider when evaluating fraud and misconduct. For example, the FDA defines falsification of data 'in proposing, designing, performing, recording, supervising or reviewing research, or in reporting research results. Falsification of data includes creating, altering, recording or omitting data in such a way that the data do not represent what actually occurred'.

It is also important to define what is considered a wrongful act. A wrongful act is defined as any act that may subvert the integrity of the review process which includes, but not limited to the following:

- Submitting a fraudulent application, offering or promising a bribe or illegal gratuity, or making an untrue statement.
- Submitting data that are otherwise unreliable due to, for example, a pattern of errors, whether caused by incompetence, negligence, or a practice such as inadequate standard operating procedures or a system-wide failure to ensure the integrity of data submissions.
- May be evidenced in a document, including informal documents such as correspondence or memoranda, or verbally, such as in telephone conversations or in one-on-one meetings.

Each suspected incident of a wrongful act should be reported and investigated to determine whether it raises significant questions regarding data integrity and reliability with respect to a regulated product.

It is important to note that overall accountability for clinical trial conduct at an investigator site level is clearly placed with the investigator. Sponsors frequently delegate their responsibilities via contracted responsibilities to contract research organizations (CROs) which are held to the same standards as sponsors for adherence to regulations. CROs contract with sponsors to perform study-related activities such as regulatory submissions, data management, biostatistics, site selection, clinical project management and monitoring, quality assurance auditing, and clinical study reports.

Historical aspects of fraud

During the last 20 plus years, there have been many historical cases in the UK which predominantly involve employees of universities and from the NHS, resulting in referral to the General Medical Council (GMC) and ultimately removal from the medical register. These cases serve as excellent test cases on understanding fraud and misconduct (Table 25.1).

The GMC's primary purpose is to protect, promote, and maintain the health and safety of the public, and ensure patient safety by ensuring proper standards in the practice of medicine. In addition, in order to be a practising doctor in the UK, the doctors must be on the list of registered medical practitioners which is controlled by the GMC, and enshrined in law, principally by the Medical Act 1983.

Table 25.1 Five examples of historical UK cases

Cases	Misconduct issues	Citation/penalties
Case 1: A landmark case for a worldwide controversy over vaccine safety was a single scientific research paper published in the *Lancet* in February 1998. Written by academic researcher, Andrew Wakefield, and co-authored by a dozen associates, the article reported on the cases of 12 anonymous children with brain disorders who had been admitted to a paediatric bowel unit at the Royal Free Hospital in Hampstead, between July 1996 and February 1997.	Case 1: Andrew Wakefield, Principal Investigator, claimed links between the MMR vaccine, autism, and inflammatory bowel disease which was published without any scientific basis. Wakefield was exposed for secretly being paid to create evidence against the vaccine and, while planning extraordinary business schemes meant to profit from the scare, he had concealed, misreported, and changed information about the children to rig the results published in the journal.	Case 1: Wakefield was found guilty of dishonesty in his research and banned from medicine by the UK GMC following an investigation by Brian Deer of the *Sunday Times*. Wakefield has publicly demanded a retraction from the *British Medical Journal*.
Case 2: John Anderton, senior kidney specialist physician in Edinburgh; former registrar and secretary of the Royal College of Physicians of Edinburgh. (1997)	Case 2: Anderton faked echocardiographic and magnetic resonance imaging data for patients and had a fake assistant, Dr Shaffick, to invent data for a clinical trial to attest to forged patient informed consents.	Case 2: Anderton was struck off by the GMC.

Table 25.1 (Contd.)

Cases	Misconduct issues	Citation/penalties
Case 3: Dr Anjan Banerjee and Professor Tim Peters published a paper in Gut (1990) whilst they were employed by King's College Hospital.	Case 3: The paper published in Gut in 1990 on drug induced enteropathy similar to inflammatory bowel disease contained falsified data. An additional abstract on induced changes in small intestine permeability in humans (Banerjee et al. Gut 1990) was asked to be withdrawn before the British Society of Gastroenterology meeting, but was published.	Case 3: Both papers were retracted in March 2001. December 2000, Banerjee was found guilty of serious professional misconduct for falsifying data and suspended. September 2002 he was found guilty of serious professional misconduct for financial fraud and struck off. March 2001 Tim Peters was found guilty of serious professional misconduct for failing to take action over the falsified research.
Case 4: Malcolm Pearce.* Edinburgh physician, senior lecturer at St George's Hospital Medical School in London. A world-famous expert on ultrasonography in obstetrics. *Pearce was an assistant editor of the Journal of Obstetrics and Gynaecology. A second author on the case report was Geoffrey Chamberlain, editor of the journal, President of the Royal College of Obstetricians and Gynecologists, Professor and Head of Department at St George's.	Case 4: August 1996 A story from a paper in the British Journal of Obstetrics and Gynecology containing a fraudulent description of successful reimplantation of ectopic pregnancy and a baby being born. A young doctor at St George's Hospital Medical School had raised questions about the two papers. The investigation showed the patient did not exist. The patients supposedly in the randomized trial could not be found.	Case 4: Among studies investigated back to 1989 – three others were fraudulent, two of them in the British Medical Journal. All the papers were retracted. Questions were raised about previous cases. Pearce was fired and subsequently struck off by the GMC. Chamberlain retired or resigned from all his positions.
Case 5: Much of Britain's legal structure concerning healthcare and medicine was reviewed and modified as a direct and indirect result of Shipman's crimes, especially after the findings of the Shipman Inquiry, which began on 1 September 2000 and lasted almost two years.	Case 5: Harold Frederick Shipman, 14 January 1946–13 January 2004. Shipman is the only British doctor found guilty of murdering his patients.	Case 5: On 31 January 2000, a jury found Shipman guilty of 15 murders, sentenced to life imprisonment. They discovered a pattern of his administering lethal overdoses of diamorphine, signing patients' death certificates, and then forging medical records indicating they had been in poor health.

Suspicion, prevention, and the reasons for fraud

In 2004, the UK Research Integrity Office (UKRIO) was established to provide access to a register of advisers who are experts to promote good conduct, and who have experience in investigating allegations of misconduct. In addition, the UKRIO provides a recommended checklist for researchers which details the key points of promoting good practice and preventing misconduct in research projects.

Competent authorities are also involved in the prevention of misconduct, in the investigation of potential cases when they occur, and in taking action or initiating action by other authorities where there is evidence of potential misconduct. This role has evolved over the years in establishment of standards and requirements for the conduct of all activities, setting out the tasks, duties, and responsibilities of all parties including the assignment of appropriate sanctions and penalties and procedures for managing confidential reports from whistleblowers.

In addition, the current systems set up the legal basis and process for sharing information between regulators within the EU and where applicable with third-country regulators. They provide transparency in cases where infringement of requirements and misconduct has been proven.

There have been significant changes to the GMC, which currently reports into the Council for Healthcare Regulatory Excellence (CHRE). The CHRE oversees GMC activity and has the authority to challenge verdicts which it considers too lenient. As a result of the Shipman case, the GMC implemented a number of reforms. One of the recent changes was a shift from simple registration of doctors to 'revalidation' of doctors' credentials (professional development and skills). The good medical practice framework for appraisal and revalidation was amended in March 2013. The Committee on Publication Ethics (COPE) was founded in 1997 as a response to questioned integrity of authors submitting studies to medical journals. This organization was founded by British medical editors, including those of the *BMJ*, *Gut*, and *The Lancet*. Through COPE's efforts, problems were discovered in the following areas:

• undeclared redundant publication or submission
• disputes over authorship
• falsification
• failure to obtain informed consent
• performing unethical research
• failure to gain approval from an ethics committee

COPE's main mission includes providing advice on cases brought by editors. It publishes an annual report describing those cases and produces guidance on good practice, encourages research, and offers teaching and training.

It is important to consider the common mistakes that can lead to the possibility of site staff taking the risk to commit misconduct or fraud. These include but are not limited to:

• inadequate supervision and GCP training of study staff
• absent investigator/lack of investigator involvement in study conduct

- inappropriate delegation of study tasks by investigator to unqualified persons (untrained/inexperienced staff)
- failure to provide adequate protection of study subjects (high number of protocol violations of inclusion/exclusion criteria, missed visits, failure to follow-up or report on adverse events, over/under-dosing of investigational product)
- overworked investigator/understaffed study (e.g. too many subjects, complex study with large data collection, too many concurrent studies)
- frequent turnover of study staff
- unusually rapid enrolment of subjects
- under-reporting/delay in submission of adverse events

It must be remembered that research misconduct/fraud does not include honest errors or honest differences in opinions. Misconduct/fraud also must not be mistaken for sloppiness or a lack of understanding, or staff taking a few short cuts inadvertently (like missing a blood pressure reading or rounding it up to the nearest 5 mmHg). When looking at fraud/misconduct cases, one needs to identify and gather evidence that shows that there was intent to deceive. The act of fraud/misconduct usually takes the form of an act of omission (i.e. not revealing all data such as reportable adverse events, concomitant medications, etc.), or an act of commission (i.e. altering or fabricating data such as laboratory values, blood pressure readings, non-existent specimens).

Financial motivation to commit fraud/misconduct is probably the most significant reason, but there may be a desire to advance one's career. Human nature will always mean that individuals sometimes behave badly without good reason, and they also suffer from temptation. If a person is overworked or overcommitted to enrol patients on to trials with unreasonable timelines, or he or she has limited staff to assist, he/she may think that falsification of data could be an easy way out. Once someone is caught up in this practice, it can be a difficult habit to kick.

The detection of fraud

Pharmaceutical companies use specific techniques in the detection of fraud (Table 25.2). For example, the use of computer programmes which run algorithms to utilize specific patterns to check:

- data which may be missing or invalid
- calendar for subject visits occurring on unusual dates (Saturday or Sunday)
- statistical outliers of data (i.e. sites with unusual number of low or high serious adverse events or unusually healthy subject population for disease being studied when compared with other investigator sites)
- performance indicator checks (number of visits/day, time of informed consent and lab collections per subject per day, identical ECG tracings for subjects, infusions or diaries filled out at same time for multiple subjects) for trending patterns

Table 25.2 Useful tips for detecting fraud

Actions	Description
Adequate systems in place	Ensure systems are in place to capture, document and deal with complaints of misconduct in a timely fashion. Follow SOPs. Helpful hint: good-quality systems eliminate opportunity for error.
Get technical	It is important to read and evaluate source documents such as X-rays, ECGs, lab results, etc., and not just to inventory them. Helpful hint: fully understand technical documents and protocol.
Fill in the blanks	Ask questions about missing dates, times, information. Offer to retrieve records yourself. Keep pulling on loose ends and see where it leads. Helpful hint: audit trails/corrections are a great place to start. Trending data can point out discrepancies as well.
Don't be intimidated	State the facts and see if the fraudster tries to cover things up. Helpful hint: obtain copies/evidence before presenting evidence.
Don't shoot the messenger	Trust information provided by the monitor. The burden of proof should be on the clinical investigator.
Be suspicious of blame shifting	Discuss with investigator the fact that he/she is responsible for the conduct of the study and is accountable for the results. Helpful hint: observe and compare what was supposed to happen on the study with what actually happened.
Cultivate whistleblowers	It is important to be approachable, use listening skills, and observe work conditions. Helpful hint: establish a good rapport with study staff.
Expect fraud	Assume that the records are bogus and the study is a fraud, and work back. Verify then trust. Helpful hint: Use systems to detect fraud (i.e., data management programs that look for data outliers, high number of queries, EDC changes that do not make sense, etc.).

The prosecution of fraud

United States

The Office of Research Integrity (ORI) website contains summaries of closed inquiries and investigations. Institutions are not required to report inquiries to the ORI if an investigation is not warranted unless the allegation had been forwarded to the institution by the ORI. There is a separate section which lists closed investigations that found misconduct, or that imposed administrative actions without a misconduct finding.

A list of all individuals currently under a PHS Administrative Action is available on the PHS Administrative Action Bulletin Board. This webpage does not maintain a listing of all persons against whom a finding of research misconduct has been made. Cases in which the debarment period has passed are removed from the online listing. The second section contains summaries of all closed inquiries and investigations that did not result in findings of research misconduct since 1994. These summaries are sanitized to protect the privacy of the individuals involved. The summaries also include cases resolved through negotiations where administrative actions were imposed without a finding of scientific misconduct (Table 25.3).

Table 25.3 Summary case listing of researcher scientific misconduct from the ORI

2011	2010	2009
Bhrigu, Vipul	Brodie, Scott J.	Afshar, Nima
Bois, Philippe	Chang, Hung-Shu	Contreras, Juan Luis
Goodwill, Meleik	Cheskis, Boris	Couvertier, Norma
Manojlovic, Marija	Goodwin, Elizabeth	Fogel, Robert
Shin, Junghee	Horvath, Emily M.	Nguyen, M.
Sanyal, Shamarendra	Linn, James Gary	Ningaraj, Nagendra S.
Solomon, Nicola	Mungekar, Sagar	Robertson, Rashanda
Wang, Sheng	Paez, Gerardo L.	Tanaka, Kazuhiro
Weber, Scott	Sezen, Bengu	Thomas, Judith
		Wanchick, Jennifer
		Van Parijs, Luk

2008	2007	Before 2007
Sperber, Kirk	Jorge-Rivera, Juan Carlos	Gelband, Craig H.
Venters, Homer	Roovers, Kristin	Kornak, Paul H.
Yang, Jusan	Sudbo, Jon	Poehlman, Eric
	Uzelmeier, Rebecca	

United Kingdom

In the UK, because no such inspectorate exists and because most of the cases thus far have occurred in industry, activity has been based on referrals by the Association of the British Pharmaceutical Industry (ABPI) to the GMC. The GMC is a statutory body whose activities are governed by the Medical Act 1983. Its decisions can be appealed to the High Court. The two other bodies in the United Kingdom that have been advocating institutional reform to address allegations of misconduct are COPE and the Association of Medical Research Charities (AMRC). In December 1997, the Medical Research Council (MRC), the major source of support for biomedical research in the UK, adopted a policy and procedure for responding to allegations of misconduct. The AMRC has advocated tighter regulations for responding to allegations of misconduct than those imposed by the MRC.

In the UK, governance rules require that a journal editor who is a practising clinician or medical researcher registered with the GMC has a duty to report to that organization any other registered member whose conduct or performance may be significantly impaired. This would include allegations of unethical research and dishonesty in any form. A finding of impaired fitness to practise owing to the previous mentioned reasons could result in the doctor's registration being affected by conditions being placed on his or her work (such as a prohibition on conducting research for a certain period or a requirement that all work be closely supervised and approved), suspension from clinical practice for up to a year (which by implication results in a heavy fine, because the doctor may not earn an income during that time), or even erasure from the register. The last of these is reserved for very serious cases and has been used in at least one case of research fraud.

The GMC has charged several doctors with serious professional misconduct as a result of alleged research misconduct. Nearly all of these cases were reported to the GMC by a private investigative body set up by the ABPI. Publication was not an issue in most of the cases but rather misconduct or dishonesty in carrying out or recording data in industry-sponsored multicentre trials.

COPE is a non-statutory voluntary organization whose members include the publishers and editors of nearly 300 journals throughout Europe, as well as some in Asia and Australasia, whose editors and publishers have adopted the COPE Code of Conduct. When editors believe patients may be at risk from the research, or when grossly unethical behavior has occurred, they may wish to report this to the national body with which the researcher is registered or which gave him/her a licence to practice. COPE's major limitation is that it is advisory and cannot apply sanctions (other than to expel a member). To date, attempts to set up a system similar to those in the US or Denmark have not succeeded, but organizations representing industry and universities, as well as COPE itself, are exerting pressure to set up a more widely based and formally constituted body.

In April 2006, the UK Panel on Biomedical and Health Research Integrity was launched. Its board includes representatives from the UK Department of Health, the NHS Executive, Universities UK, MRC, ABPI, COPE, and other interested parties. When the UKRIO was established in 2006, it set up a telephone hotline for individuals to report misconduct or confirm whether certain actions are misconduct. However, the hotline has no investigative powers; therefore, it has not been universally welcomed by the scientific community.

The UK Fraud Act 2006 creates a new statutory offence of fraud and defines the three possible ways of committing it. The greatest penalty imposed for the offence is a custodial sentence of 10 years which is the same as for the main existing deception offences and for the common law crime of conspiracy to defraud.

Consequences for those who expose misconduct

The potentially severe consequences for individuals who are found to have engaged in misconduct also reflect on the institutions that host or employ them and also on the participants in any peer-review process that has allowed the publication of questionable research. This means that a range of actors in any given case may have a motivation to suppress any evidence or suggestion of misconduct. Persons who expose such cases, commonly called 'whistleblowers', can find themselves open to retaliation by a number of different means. These negative consequences for exposers of misconduct have driven the development of 'Whistleblowers Charters', designed to protect those who raise concerns. In July 1998, new legislation came into force in the UK to protect employees who exposed wrongdoers known as the Public Interest Disclosure Act, designed to protect whistleblowers and legislation. The Protected Disclosures bill 2013 was published on 3 July 2013 and is part of the Programme for Government, and aims to provide comprehensive whistleblower protection across all sectors of the economy.

A whistleblower almost always acts alone. His or her career becomes completely dependent on the decision about alleged misconduct. If the accusations prove false, his or her career is completely destroyed, but even in the case of a positive decision, the career of the whistleblower can be placed under a cloud, his or her reputation of 'troublemaker' will prevent many employers from hiring him or her. There is no international body where a whistleblower could vent concerns. If a university fails to investigate suspected fraud or provides a fake investigation to save its reputation, for example, the whistleblower has no right of appeal (Figure 25.1).

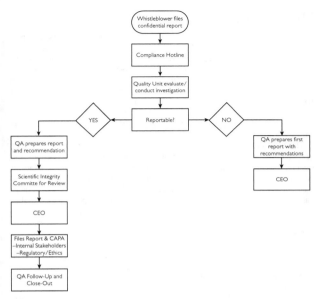

Figure 25.1 Typical process flow in whistleblowing.

Sharing information

There are many options available to regulators regarding sharing information. Most focus on the need for harmonizing efforts and resources.

The FDA–EMA Good Clinical Practices (GCP) initiative was designed to ensure that clinical trials submitted in drug marketing applications in the US and EU are conducted uniformly, appropriately, and ethically. The 18-month pilot began on 1 September 2009, and is focused on collaborative efforts to inspect clinical trial sites and studies involving pharmaceutical products. Since the pilot began, the FDA and the EMA have shared inspectional information on dozens of applications and have collaborated on joint and observational inspections.

The FDA's Disqualification/Debarment Actions have increased transparency to ensure that sponsors and IRBs involved in the development and oversight of new medical products have ready access to information about what actions the FDA has taken in these regards. FDA has developed a webpage where links to all pending and completed disqualification proceedings can be found. For debarment proceedings, the FDA lists proposals to debar (on the same website as proposals to disqualify) and debarred persons.

The UK MHRA, through the Freedom of Information (FOI) Act releases some information, which is typically updated on a monthly basis. For releases which have not been posted directly, the MHRA provides a fully searchable pdf document, which lists all FOI requests which have been answered in full, or in part, as a result of requests made under the Act.

By improving access to information about all debarment and disqualification proceedings and by sharing of information across the various inspectorates, those who commit acts of fraud/misconduct will become publicly known. This will help in the protection of public health. However, there is still some way to go, especially in the UK, with regard to sharing this information with those who wish to run clinical studies.

Summary

It is vital to acknowledge that mistakes do happen. Investigator sites can prevent fraud by identifying, acknowledging, and correcting their mistakes. This will involve documenting and reporting to the sponsor, ethics committee, and regulatory authorities as appropriate. There is no shame in making an honest mistake; it is better to admit to making one than to try and cover it up. However, it is worth noting that this concept may be difficult to accept, especially if one is eminent in one's field.

Clinical investigators play a critical role in ensuring high-quality studies. Good care of patients is not the same as GCP in research. It is important that all staff have a clear understanding of responsibilities under the research regulations. At stake is public confidence and participation in clinical trials and ultimately the availability of safe and effective products.

To ensure high-quality data and research subjects who are safe when participating in a clinical trial, high standards must be built into the study at every step. Systems must be implemented to detect and correct errors in real time, and processes must be created that limit opportunity for errors. Particular attention must be paid to monitoring queries, and responses must be prompt. Do not place needless requirements or unreasonable demands on the site, ensure protocols and outcomes assessments are simplified, restrict the number of protocol amendments, and check CRFs and consent forms against each change.

All staff involved in clinical research must have high-quality training. It is important to make sure that all staff have the necessary resources and support needed to accomplish their tasks and ensure they are monitored or supervised closely. No staff member must perform tasks he or she is not qualified to do.

Finally, look at disaster planning (e.g. backups if key study staff leave or a site experiences flood or disaster) and perform initial and continuing risk assessments to ensure fraudulent behaviour will always be detected and reported.

Reference

1. Wells F, Farthing M, eds. *Fraud and Misconduct in Biomedical Research*. 4th edition London: RSM Press, 2008.

Further reading

Presentation posted on FDA website by Stan W. Woolen, Former FDA Associate Director for Bioresearch Monitoring. 'Misconduct in Research—Innocent Ignorance or Malicious Malfeasance?' ℘ www.fda.gov/downloads/AboutFDA/CentersOffices/.../UCM196495.pdf

Ball, LK (2010). Investigator Responsibilities—Ensuring Data Quality in Clinical Trials - Office of Compliance, CDER/FDA-UCM Presentation: 08 November 2010.

A Report of the Royal College of Physicians, Fraud and Misconduct in Medical Research, Causes, Investigation and Prevention. London: Royal College of Physicians; 1991:3.

The UK Research Integrity Office (UKRIO). Procedure for the investigation of misconduct in research, August 2008.

MRC Policy and Procedure for Inquiring into Allegations of Scientific Misconduct (Medical Research Council, 1997).

Authorship

What is an author?

This simple question causes much confusion among researchers and can result in disputes and publication delays. Authorship should be considered at the very start of study planning. Gather the views of all contributors and team members early on and consult the department's authorship policy. The proposed rapid review checklist for authors (the 5Ds) may be useful for this purpose (Box 26.1).

> **Box 26.1 Proposed rapid review checklist for authors (the 5Ds)**
> 1. Design in whole or part
> 2. Data collection in whole or part
> 3. Data analysis in whole or part
> 4. Discussion of findings and/writing in whole or part, and ability to
> 5. Define the paper and its message in whole or part

Most medical journals subscribe to the model proposed by the International Committee of Medical Journal Editors (ICMJE).[1] The ICMJE statement requires authors meet *all* of the following criteria:
- substantial contributions to conception and design, or acquisition of data, or analysis and interpretation of data;
- drafting the article or revising it critically for important intellectual content; and
- final approval of the version to be published.

However, this definition was challenged in the 1990s for two reasons: the amount and scope of support required in conducting clinical studies was increasing, and authors failed to appropriately report contributions. The ICMJE statement does not make it obvious who has contributed what to the research, nor does it clarify who is responsible for the overall content, and so, not surprisingly, finding this definition inadequate, journals such as the *British Medical Journal* began listing contributors in two ways:
1. by list of authors' names at the beginning of the paper; and
2. by contribution, at the end of the paper, detailing who did what.

Collaborations

When a group of researchers has collaborated on a study, their results are published as a multi-authored paper. At multicentred sites it may be difficult to ascertain all group members—some may not meet ICMJE authorship standards. Authors should consider how best to report contributions and who will take responsibility for content. In its *Manual of Style*, the *Journal of the American Medical Association* describes two multi-authorship models:[2]
- 'Authorship in which each person in the group meets authorship criteria, in which case the group is listed as the author, with the caveat that editors may require at least one co-author to assume the role of content guarantor.
- Authorship in which a select subgroup of the whole is listed in the byline on behalf of the whole.'

In 2009, Whellan and colleagues proposed a method of describing author-ship within the HF-ACTION (Heart Failure: A Controlled Trial Investigating Outcomes of Exercise Training) trial.[3] HF-ACTION was a multicentred trial involving nearly 100 investigators from 82 international centres. The method involved two steps:

- Collecting personnel interests regarding potential future manuscripts; and
- Ranking site personnel to assign authors.

The HF-ACTION method established whether a contributor qualified and led the authorship position, based on trial participation.

First and last authors

There has been much discussion surrounding the importance of the order of names in a paper's authorship citation. The most prestigious position in the author listing is the first, namely due to citation referencing in the text being shortened to the first author 'Lang et al.', 'Lang and colleagues' etc. The last author listed is commonly the project supervisor, although some assume this position is an honorary listing, which may give rise to suspicions of inappropriate authorship models.

Joint first authors are usually qualified with a footnote such as: 'authors Lang and Whelan contributed equally to this project'.

There is no general rule for the order of authors listed, however it should be a joint decision, made prior to write up, and agreed in writing. Authors should refer to the instructions for authors for the individual journal for guidance.

Inappropriate authorship models

The following models are considered bad practice and should be avoided at best, or at least discussed with the editor and properly acknowledged.

Ghost authorship

Ghost authors are professional writers, often funded by the pharmaceutical company, who write up the research findings. While they can improve the quality of the manuscript and the speed at which it passes through peer review, there is potential for pharmaceutical companies to influence the interpretation of the results because the companies themselves and their involvement in the authorship are typically undisclosed and unacknowledged. It is essential that those listed as named authors maintain full control of the content of their paper.

Medical writers have a responsibility to ensure that the papers they write are scientifically justifiable and the EMWA guidelines should be followed. The BMJ's Good Publication Practice (2009) also offers good advice.

If a medical writer meets authorship criteria, then he or she absolutely must appear in the author byline. If he or she does not but made some contribution then the individual should be mentioned in the Acknowledgements section, with a note on the source of funding (who paid them).

Guest and honorary authorship

Guest author is an honorary title given to someone who makes no real contribution to the project, and so meets none of the IJCME criteria for authorship. This title may be offered to non-authors on the prospect that inclusion of a high-profile specialist will improve the chances that the study will be published, or increase the perceived status of the publication.

'Of 499 newly qualified medical doctors surveyed found that "In 30 percent of the dissertations, there were 'authors' who had not made any significant scientific contribution . . . Very junior researchers also seem to be encouraged into a behaviour that may continue for the rest of their careers."'

Other surveys back up the *Lakartidningen* report. Wisler and colleagues presented results of an anonymous online survey at the International Congress on Peer Review and Biomedical Publication in Vancouver, Canada in September 2009. It emerged that in 545 usable responses on honorary authorship, 21% of articles published in top tier medical journals in 2008 suggested incidence of guest authorship.

Most authors (and groups) do not adopt poor practices in this regard. The potential negative outcomes of guest authorship for the authors themselves include personal liability for guest authors and devaluation of the legitimate contribution of the true co-authors. Supervisors clearly have a role to play in facilitating discussions on this subject.

Anonymous authorship

Because scientific reporting requires accountability, undisclosed authorship is not acceptable in scientific, technical, and medical publishing. Anonymous authors lack accountability, throwing in doubt the credibility and authority of the research. Without knowledge of an author's expertise the reader is unable to confirm the appropriateness of the interpretation of their study.

Confirming authorship and avoiding disputes

Before writing up starts it is a good idea to agree on the responsibilities of each of the team members, ideally at a meeting. This will prevent potential disputes occurring later. Albert and Wager[4] provide insightful advice for researchers on how to avoid conflict with colleagues in this regard.

Intellectual property and copyright

The legal rights that result from intellectual activity are contained within intellectual property law. In copyright law, an 'author' is the person whose *creativity* led to the work being created. Intellectual property is traditionally divided into two branches: 'industrial property' and 'copyright'. Scientific works belong to the copyright branch of intellectual property.

Rights of the author/copyright holder

In medical publishing, authors are required to assign copyright or licensing rights to the journal publishing their study. This ensures that requests from third parties to reproduce articles are handled consistently and will also allow the relevant paper to be as widely disseminated as possible. Although individual arrangements vary, these agreements allow the authors to retain certain rights to the material, such as patent rights described in the study. Depending on the version of the paper (pre peer review vs post peer review vs published pdf), authors are allowed some sharing and self-archiving rights.

Work for hire/employer owned

If the study was written up while the author was employed (as a 'work-made-for-hire'), the published work is owned by the employer. In these cases, the employer signs the agreement form *in addition* to the author. The employer retains the same right to transmit the work as the author.

Government contracts/civil servants

UK government employees (including civil servants) publishing work as part of their official employment do not own the copyright to their work. It belongs to the Crown.

Multi-author/centre papers

The corresponding author is responsible for warranting and signing on behalf of co-authors, that the work is original and that all individuals identified as authors actually contributed, and all individuals who contributed are included.

Author responsibilities

An author's overarching duty is to report an original, accurate, focused, repeatable account of the study as well as an objective discussion of its significance. Negative reporting is as important as presenting a positive outcome.

Originality

Originality is an essential part of science reporting; reproducing studies in previously published work that pose no new questions wastes everyone's time. This kind of publication can also expose patients to experimental risks when there is no need. Submissions are more often rejected without review if the editor can find no novelty or new creative insight.

Plagiarism

Plagiarism is research misconduct. Centres will discipline and may even take legal action against investigators who are found guilty of serious misconduct.

The effects of plagiarism are twofold: not only does plagiarism misrepresent another's work, it also fails to credit and acknowledge the true source of that work. Journals are transferring onus to the author in this regard. For example, in common with other biomedical titles, *Pediatric Anesthesia* mandates authors screen their manuscripts for plagiarism before submission.

There are many websites that offer free basic screening that authors can use. This has been criticized by some editors as not actually preventing plagiarism but instead merely highlighting the most obvious cases, and encouraging paraphrasing. Pre-screening is not a new concept; turnitin, on online plagiarism-checking programme, has been available for some time, and it checks against text of published work, internal reports, dissertations, etc., submitted at many different institutions ℘ http://turnitin.com.

Dual publication

Dual publication. Duplicate or redundant publication takes many forms and can be genuinely confusing for authors. It may also have copyright violation considerations.

Submissions that violate dual publication policy
Concurrent submission

Because peer review takes a considerable amount of the time from submission to publication, it can be tempting for authors to take a scatter-gun approach to submission. However, it is unethical for an author to submit identical or significantly similar research in more than one journal concurrently.

Self-plagiarism

Editors find this unacceptable as it not only wastes reviewer and editor time, it also inaccurately presents the author's list of publications as greater than it really is.

Submissions not (widely) considered dual reporting

Although the following may not be inappropriate dual publication, authors need to be sure they follow appropriate steps and should consult the editor of the journal before embarking on a submission.

Abstract publishing

It is common for journals to publish the poster abstracts or conference proceedings from specialist societies. Authors may then submit the full paper sometime after (or even before) the abstract is actually published. This is not considered dual publication because abstracts do not present full results or analysis.

Republished papers

Papers may be republished in a different context if the results have potential consequences or benefit to a wider audience, but only if appropriate permissions are granted and acknowledgements are made. The original source should be referenced in the abstract, main text, as a reference, and as a footnote.

To prevent possible redundant publication, authors should at the time of submission bring to the editor's attention any similar papers reporting the same results.

Permissions

Repurposing previously published images and other copyrighted material requires approval from the original publisher, even if the author wishes to use *his or her own* previously published figures. Getting approvals is a relatively simple procedure and is commonly transacted online within a few days.

References

1. International Committee of Medical Journal Editors (ICMJE). Uniform requirements for manuscripts submitted to biomedical journals. II.A. Authorship and contributorship. ℵ www.icmje.org/#author
2. *American Medical Association Manual of Style: A Guide for Authors and Editors*, online edition. Oxford: Oxford University Press. ℵ www.amamanualofstyle.com
3. Whellan DJ, Ellis SJ, Kraus WE, et al. Method for establishing authorship in a multicenter clinical trial. *Ann Intern Med* 2009;151:414–20.
4. Albert T, Wager E (2003) How to handle authorship disputes: a guide for new researchers. The COPE Report 2003. ℵ http://publicationethics.org/files/u2/2003pdf12.pdf (accessed 17 August 2011).

Further reading

Council of Science Editors (2009). CSE's White Paper on Promoting Integrity in Scientific Journal Publications, 2009 Update. Available here: http://www.councilscienceeditors.org/i4a/pages/index.cfm?pageid=3331 (accessed 27 June 2011).

Publication process

Dissemination of research

Introduction

The purpose of this chapter is to provide guidance to assist in dissemination of research findings by poster and paper presentation.

An important aspect of the research process is dissemination and sharing of the research findings and releasing them into the public domain. Research dissemination involves the process of extracting the main messages or key implications derived from the research results and communicating them to targeted groups in a way that encourages them to factor the research implications into their work.

With respect to clinical trials involving human subjects, the public dissemination of results must comply with the Declaration of Helsinki. Principle 36 states: 'Both authors and publishers have ethical obligations. In publication of the results of research, the investigators are obliged to preserve the accuracy of the results. Negative as well as positive results should be published or otherwise publicly available.'

Failure to disseminate research results, positive or negative, can adversely affect the relevance of other trials and may expose future patients to inferior interventions. Publication bias can impact on the utility of systematic reviews and meta-analyses of trials.

The targeted groups for research dissemination include health professionals as well as research participants, patients, and policy makers. Research participants, whose enrolment made the clinical trial possible, are entitled to know the results of the trial and the implications of the results for their health.

In the dissemination plan, consider the following:
• The message to be disseminated
• Methods for dissemination
• Who is the target audience?
• How will the message be delivered?
• Where will the message be delivered?
• Time frame for the dissemination activities?
• Numbers of the target audience that the dissemination activity is expected to reach.

The traditional vehicles for dissemination of research at academic conference presentations are poster and oral presentations. It is beyond the scope of this chapter to include other modes of research dissemination such as press releases to the mainstream media and more novel methods such as podcasts, but these should also be considered.

Poster presentations

Poster presentations are generally undertaken at conferences and are an ideal way of disseminating research findings through visual and informal means. A successful poster presentation requires careful preparation which should include the following elements (Table 27.1):

Table 27.1 Poster presentation preparation

Before you begin	Respond to a 'call for abstracts'. Read carefully and adhere to the criteria
Preparation	<ul><li>Allow sufficient time to prepare the poster (remember to allow sufficient time for printing)</li><li>Establish a budget for the poster</li><li>Determine the key message(s) of the poster</li><li>Review the poster with co-investigators and principal investigator</li><li>Check which document formats the printing company supports (common ones include Adobe Acrobat, Adobe Illustrator, Microsoft Publisher)</li></ul>
Content	<ul><li>Title and the researchers</li><li>Effective headings</li><li>Research questions and purpose</li><li>Methods used and data analysis</li><li>Results</li><li>Implications and conclusions</li><li>References</li><li>Meticulously check content for typos, extra spaces, misaligned text, poor-quality images. What looks good on-screen or on A4 paper does not necessarily work when printed on a larger scale. Ask the printer if a proof copy can be supplied</li></ul>
Visual impact	Enhance delivery by:<ul><li>Using effective fonts</li><li>Using pictures (the higher quality the better, particularly for logos), graphs, charts</li><li>Keeping information simple with limited narrative</li></ul>
Design features	<ul><li>Consider effective colour coordination for the poster</li><li>Adhere to recommended size of posters</li><li>Aim for it to be possible to read the poster from a distance of 2–3 metres</li><li>Design the poster for easy transportation</li></ul>
At the conference	To maximize impact:<ul><li>Give yourself plenty of time to set up</li><li>Engage with those looking at the poster</li><li>Make a note of names and addresses for post-conference contact</li><li>Consider distribution handouts</li></ul>

Oral presentations

Being well prepared helps to allay anxiety, so start preparations well in advance of the presentation (see Table 27.2).

Table 27.2 Oral presentation preparation

Submission of an abstract	Most conferences ask for 'abstracts' and these are then reviewed for acceptance, therefore it is imperative to follow the guidelines. An abstract needs to be succinct and describe aspects of the research process, conclusions, and findings.
Length of presentation	Often conference presentations are limited to 10 minutes. Five minutes of this time may be allocated to questions. Practice the presentation to ensure it fits within the allotted time.
Content	Limited time dictates that the presentation should be succinct and contain: • A title. • A brief overview of the purpose of the study. • A sentence or two about the design. • A concise description of the sample and methods. • The findings and conclusions. • Correct attribution of slides, particularly if reproducing tables/graphs from journal articles—many conferences now allow audiences to review slides at a later date and it is important that they are properly referenced.
Technical aspects	• Microsoft PowerPoint and Apple Keynote both have their strengths and weaknesses; it is equally possible to create an excellent or terrible presentation in both of them! Double-check what software will be available on the day: it is normally PowerPoint, but be aware that some places may use other packages such as Open Office. Be aware that the programme available may mean that slides may not always appear quite as planned. • Video can add a great deal to a presentation but unfortunately leads to large file sizes and complexity. Try to compress video files or use a more modern format as this generally leads to smaller file sizes, making presentations easier to load and present. The more recent versions of presentation software also tend to be better at handling video. Have backup options in case things don't work (e.g. have the videos as separate files so that if the versions embedded in the presentation are not working, the presentation can still be made). In general, it is better to be able to run presentations with embedded video on a personal laptop (where you've had a chance to make sure it works), but not all conference venues provide for this. • It is important to have a consistent layout to slides, particularly if creating a talk using slides from previous talks. Make use of Slide Master functionality in the presentation software to give a consistent theme. • Stick to a small palette of colours and just one or two fonts. • Minimize transitions between slides and animations within slides; often displaying the whole slide at once can be just as effective.

Table 27.2 (*Contd.*)

Preparation	• Find out who the audience will be and how many people will attend so that you can prepare accordingly. • Know your subject well. • 10 pages equals to about 12 minutes oral. • Consider using effective audiovisual (AV) material. • Do not overcrowd slides, check spelling, and make sure the print is large enough to be seen by all the audience. • Practice presenting the paper with colleagues for critical feedback. • Prepare for the worst! Take the presentation file in multiple file formats and on more than just a USB stick. Consider e-mailing a back-up copy to yourself or storing it in an online/cloud storage service such as Dropbox ✍ www.dropbox.com. Many conferences will ask for slides to be submitted in advance, which at least takes the pressure off in this regard.
At the conference	On arrival at the conference: • Locate the speaker presentation room to run through slides to see if they are compatible with the AV equipment. • Locate the room where presentation will take place. • Get an idea of the room arrangement and its size. • Check, if possible, that the visual aids work.

Summary

Dissemination refers to the sharing of research findings by researchers who have been involved in the research process. A good presentation can be an effective way to share the results of research with peers. Feedback received during a presentation can be invaluable in refining the research and preparing for publication.

Aspects of research ethics to be addressed in a publication

Registration of clinical trials

Registration of clinical trials in publicly accessible databases has been a condition of publication for most medical journals for the past five years. All randomized clinical trials should include a flow diagram and a completed randomized trial checklist and a trial protocol.

Publications of clinical trials sponsored by pharmaceutical companies should follow the guidelines on good publication practice. In June 2011, the International Federation of Pharmaceutical Manufacturers and Associations released a statement on its current policy for phase 3 trials, committing its member associations to this.

Patient consent

Human subject protection is a critical part of research conduct. Manuscripts concerned with human studies must contain a statement of informed, written consent, that studies have been performed according to the World Medical Association's Declaration of Helsinki and evidence of independent ethics committee (IEC) or institutional review board (IRB) approval.

Authors wishing to publish in US journals should note that the US Food and Drug Administration (FDA) rejected amendments of the Declaration, and in 2008, replaced the declaration with the GCP Guidelines.

If individuals could be identified from a publication (e.g. from images or from details), authors must *also* obtain explicit consent from the individual. Parental or guardian consent should be obtained for the vulnerable such as infants and children.

Disclosures

Conflict of interest

A conflict of interest may arise when an author has financial or personal relationships or affiliations that could be perceived to have the potential to influence his or her decisions, work, or manuscript.

Every author named on a paper must cite any potentially competing interests. These include financial interests, research support in related areas, and recent, present, or anticipated employment of the author which may be influenced by the publication of the paper.

Funding

Authors should disclose all sources of funding (government, corporate, charity, private) and any products or services (materials and equipment, statistical analysis, and scientific writing) provided by third parties. The author who arranged payment (regardless of who supplied the funding) should state this on his or her declaration too.

Journal impact factors—what you need to know

Appraising the quality of scientific and medical research can be difficult. Criteria that have been used include journal prestige, author reputation, the prestige of the institution from which the research derives, and perceived importance and relevance of the research field. However, these factors are both qualitative and subjective. There is demand for quantitative and objective indicators to evaluate research related to published science. The journal impact factor is the most widely used indicator of the impact or quality of scientific journals.

What is an impact factor?

More than 7350 science journals receive an updated journal impact factor each year in the new edition of Thomson Reuters ISI Journal Citation Reports.

The ISI has created three standardized measures to assess the way a journal receives citations to its articles over time (Figure 27.1):

- The impact factor. The impact factor represents the average number of citations per article the journal received during the previous two years.
- The immediacy index. The immediacy index gives a measure of the way in which the curve is skewed; that is, the extent to which the peak of the curve lies near to the origin of the graph. It is a fraction, where the citations a journal receives in the current year is the numerator and the number of articles it publishes in that year is the denominator.
- The cited half-life. The cited half-life is a measure of how long articles in a journal continue to be cited after publication.

Citations to articles published in a given year often peak between two and six years after publication. After this peak, citations tend to decline over time.

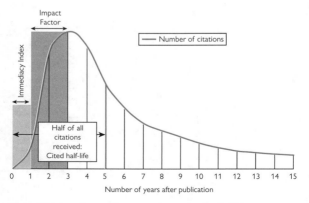

Figure 27.1 Journal impact factor, immediacy index, cited half-life.

Impact factor is a ratio, calculated by taking the number of times a journal article is cited in the reference lists of other journal articles (citations) and dividing this by the total number of major articles that the journal publishes (source items), albeit with a few refinements, including that:

- not all the articles published by a journal are classified in journal citation reports as source items (e.g. editorials and letters)
- all the citations recorded in the journal citation reports, whether they are citations to source items or to other articles like editorials and letters, contribute to journal impact factors
- the only citations that count towards impact factors are those received in the two years following the year of publication, but not in the year of publication or the years following this two-year window (there are other measures in the journal citation reports that look outside this two-year window, including immediacy index and five-year impact factor)

As one might expect, journals typically publish a small number of 'blockbuster', highly cited articles, a small number of articles that are cited few times, and a large number of articles with citation profiles that are reasonably close to the journal's impact factor (Figure 27.2).

Citation profiles, and therefore journal impact factors, vary between research areas. Where there is more research activity, citations to journal articles accrue in greater numbers and more quickly. Journal Citation Reports accommodates these variations by presenting (and ranking) impact factors in categories. For example, using the 2009 edition of Journal Citation Reports, a journal just inside the top quarter of the list of 133 journals in the 'Medicine, General and Internal' category, like *International Journal of Clinical*

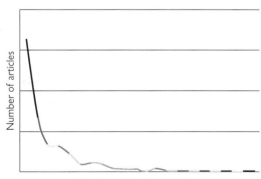

Number of citations received

Figure 27.2 Spread of citations received by articles (all articles, including source items and non-source items) published in 2009 in *International Journal of Clinical Practice*; Journal Citation Reports category: Medicine, General and Internal; 2009 impact factor: 2.245; 2009 Rank 31/133.

Data extracted from ISI Web of Knowledge on 28 June 2011.

Practice, could expect to have an impact factor of 2.245. A journal just inside the top quarter of the list of 166 journals in the 'Oncology' category, like *Molecular Cancer Research*, could expect to have an impact factor of 4.162.

Why should you care about impact factors?

Researchers can be confident that some of the people they work with (e.g. other researchers, teachers, librarians, research administrators, research funders) are using impact factors to '[e]valuate and document your institution's research investment. Identify the most appropriate, influential journals in which to publish'.

There are also incentives for academics to publish in journals with an impact factor, for example:

- Career incentives—promotion and tenure may depend on a faculty member's publication record
- Government-initiated incentives—the Research Excellence Framework (REF) replaces the Research Assessment Exercise (RAE) to assess the quality of research in UK higher education institutions and allocates national funds to departments on the basis of past performance and peer review.
- Cash incentives—some countries (China, Korea) may have introduced a system of cash bonuses to individuals for each article published in high-impact journals.

Other metrics

Immediacy index

Like the impact factor, the immediacy index is a bibliometric tool produced by Thomson Reuters ISI. An immediacy index calculates the quality of a journal by the citations it receives from a subset of journals indexed by Thomson Reuters over a single calendar year.

For example, *The Journal of X* receives 50 citations in 2008, while the number of source articles in *The Journal of X* in 2008 is 175. The 2008 Immediacy Index: $50/175 = 0.28$.

h-index

The h-index focuses specifically on the individual researcher, quantifying the output and impact of his or her work. The calculation is cumulative and based on the distribution of citations across the number of publications of an individual researcher. The metric was introduced by Jorge E Hirsch, who explained that a 'scientist has index h if h of his/her Np papers have at least h citations each, and the other (Np-h) papers have ≤ h citations each'.

As an example, Professor X published 100 papers over his lifetime, and had an h-index in 2005 of 17. This would mean that in 2005, out of Professor X's 100 papers, at least 17 had received 17 citations.

The advantage of the h-index is that it is less reliant on the number of citations or number of papers where the total number of citations can be skewed through the publication of a single influential or popular paper, and where the output of a researcher does not reflect the quality of that research. The h-index was intended to be the balance, calculating the quality as well as impact over time.

Eigenfactor

The Eigenfactor is calculated from the number of citations a journal receives, but it also weights these citations. Higher rankings are given to citations from journals that are highly ranked and more influential. Eigenfactor is free to access at: ॐ http://www.eigenfactor.org/

Five-year impact factor

As the name indicates, the five-year impact factor looks at a journal's citations and publications over five years rather than the standard two-year period. The calculation follows the same pattern as the regular impact factor, with citations in one year from articles published in the previous five, divided by the number of source items published in those five years.

The advantage of the five-year impact factor is that it provides a longer timescale on which to judge the impact of a journal. While an impact factor may rise or fall dramatically between two given years, a five-year impact factor, while still shifting, can offer a more stable view. It is especially useful for journals whose research may take longer to be cited, or where citations are small and comparison over the longer term is more meaningful.

Ensuring your article can be found and cited

The life of a paper does not stop once it has been accepted and published. It must be found, read, and hopefully cited. In the online world this can be a complex task, due to the volume of research output combined with the amount of information available on the web. There is a simple set of rules that can help to ensure that a given paper has the best chance of being found.

Optimizing your title and abstract

The title and abstract of your article are freely available online, and search engine generally find papers based on the words contained in these two parts of an article. As readers will search for specific keywords and terms, it is essential that the title and abstract contain words that accurately reflect the article. A title especially is important as in many ways it will carry the weight of the article on its shoulders. A search engine will assume that the words within a title summarize the most important elements of an article. Authors should reflect on what an article is about and what terms readers may use to find it online.

Rules of publishing

Research can be disseminated in many forms but publication in a peer-reviewed journal has the most prestige.

Writing for publication

Writing for peer-reviewed journals is an invaluable skill that can be difficult to acquire and it requires practice. Several resources are available and may be subject-specific. Advice on writing manuscripts can be found at ℒ www.oxfordjournals.org/for_authors/ and subject-specific advice for rheumatology ℒ http://rheumatology.oxfordjournals.org/. The SQUIRE (Standards for Quality Improvement Reporting Excellence) guidelines offer clear advice on writing a healthcare manuscript ℒ http://squire-statement.org.

A manuscript must be well written, clear, and concise, and the content presented in a logical manner using plain language. The format of manuscripts will depend on the specialist field and journal; most follow the IMRAD format (Introduction, Methods, Results and Discussion). A manuscript should contain something original that will interest readers; originality is the key to getting the manuscript published. Always get a manuscript peer-reviewed before submission by experienced colleagues who will give constructive and honest criticism; revise the manuscript accordingly. If the journal is not in your native language, ask a native-language speaker to read the manuscript. A well laid-out manuscript will help the editor and reviewers come to a judgement about whether or not to accept for publication; consider font, font size, line spacing, and justification.

No matter how well-written or original a manuscript is, its impact will also depend on how accessible it is in literature databases. Table 27.3 shows factors that will influence retrieval.

Table 27.3 Factors that will influence retrieval of an article from a literature database

Title	Precise, accurate, not too long, and appealing
	Do not use multiple clauses
Key words	Keywords are vital for correct retrieval of the article—databases use keywords as search terms. If you use the wrong keywords the article will not be retrieved in the database.
	Use the keywords already in the journal's system if possible.
	Highly specific or novel keywords may not be retrievable.
Abstract	The abstract must tempt the reader to read the full article.
	Journals will specify required length.
	Be clear and concise; give detail and actual results rather than vague statements.

Publication

Choosing the journal

It is important to submit the manuscript to the most appropriate journal. Factors that may influence this decision are shown in Table 27.4. Information is available on the journal website or from the editorial office.

Table 27.4 Factors that will influence journal choice

Factor	Comments
Subject area	Who is the target audience?
	Where will the research have the most impact?
Impact factor (IF)	Does the journal have an impact factor?
	Is it in the range that is acceptable to you, your colleagues, and your institution?
Literature database listing	Is the journal listed on the most appropriate searchable database, e.g. Medline, CINHAL?
Rejection rate	Rejection rate will often ↑ with ↑ IF.
Review time	This is highly variable and will depend on many factors including the efficiency of the editorial office, availability of reviewers; three months is not unreasonable.
	N.B. The number of resubmissions is a major determinant.
Production processing time	The time from acceptance to online publication will vary; authors can speed this up returning corrected proofs quickly.
Time to print if applicable	There may be a long wait until manuscript is in print.

The review and publication process

An example of the review process is shown in Figure 27.3. Before submitting a manuscript it is essential to read and comply with the instructions to authors (available on journal website). A link to the manuscript-handling website is usually available on the journal website (e.g. Manuscript Central), and it usually includes an automated system that generates reminders, receipts, and notices. Many journals expect the manuscript to be submitted as a series of files as shown in Table 27.5. It is important to check the journal requirements and have the files in order before starting the submission process. This is particularly important if the review process is blinded.

The author is guided through the submission process; copy and paste details into the spaces to maintain accuracy. The files are converted into a proof, which must be reviewed by the submitting author. N.B. Check the proof carefully to ensure that all the files have been converted. If the process is anonymous, the title page will not be included in the proof. It is the proof that will be sent to the reviewers rather than the original documents. Remember to press the submission button!

The review process can be monitored online by the authors.

Table 27.5 Example separate documents required for manuscript submission

Document	Details
Title page	Title
	Authors—names, affiliations, addresses
	Corresponding author's contact details
	Author roles
	Conflict of interest statement
	Funding sources if applicable
Manuscript	If the review is anonymous remember to include the manuscript title
	The abstract should be at the start of the manuscript
	Page numbers are essential
	Line numbering may be useful
Tables	Numbered and titled—tables should stand alone
Figures	Numbered and titled—figures should stand alone
Covering letter	Addressed to the editor in chief
	State the importance of the study without hyperbole.
	Confirm that the work is original and not under consideration by another journal
Completed copyright form	

Editorial office
The editorial process will vary between journals and editors, therefore the following details will also vary. The manuscript will be checked to ensure the proof has loaded correctly, the files are in the correct format (e.g. Word), the necessary details are on the title page, an ethics statement is present if required, and the author's instructions have been followed including referencing style. Once the checklist is complete the manuscript is available to the editor, who may be the editor in chief (EIC), regional editor (RE), or subject editor (SE), depending on the journal configuration.

Role of the editor
The editor wants to publish articles that enhance the reputation of the journal, increase readership, subscriptions, and citations (and therefore IF). Most spend a lot of time looking at poor-quality papers and trying to improve them; they look for reasons to accept rather than reject a manuscript. The editor will consider the following factors when deciding whether or not to send the manuscript to be reviewed:
- Does it fit the scope of the journal?
- Presentation
- Language
- Writing style
- Rigour
- Originality

- Contribution to knowledge
- Other factors relating to the journal

Reviewers

The editor will select reviewers (usually two) based on their expertise, experience and expertise at reviewing (including punctuality and reliability) and availability. Some journals allow authors to give preferred and non-preferred reviewers. The editor may or may not comply with these wishes.

N.B. This process can be time-consuming and several reviewers may be invited before two are identified. The manuscript handling website may be misleading on this count; it may show that reviewers have not been invited rather than have not agreed to review.

Editorial decision

The editor reviews the reviewer's comments and decides to accept without further revisions, request minor or major revisions, or reject the manuscript. The authors will be notified of the decision with reviewers' and editor's comments. If the study is interesting but the manuscript is not acceptable, authors may be asked to rewrite and resubmit. This will be dealt with as a new submission and NOT a resubmission.

Resubmission

The revisions should be shown as tracked changes or highlighted. Responses to the review comments should be polite and specific, detailing changes. At the discretion of the journal and editorial office the revised manuscript may be reviewed by the editor or sent for further peer review. Some manuscripts require more than one resubmission before acceptance. Do not be afraid to rebut comments, but a rebuttal should be made using good arguments and remember that other literature may support your arguments.

N.B. It is important to revise and resubmit the manuscript as soon as possible. Most journals give a specified period for resubmission. Before resubmitting, check that the literature review is still current.

Production

Once the manuscript has been accepted, the manuscript will pass to the production editor who will organize copyediting and proofing. Once finalized, the article will usually be published online before print publication, if applicable.

Publishing ethics

Most healthcare journal editors are members of the Committee on Publishing Ethics (COPE ℘ http://publicationethics.org) and conform to their code of conduct. Publishers also have an ethical code of conduct.

Authors

Authorship is discussed earlier in this chapter. It is unethical to submit a manuscript without the agreement of ALL authors and many journals insist that all authors sign the submission letter; multiple submission letters are usually acceptable.

Plagiarism

The manuscript must be original and the text not plagiarized from any other publication, including Internet resources. Increasingly, specialized software is being used to detect plagiarism. It is also important not to self-plagiarize; each article must be original even if written by the same author(s).

Multiple (redundant publishing) submissions

It is not acceptable to submit a manuscript to more than one journal at the same time. The submission letter must state clearly that the manuscript is not under consideration by another journal. If a manuscript is rejected it can be submitted to another journal, but remember to change the manuscript according to the author instructions for the new journal and re-address the submission/covering letter (Table 27.5).

Copyright

Before an article can be published, a completed copyright transfer form (exclusive licence form) must be submitted to the editorial office and/or production office. The completed form can be uploaded on to the manuscript handling website. Copyright protects the use of the published material against plagiarism, libel, or infringement. The publisher holds the copyright to the published article. Authors should contact the publisher for full details of authors' rights.

Reporting guidelines

Reporting guidelines have been produced in order to improve the quality of research reporting and are available from the Equator Network ℘ www.equator-network.org (Table 27.6). Authors are increasingly being asked to use reporting guidelines, and they should be seen as an aid to writing not an obstacle.

Table 27.6 Examples of publishing guidelines

Guideline		Type of reporting
CONSORT	Consolidated Standards of Reporting Trials	Randomized trials
PRISMA	Preferred Reporting Items for Systematic Reviews and Meta-Analyses	Systematic reviews, meta-analyses
STROBE	STrengthening the Reporting of OBservational studies in Epidemiology	Cohort, case-control, cross-sectional studies
SQUIRE	Standards for QUality Improvement Reporting Excellence	General guidance on healthcare writing articles

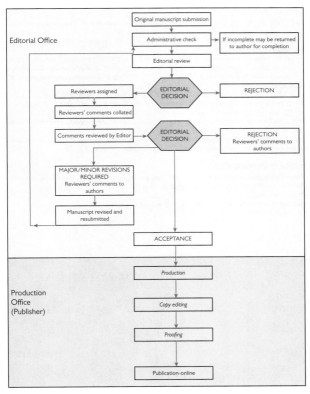

Figure 27.3 Example of the manuscript review process for a peer-reviewed journal.

Transparency

Since May 2011, all clinical trials authorized in the EU are published in an official EU register of clinical trials which is available at ℘ www.clinicaltrialsregister.eu. This website also contains information on whether recruitment for a clinical trial is still ongoing. Importantly, transparency in clinical research ensures that the results of all clinical trials are made public irrespective of whether the findings are favourable, thereby avoiding publication bias. Further details on how to manage the disclosure of clinical trials and a disclosure toolkit can be found online (please refer to the useful links section).

Further reading

HF-ACTION *(Heart Failure: A Controlled Trial Investigating Outcomes of Exercise Training)* trial. Ⓢ www.clinicaltrials.gov registration number: NCT00047437

Bonita RE, Adams S, Whellan DJ. Reporting of Clinical Trials: Publication, Authorship, and Trial Registration. *Heart Failure Clin* 2011;7:561–7.

Bhandari M, Busse J, Kulkarni A, et al. Influence of Authorship Order and Corresponding Author on Perceptions of Authors' Contributions. Abstract presented at the International Congress on Peer Review and Biomedical Publication 2009. Ⓢ http://www.peerreviewcongress.org/abstracts_2009.html

Harden RM. Death by Powerpoint – the need for a 'fidget index'. *Med Teach* 2008;30:833–5.

Miller JE. Preparing and presenting effective research posters. *Health Serv Res* 2007;42:311–28.

Smith R. How not to give a presentation. *BMJ* 2000, 321:1570–1.

Woolsey JD. Combating poster fatigue: how to use visual grammar and analysis to effect better visual communications. *Trends in Neurosciences* 1989; 12:325–32.

Zerwic JJ, Grandfield K, Kavanaugh K, et al. Tips for better visual elements in poster and podium presentations. *Educ Health* (Abingdon). 2010 Aug;23(2):267. Epub 2010 Jul 23.

Useful internet sites

Ⓢ http://www.posterpresentations.com/html/free_poster_templates.html. This is a useful website for downloading templates for poster presentations.

Ⓢ www.clinicaltrialsregister.eu

Ⓢ www.abpi.org.uk/our-work/mandi/Pages/clinical-trial-transparency.aspx

Start-up toolkit:
from funding an idea,
through implementation,
to achieving an impact

Starting out in research

Introduction—thinking of doing research?

Research underpins almost every aspect of clinical and healthcare services and it is never too early or too late to consider being involved in a good research project. However, in order to do this it is important to have adequate time, resources, and support within a studentship or job role to undertake research as it is a serious business. For some, this will mean actively finding a way to build in protected research time into their existing role or find a role that will allow good research to be undertaken.

Undergraduate and Masters degree projects

Most undergraduate degrees will have a specified requirement for a research project that is undertaken towards the latter stage of the degree. This ensures that there is already core knowledge in a subject area and projects can be on 'hot topics' or pieces of work that are part of bigger projects involving supervisors. When undertaking an undergraduate dissertation, it is more important to try and choose a project that will give a good flavour of a particular area or type of research, than to pick the most in-depth or cutting-edge project on offer. This can then serve as generic experience to guide future career choices.

Masters degrees on the other hand, can be either taught, incorporating a time-limited and circumscribed dissertation project, or can be undertaken purely by research where a more substantial, supervised piece of research can be undertaken over one to two years (in the UK, this is normally one year full-time if a science or research degree, and usually two years full-time if a doctorate). This results in a more in-depth dissertation along with the understanding of core concepts in the subject area. In choosing a project for a dissertation within a taught degree, because time is very limited, often secondary analyses of data or literature-based projects will be more suitable than those involving set-up and approvals from scratch as well as real-time data collection and analysis. Both secondary data analysis and synthesis of data or information from existing literature are cardinal research skills, useful to have under the belt either for further research or simply approaching clinical and healthcare evidence with a 'research-aware' approach. Similarly, the experience gained from undertaking a Masters by research need not be constrained by the subject area itself; this can be a very good way to develop a range of generic skills that can be applied in other subject areas.

Undertaking a PhD and other doctoral-level studies

The decision to undertake a PhD should not be taken lightly. Doctoral studies are a major undertaking, ranging from three to four years full-time to over five years for part-time degrees. Healthcare professionals often choose to undertake doctoral studies part-time alongside clinical work and often their studies will complement their job roles. Medical doctors and dentists (particularly in the UK) can choose to undertake a medical doctorate by research (MD or DM), usually in a subject area allied to their postgraduate specialty. Similarly, public health professionals in various parts of the world can undertake a professional doctorate in public health (DrPH) which combines taught elements with substantial research. For very experienced researchers, a PhD or MD can be awarded on retrospective assessment of a range of related peer-reviewed publications in a certain area. However, the classical PhD studentship usually starts off as an MPhil in the first year, during which time projects within the PhD are successfully developed, leading to progression on to full PhD studies from the second year.

The hallmark of a good PhD is original thinking and the ability to tell a story at the end which demonstrates a genuine and substantial effort (of publishable standard) towards progress in a given area of scientific research. Having a keen interest in the subject area of a PhD is essential as it is a journey that requires a good measure of passion for the topic, which can help overcome obstacles as well as drive innovation. However, it is not necessary for PhD studentship to result in a new discovery or a plethora of high-impact peer-reviewed papers unless undertaking a portfolio PhD by publication! What is more important is that a PhD demonstrates a robust and systematic approach that adds significantly to the learning, development, and expertise of the candidate, possibly in a specialized scientific area, complemented by related but transferrable knowledge and research skills.

Research 'tasters', professional training, and projects alongside clinical or healthcare jobs

Starting out in research doesn't have to involve undertaking a prescribed course of study through a degree programme. A number of formal and informal research 'taster' opportunities and more structured internships are offered by a number of research organizations. These can take days, weeks, or several months to complete, depending on the area of research, the level of the opportunity, and the organization type (e.g. university departments, government or independent research units/institutes, healthcare institutions including hospitals, contract research organizations (CROs), the pharmaceutical industry, and manufacturers of food, beverage and healthcare products). These opportunities may at times be relatively informal and possibly *pro-bono* but are a very useful way of gaining rapid insight into the workings of a well-established set of research machinery and they can also help to decide what type of research might be good as a future career choice.

Doctors and other healthcare professionals can hold clinical jobs which offer protected time as well as a limited amount of resource to undertake research projects allied to their clinical practice. In the UK, early-career doctors and allied healthcare professionals can obtain about 25% research time through 'integrated clinical academic training' positions within the National Health Service which can lead on to a successful application for a full-time funded clinical PhD. Various similar models exist in other countries.

Another training-led route to becoming a career researcher can be via professional training and quality-assured examinations such as the benchmark professional certifications/diplomas required to discharge key roles relating to clinical trials. A number of other vocational training and benchmarking routes exist across the globe.

However, beyond these formal arrangements, healthcare professionals often come across unanswered clinical problems which instigate research and innovation with patient or public benefit as a potential outcome. In recent years, a number of countries have broken down some of the traditional barriers of academic research by upholding the aspirations of developing research-friendly healthcare institutions that can support good research ideas, particularly those with direct clinical interface or impact.

Asking a research question

Asking questions is a straightforward process and goes with the premise of scientific curiosity that fuels research. However, formulating the right research question can be tricky, and if the wrong questions are asked, then however well-designed or conducted a study might be, it is unlikely that the right answers will be found.

A research question needs to be focused and specific and can determine the choice of study design. For instance, if we wish to find out the current prevalence of carotid stenosis in UK adults, a cross-sectional study design would suffice. However, if we want to find out what the aetiological determinants or risk factors of carotid stenosis are, a case-control study would be appropriate. Shifting gears slightly, if we want to know whether tackling these risk factors actively reduces the prevalence of carotid stenosis, then a randomized controlled trial would be appropriate. Finally, if we want to find out if trends over the life course influence the development of carotid stenosis then we would employ a cohort study.

In asking a research question it is important to check whether it is supported by available literature and whether the question has already been asked or answered before. If a literature search confirms that this is a question that is still worth asking then the next thing to check is whether the question is actually answerable in a practical way and whether the fact that there are no existing studies based on this question might be due to lack of feasibility. For clinical trials, due to the need for transparency, current but as yet unpublished trials can be found on a number of different open-access trials registers. These can highlight unanswered questions which still need to be interrogated. For other types of studies and in general, when reviewing the literature, a good rule of thumb is that if there are scores of articles found to review, then the question may need to be narrowed down to lead to meaningful results.

When asking a research question, methods and resources are equally important to consider as well as the ethical implications of asking a research question and ascertaining whether an 'experiment' would be permissible in the current regulatory landscape. Another key consideration when asking a research question is to begin with the end in mind; visualize possible outcomes and consider how these may affect the study population or clinical and healthcare practice more widely.

The research question is usually framed to test a hypothetical outcome of a piece of research, that is, a central hypothesis and a primary research question usually provide the 'main answer'. Whilst any given study can also seek to answer a number of secondary or related questions, it is important that the primary question is not lost. Moreover, a study design will often support the robust testing of only a single hypothesis and any secondary questions will be purely exploratory.

All of the above said, formulating a research question need not be a daunting task and one can appear more naturally than one might think. Every time we have a good idea and ask ourselves in a clinical or healthcare context 'why don't we do it *this* way rather than *that* way', or 'could we be doing a better job for patients or the population at large', these sow the seeds of what could become a paradigm-changing research question.

Finding research funding

Having formulated the research question and thought through the steps of implementation of a research project, there is just one small hurdle to overcome: finding research funding.

For those undertaking research as part of a studentship or degree programme, it is important to ensure that adequate funding is already in place within the hosting department. For those wishing to conduct *de novo* research from scratch, a grant application is the next thing to tackle. Examples of the key questions that major research funders are looking for applicants to address are as follows:

- Does the proposal fit well within the objectives and scientific remit set out in the call specification?
- Is there a good medical or scientific rationale for pursuing the questions or gaps in knowledge that are being addressed? Is success likely to lead to significant new understanding?
- To what extent will this project contribute, directly or indirectly, to relieving the burden of disease?
- Is there added value in pursuing this work through research links with other countries?
- Is there similar or complementary research underway elsewhere?
- Has the individual or group established a high-quality track record in the field?
- How innovative are the proposals?
- Are the proposed methods appropriate and feasible for the delivery of the research question?
- Are the experimental plans realistic, given the aims of the research and the resources?
- Are the methods and study designs competitive with the best in the field?
- Have major scientific, technical, or organizational challenges been identified, and will they be tackled well?
- Is it feasible that the outputs of the research could be scaled up? For example, (where appropriate) is the level of involvement of clinical and non-clinical (community) health workers, other elements of civil society, industry, policy/decision makers, and patient groups/families adequate to increase the likely opportunities to scale up the findings of the research?

In the UK, major research funders include member organizations under Research Councils UK ℘ www.rcuk.ac.uk, such as the Medical Research Council ℘ www.mrc.ac.uk and the Biotechnology and Biological Sciences Research Council ℘ www.bbsrc.ac.uk, as well as funding organizations under the UK Clinical Research Collaboration ℘ www.ukcrc.org. In addition, the National Institute of Health Research in England ℘ www.nihr.ac.uk, as well as its devolved counterparts, is a major funder of applied healthcare research. Many of these funders not only support research but also build capacity by providing training posts to early- and mid-career researchers. There also are also a number of charities which provide small-scale to programme-level funding and fall under the Association of Medical Research Charities ℘ www.amrc.org.uk. Well-known charities in the UK include the Wellcome Trust ℘ www.wellcome.ac.uk, the British Heart Foundation ℘ www.bhf.org.uk, Diabetes UK ℘ www.diabetes.org. uk and Cancer Research UK ℘ www.cancerresearchuk.org, to name a few. The NHS also has a number of local and regional funding schemes available particularly to its staff. Professional membership organizations and other postgraduate training bodies also offer their members or trainees small to medium-sized grants to help pump prime research (e.g. British Medical Association ℘ www.bma.org.uk and the Academy of Medical Sciences ℘ www.acadmedsci.ac.uk). Other countries have a range of similar organizations from which research funding can be sought (e.g. European Research Council, National Institutes of Health in the US, the National Health and Medical Research Council in Australia, and the Indian Council of Medical Research in India). The pharmaceutical industry is also a significant source of funding, particularly for clinical trials and associated studies across various parts of the globe.

Looking for grants can be daunting. A good start is to take an 'evolutionary' approach, starting small with a well-designed feasibility study or a potentially scalable pilot which can be funded by a small to medium-sized grant perhaps won at a local or regional level. The results obtained from this preliminary work can then guide a larger piece of follow-on research. Funders can thus judge how well the initial research is conducted, and have confidence that the larger project would be run on equally competent grounds. Many of the initial teething troubles will have already been addressed and the research question and design would have been informed by preliminary findings. The 'revolutionary' approach seeks a major grant in the first instance. An inexperienced applicant would be wise to get as much advice from more experienced researchers as possible before venturing down this line. However, major research funders often see this as an opportunity to support capacity building of the next generation of researchers, something that attracts tremendous kudos.

Resilience is critical in applying for funding as the competition is extremely high and at times multiple re-applications are needed before a proposal is funded. However, each successive iteration of a proposal can lead to improvement. Beginners' luck may prevail as it sometimes does, and occasionally the brilliance of an original idea will be immediately obvious to the funding body. However, these scenarios apart, persistence pays off. A good idea is likely to gain funding eventually. If an idea does not attract funding, might a different idea work?

Developing an idea and designing a study

A good study starts with a good hypothesis that is based on comprehensive review of the available evidence. Whilst a badly analysed study can potentially be re-analysed, a badly designed study is difficult to rescue at the analysis stage.

The following are basic considerations in study design:
- Carefully choose and frame a research question
- Identify a target population
- Decide on type of study
- Define an intervention/exposure of interest
- Specify inclusion/exclusion criteria (if relevant)

- Outline recruitment strategies (if relevant)
- State primary and secondary endpoint(s)/outcome(s)
- Choose valid and reliable measures
- Outline a measurement schedule
- Estimate sample size and power of detection
- Take steps to minimize chance, confounding, and bias

Deciding on the type of study can be guided by the following questions:
- What is the aim of the study?
    - Descriptive
    - Analytic
- Any randomization?
    - Experimental
    - Observational
- When are the outcomes determined?
    - Cohort
    - Cross-sectional
    - Case-control

Some of the most critical mitigating factors in study design are as follows:
- Validity
    - Internal: results not due to chance, bias, or confounding factors
    - External: generalizability
    - Symmetry: groups are similar
- Confounding: distortion of the effect of one risk factor by the presence of another (see Figure 28.1)
- Bias: any effect from design, execution, and interpretation that shifts or influences results
    - Confounding bias: failure to account for the effect of one or more variables that are not distributed equally
    - Measurement bias: measurement methods differ between groups
    - Sampling (selection) bias: design and execution errors in sampling
- Sample size calculation
    - To determine the number of subjects needed to detect a clinically relevant intervention effect if a test of hypothesis is relevant
    - Small sample size may not be able to detect an effect
    - Large sample size is wasteful and potentially unethical
    - For studies recruiting a fixed number of subjects, power calculation can estimate the statistical power

As part of developing a research idea, it may be helpful to refer to the resources and toolkits provided by the National institute of Health Research

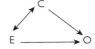

Figure 28.1 Confounder (C) e.g. coffee drinking, and Exposure (E) e.g. smoking, both associated with one another and independently associated with outcome (O) e.g. lung cancer.

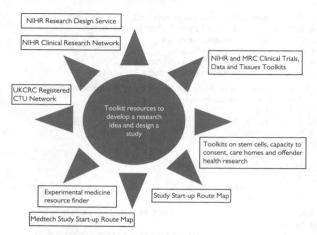

Figure 28.2 NIHR resources and toolkits.

(NIHR). These incorporate good research practice and provide documents and links that can inform research design (Figure 28.2). These toolkits also provide tailored guidance to help steer researchers through parts of the relevant regulatory approvals process.

Developing a protocol

When starting a research study, the first document that is required is the research protocol. The protocol is an essential part of any research ethics application.

A study protocol should describe the research plan in detail (Figure 28.3). It should be written in such a way that other people reading the protocol will be able to repeat the experiment without ambiguity. Creating a robust study protocol is at the heart of ensuring that research is of the highest standard.

The protocol also forms part of the official research documentation and should be kept as part of the trial master file or investigator site file. All these documents are formal documents and must be kept and managed according to best practice. This means that any changes made to them are validated and recorded with appropriate version control.

Protocol content

The first stages of the protocol will involve discussing research ideas with others, usually including the candidate's supervisor or department head. At this stage, ideas are being turned into a research question.

Once a research question has been established, aims and the specific hypothesis can be developed. The research proposal must be put into context of existing knowledge, which will involve a literature search and sourcing of systematic reviews.

Protocol structure

Layouts and headings may vary slightly but the basic elements remain the same for any protocol: title, summary, aims, background, design of the study, ethical considerations including risk and benefits to participants, consideration must be given to describing how the research question will be addressed, and how the collected data will be analysed and the findings disseminated (Chapters 2 and 27).

Approvals and successful ethics applications

Before proceeding with any study idea or developing a proposal into a funding application and subsequently into a protocol, it is important to ensure that full institutional approval is in place for the project and that key designated individuals have signed off on both scientific and governance aspects of a proposal. This can range from a relatively quick and informal process (e.g. student projects) to a multilayered process involving a number of different key organizations (e.g. university departments, NHS R&D, main sponsors, funders, the Medicines and Healthcare products Regulatory Authority (MHRA) for CTIMPs as well as borderline studies). Each organization may have its own internal approvals processes. However, two of the central requirements prior to a protocol being submitted for external approval by an independent ethics committee are the requirements for robust scientific peer review as well as the study sponsor(s) agreeing to take on a study. It is important to build sufficient time into the set-up phase of a study to ensure that these basic approvals are in place prior to submitting an ethics application. The steps towards a potentially successful ethics application are outlined in the following.

The role of the research ethics committee

Ethics committees exist to safeguard the well-being of human subjects of research. Any organization that follows good research practice will expect all research to be carried out under appropriate external ethical approval.

The purpose of an ethics committee is not to review the scientific value of the research but to look at its impact on volunteers/patients and decide if the question answered by the research is, in its opinion, worth the discomfort volunteers/patients will endure.

1. Research ethics committees follow the principles outlined in two major guidance documents: The Belmont report—created by the National Commission for the Protection of Human Subjects of Biomedical and Behavioural Research, first issued in 1978. This document promotes three basic principles for research on human subjects, autonomy, beneficence, and justice.

2. The Declaration of Helsinki—developed by the World Medical Association (WMA) as a statement of ethical principles for medical research involving human subjects, including research on identifiable human material and data.

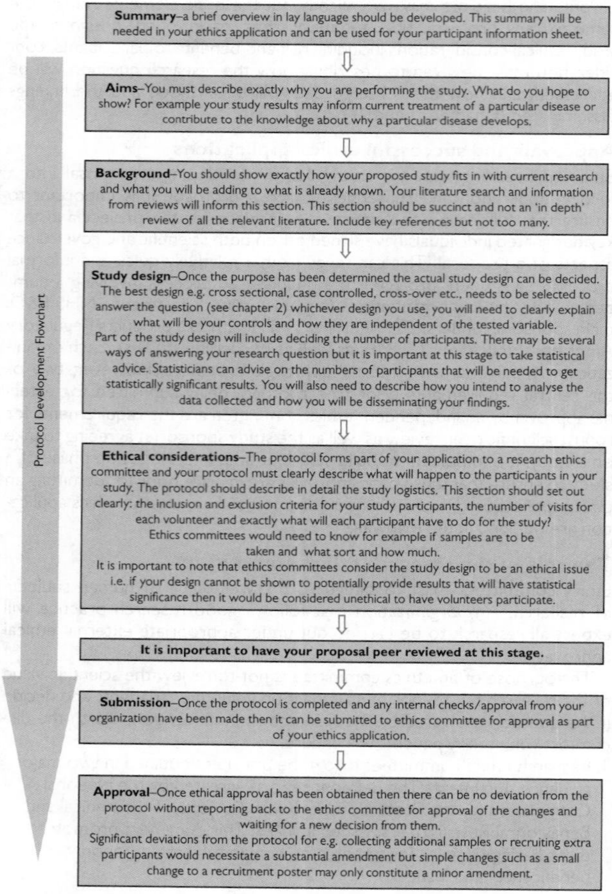

Protocol Development Flowchart

Summary–a brief overview in lay language should be developed. This summary will be needed in your ethics application and can be used for your participant information sheet.

⇩

Aims–You must describe exactly why you are performing the study. What do you hope to show? For example your study results may inform current treatment of a particular disease or contribute to the knowledge about why a particular disease develops.

⇩

Background–You should show exactly how your proposed study fits in with current research and what you will be adding to what is already known. Your literature search and information from reviews will inform this section. This section should be succinct and not an 'in depth' review of all the relevant literature. Include key references but not too many.

⇩

Study design–Once the purpose has been determined the actual study design can be decided. The best design e.g. cross sectional, case controlled, cross-over etc., needs to be selected to answer the question (see chapter 2) whichever design you use, you will need to clearly explain what will be your controls and how they are independent of the tested variable. Part of the study design will include deciding the number of participants. There may be several ways of answering your research question but it is important at this stage to take statistical advice. Statisticians can advise on the numbers of participants that will be needed to get statistically significant results. You will also need to describe how you intend to analyse the data collected and how you will be disseminating your findings.

⇩

Ethical considerations–The protocol forms part of your application to a research ethics committee and your protocol must clearly describe what will happen to the participants in your study. The protocol should describe in detail the study logistics. This section should set out clearly: the inclusion and exclusion criteria for your study participants, the number of visits for each volunteer and exactly what will each participant have to do for the study? Ethics committees would need to know for example if samples are to be taken and what sort and how much.
It is important to note that ethics committees consider the study design to be an ethical issue i.e. if your design cannot be shown to potentially provide results that will have statistical significance then it would be considered unethical to have volunteers participate.

⇩

It is important to have your proposal peer reviewed at this stage.

⇩

Submission–Once the protocol is completed and any internal checks/approval from your organization have been made then it can be submitted to ethics committee for approval as part of your ethics application.

⇩

Approval–Once ethical approval has been obtained then there can be no deviation from the protocol without reporting back to the ethics committee for approval of the changes and waiting for a new decision from them.
Significant deviations from the protocol for e.g. collecting additional samples or recruiting extra participants would necessitate a substantial amendment but simple changes such as a small change to a recruitment poster may only constitute a minor amendment.

Figure 28.3 Protocol development flow chart.

Researchers conducting studies that involve human participants have a legal responsibility to follow best practice and only conduct studies that have been ethically approved. Approval from an ethics committee is a formal process; it takes time and must be acquired before any study can begin. Factor this in and aim to submit an ethics application well ahead of your start date.

Most applications will be submitted to the National Research Ethics Service (NRES) and reviewed by NHS Research Ethics Committees (RECs). Some ethics committees may be organized differently, such as university ethics committees.

Who sits on ethics committees?

Probably the most important fact to remember about ethics committee members is that they come from a variety of backgrounds. Any ethics application will not be reviewed solely by scientists or medical professionals. Committees will always have lay members with little or no understanding of scientific or technical details. This is important to keep in mind when submitting an application. The committee is there to look at the ethical aspects of the study and review the potential outcome and importance of the research, weighing this up against the burden to the participant.

For example, a committee may give approval to a study which involves intensive blood sampling from participants if the outcome of the study will inform future cancer therapies, but not if the outcome has less direct beneficial results.

The application—NRES via IRAS

In the UK, an application to a research ethics committee must be submitted online. The process for submitting the application is continuously changing and improving. The Integrated Research Application System (IRAS) ℜ www.myresearchproject.org.uk allows researchers to log on and generate the appropriate forms for submission to NRES.

IRAS can generate many difference forms, some of which will have no relevance to the particular piece of research planned. The filter system will generate only those forms that are needed: NRES/NHS/HSC Research Ethics Committee.

The ethics application process in other countries will be different. This is something researchers must be aware of, not only in the case of studies to be conducted in other countries but also those involving multinational collaborations. Under the requirements of the Clinical Trial Regulation there will be a single portal for submissions thus standardizing the process in the EU. Some countries have similar research ethics processes to the UK (e.g. Australia ℜ www.nhmrc.gov.au/health-ethics/australian-health-ethics-committee-ahec, the Netherlands ℜ http://www.ccmo-online.nl/main.asp?pid=1&taal=1), but some countries may have very different procedures and requirements. Guidance can be easily found via an online search.

Filling out the form

In order to ensure that IRAS is generating the correct form, it is important not to guess at answers.

Researchers should ensure that they understand what is being asked before committing to an answer. Employers will have standard responses to questions such as indemnity, and who the sponsor is, for example.

Some sections require some answers to be in language suitable for a lay-person to understand. Scientists used to writing complex technical documents often find this difficult. However, it is vital to the application that these sections are clear. Lay members of the committee will not understand technical detail. It is useful to give these sections to other people not in your field of expertise to look at before submission and check that they can understand them.

Main application questions

The IRAS online form for obtaining ethical approval will cover all aspects of the study.

Be well prepared before starting to complete the form and have in place an internally reviewed robust protocol prepared (this will need to be submitted in addition to the IRAS form).

Purpose and design

These questions should have already been addressed in the study protocol. It is particularly important that statistical advice with regard to the number of intended volunteers has been taken. It would be considered unethical to recruit volunteers or patients to a study that is statistically underpowered.

Recruitment

There will be questions about recruitment. How will this be done? Who will be conducting it? Answers to these and other questions, and examples of any documents that will be using (e.g. advertising posters and approach letters to volunteers) will need to be submitted. These should be clearly understandable and not coercive in any way.

Inclusion/Exclusion

A particular type of person will probably need to be recruited in order to minimize variation. The committee will need to know what the inclusion/exclusion criteria will be (e.g. only males, only those under 60 years). There may be more specific requirements such as people without diabetes or people who are overweight. Researchers will be asked why they need a particular type of participant, and recruitment posters/letters must cite this clearly. Think carefully about this and remember that all documents submitted are the ones that will be used for the study; alterations will not be possible without renewed application to the ethics committee for approval of a substantial amendment, and this will take time. Often researchers regret putting restrictive criteria in when they start the study and find they cannot get enough volunteers unless they recruit more widely.

In addition, if screening of participants before they start the study for conditions such as diabetes, raised blood pressure, etc., then procedures must be in place to report clinically abnormal results. Usually templates for standard letters written to participants' GPs reporting clinically relevant results will be submitted with an application.

Risks, burdens, and benefits

Perhaps the most import questions are those about risks, burdens, and benefits to the participant. These are central to the ethical decision to be made. It is vital to be clear and honest about what will happen in the study. If no direct benefits will accrue to participants this must be stated, but if the information gained as a result will benefit others, state this. The committee will look at the research as a whole and make a judgement about its worth. It may be considered that the study burden to the participant is too excessive to answer the research question. Similarly, the study may ask a great deal of participants but the committee may look at the potential outcome and decide that the burden is justified.

Consent

Consent is central to any ethics application (see Chapter 9), and is a legal obligation. The application will ask questions about how consent is to be obtained. This is a vital part of the application, which must show that the consent process has been properly followed. Copies of the proposed consent form and participant information sheets must accompany the application. Remember that all documents for participants will have to be written in lay language (it is suggested that the volunteer information sheet is aimed at the level of someone with a reading age of 10 years).

Confidentiality

All information/data gathered during the study must be treated appropriately and researchers will need to offer evidence that this will be the case. Questions regarding storage and use of personal information will be asked, and compliance with the Data Protection Act assured. Participants are usually given code numbers and only these codes may be used to identify data and samples. The study investigator will then hold a key for linking the participant's name and personal details to the codes. This link must be kept securely protected either in a locked cupboard, or password-protected electronically. The code can be accessed in the event that clinical results need to be reported. The committee will also ask how long the study data will be retained after the study has finished. Will the data be shared with other researchers? These are questions that are worth discussing with the researcher's employer, and bear in mind that restrictive answers have consequences for the conduct of the existing as well as future trials. For example, if it is stated that data will only be used for this study, then it cannot be used as part of another study without new ethical approval being granted.

Samples

Consent must be correctly obtained to ensure compliance with the Human Tissue Act. What will happen to residual samples collected? Will samples be stored for later research?

All these questions should be considered carefully and with a view to the post-study analyses. What is intended here must be written in the application; additional tests or ideas cannot be added without ethics committee approval.

Time taken

It takes a maximum of 60 days (legal requirement) from submitting an application for a standard product to approval. Extra time will be needed if there are questions and modifications asked by the ethics committee.

Researchers are told when their application is being reviewed and they may attend the meeting. It is highly advisable that they do so as they then can answer any questions about the research directly, thus avoiding delays in the application if queries come back via letter.

Proportionate review is now used in practice if the study does not present any major ethical concerns, and here the ethics process is considerably shortened.

Safety and regulatory considerations

Collection of safety information is fundamental to research studies involving human subjects. This includes detection and management in line with the duty of care. It is vital to understand the terminology and ensure excellent record keeping, follow-up, and reporting.

Terminology

Adverse event (AE) (or adverse experience): any untoward medical occurrence in a subject to whom a medicinal product has been administered, including occurrences which are not necessarily caused by or related to that product.

Adverse drug reaction (ADR): any untoward and unintended response in a subject to an investigational medicinal product which is related to any dose administered to that subject.

Unexpected adverse reaction: an adverse reaction the nature and severity of which is not consistent with the information about the medicinal product in question set out:
- in the case of a product with a marketing authorization, in the summary of product characteristics for that product
- in the case of any other investigational medicinal product, in the investigator's brochure relating to the trial in question.

Serious adverse event (SAE) or serious adverse drug reaction (SAR) or suspected unexpected serious adverse reaction (SUSAR): any adverse event, adverse reaction, or unexpected adverse reaction, respectively, that:
- results in death
- is life-threatening
- requires hospitalization or prolongation of existing hospitalization
- results in persistent or significant disability or incapacity
- consists of a congenital anomaly or birth defect.

Important medical events that may not be immediately life-threatening or result in death or hospitalization but may jeopardize the patient or may require intervention to prevent one of the other outcomes listed in the definition above should also be considered serious.

Further guidance on safety reporting can be found in the Detailed guidance on the collection, verification and presentation of adverse reaction reports arising from clinical trials on medicinal products for human use, June 2011 ℘ http://ec.europa.eu/health/files/eudralex/vol-10/2011_c172_01/2011_c17201-en.pdf

Investigator responsibilities

The investigator shall report any serious adverse event (SAE) which occurs in a subject immediately to the sponsor.

The immediate report may be made orally or in writing and shall be followed by a detailed written report on the event. Where the event reported consists of, or results in, the death of a subject, the investigator shall supply the sponsor with any additional information requested by the sponsor. Where the death has been reported to the relevant ethics committee, the investigator shall supply any additional information requested by that committee.

Sponsor responsibilities

The sponsor shall keep detailed records of all adverse events relating to a clinical trial which are reported to him or her by the investigators for that trial. The licensing authority may require the sponsor to send those records, or copies of such records, to the authority.

A sponsor shall ensure that all relevant information about a SUSAR which occurs during the course of a clinical trial in the UK, and is fatal or life-threatening, is reported as soon as possible to the MHRA, the competent authorities of any European Economic Area (EEA) state, other than the UK, in which the trial is being conducted, and the relevant ethics committee.

It is a statutory requirement that this is done no later than seven days after the sponsor was first aware of the reaction. Any additional relevant information should be sent within eight days of the report.

A sponsor shall ensure that an SUSAR which is not fatal or life-threatening is reported as soon as possible, and in any event not later than 15 days after the sponsor is first aware of the reaction, to the MHRA, the competent authorities of any EEA state, other than the UK, in which the trial is being conducted, and the relevant ethics committee.

Further information is available in: Detailed guidance on the collection, verification and presentation of adverse reaction reports arising from clinical trials on medicinal products for human use—2011.

The key points relating to pharmacovigilance are included in Part 5 of The Medicines for Human Use (Clinical Trials) Regulations 2004: SI 2004/1031 ℘ www.legislation.gov.uk/uksi/2004/1031/contents/made

What to include in an SUSAR report

The data elements expected in an SUSAR report are listed in detailed guidance on the collection, verification, and presentation of adverse reaction reports arising from clinical trials on medicinal products for human use—June 2011, ℘ http://ec.europa.eu/health/files/eudralex/vol-10/2011_c172_01/2011_c172_01-en.pdf and there is excellent step-by-step guidance on the EudraVigilance website ℘ https://eudravigilance.ema.europa.eu/human/index.asp

Where incomplete information is available at the time of initial reporting, all the appropriate information for an adequate analysis of causality should be provided as follow-up reports as it becomes available. All SUSARs must be reported electronically via the EudraViglance website.

Urgent safety measures

The sponsor and investigator may take appropriate urgent safety measures to protect clinical trial subjects from any immediate hazard to their health and safety. The measures should be taken immediately. There is no need to wait for licensing authority approval before implementing urgent safety measures; however, the regulators (MHRA) must be informed in writing in the form of a substantial amendment within three days.

Temporary halt of a trial

When a sponsor halts a trial temporarily, he or she should notify the regulatory authority (MHRA) and ethics committees immediately and at least within 15 days from when the trial is temporarily halted. The notification should be made as a substantial amendment using the notification of amendment form and it must clearly explain what has been halted (e.g. stopping recruitment and/or interrupting treatment of subjects already included) and the reasons for the temporary halt.

Premature trial closure

If a trial is terminated before the date specified for its conclusion (in the application), the sponsor should notify the licensing authority and the ethics committee within 15 days of the date of termination by submitting a declaration of the end of a clinical trial form.

Toolkit for IMP

This guidance has been prepared by MODEPHARMA ✆ www.modepharma.com to codify good practice in publicly-funded clinical trials and the advice is offered in that spirit.

Table 28.1 highlights some common IMP-related challenges seen across the initial stages of a clinical trial lifecycle. These challenges can be avoided with diligent planning and awareness of the underlying issues.

Trial supplies checklist

This checklist highlights key questions that must be considered when arranging trial supplies. The objective is to consider as many of these as early as possible to (a) establish the most optimal trial medication solution, and (b) avoid funding shortfalls during the conduct of the trial.

(A) Regulatory considerations
- Is it a clinical trial of a medicinal product?
  - Does the study fall under the Clinical Trials Directive?
  - Is the product an investigational medicinal product (IMP) or a non-investigational medicinal product (NIMP)?
  - Can the reduced requirements from the MRC/DH/MHRA Joint Project on risk-adapted approaches to the management of clinical trials of IMPs apply?
- Does the trial involve multiple countries?
  - What are country-specific IMP requirements?

(B) Product considerations
- What medicinal products and dosage form will be used?
  - Existing commercial products with marketing authorizations in an EU member state?
  - Commercial product with marketing authorization in non-EU country?
  - Novel substances and products (new product)?
  - Placebos (new product) required?
- Source of products?
  - Sourced directly from marketing authorization holder?
  - Purchased via commercial wholesale/hospital channels?
  - New manufacture via one or more contract manufacturers?
  - Imported from a non-EU country?

Table 28.1 Common IMP-related challenges

Challenge	Common risks
Protocol development phase	Non-compliance or high withdrawal rate
• Insufficient consideration of patient population factors • Sub-optimal choice of active/placebo dosage forms • Lack of awareness on regulatory requirements for IMP manufacturing • Inaccurate budgeting of IMP costs	• Non-compliance or high withdrawal rate • Poor trial design/wastage of drug • Regulatory approval delayed/failed • Insufficient funding for the trial to continue
Trial set-up phase	
• Little or no experience with contract manufacturers • Hidden costs in quotes making them difficult to interpret and compare • Incomplete and/or poorly understood manufacturing specifications • Missing technical agreements • Inadequate project planning	• Poor IMP quality and design • Paying more than expected • Sponsor's responsibilities not adequately covered • Manufacturing delays
Trial implementation phase	
• Insufficient blinding of IMPs • Inadequate labelling of IMPs • Poor quality IMP and packaging • Inappropriate supply chain or processes • IMP adversely affected during storage and transport • Failure to monitor product quality issues including recalls	• Credibility of results • Patient safety risk/regulatory noncompliance • Interruption to treatment • Patient loss of confidence and drop-outs • Early trial stop by sponsor or competent authority

- What is the approach to blinding?
  - How will comparator products including placebos be made to match in appearance, packaging, and labelling?
  - Is the blinding approach suitable for the trial's patient population?
  - What are the randomization arrangements?
  - What are the emergency unblinding arrangements?

(C) GMP manufacture considerations
- Is IMP manufacture required?
  - Where will manufacturing of IMP take place?
  - Can Regulation 37 for 'assembly' work be applied?

- What pharmaceutical development work is required?
  - Development of blinded products?
  - Analytical method development and validation?
  - Stability testing to establish shelf-life?
- Where will the products be manufactured and/or where will the products be released for clinical trial use?
  - Are all IMPs including placebos manufactured by an MIA(IMP) holder?
  - How will the sponsor assess that manufacturer is suitable for the planned works?
  - Will the manufacturer of the marketed product provide the placebo or is placebo manufacture required?
  - Is the placebo identical in appearance and packaging?
  - In the case of non-EU imports, is an audit necessary?
  - What analytical work is required for QP release?
- CTA application manufacturing information available?
  - Has the final QP releasing site in the EU been selected?
  - IMPD: full/simplified required, or will the SmPC suffice?
  - Labelling requirements fulfilled?
  - Shelf-life: are sufficient data available for the IMP in its final packaging to justify the proposed shelf-life or is a stability study required?
- Standards, specifications, and manufacturing scope agreed with the manufacturer?
  - Blinded product specifications agreed?
  - Agreement on number of manufacturing campaigns required to cover the duration of the trial agreed under consideration of the product shelf-lives?
  - Manufacturing scope and timeline agreed?
  - Technical agreement (table of responsibilities) agreed?
- Documentation requirements?
  - Documentation system for full IMP accountability in place?
- Storage and distribution arrangements considered?
  - Who will undertake storage of trial supplies and patient returns?
  - Under what temperature conditions?
  - Has this cost been considered for the duration of the trial?
  - Where will reconciliation and destruction be performed?

(D) Costing considerations
- Have all IMP-related costs been considered?
  - Regulatory costs?
  - IMP sourcing, manufacturing, storage, distribution, returns, and destruction costs?
  - Is VAT applicable?
  - Dispensing costs?
  - Prescription charge applicability?

More detailed considerations and further explanation may be found within Chapter 17 of this book.

From data to dissemination

There is a well defined process for the flow of data through the clinical trial life cycle. Figure 28.4 shows the steps from protocol to marketing approval. Alongside the reporting of data in an analysable form, it is important to consider which statistical tests will be used. The choice of statistical test depends on the following factors:

1. Aim of the study (comparing two independent samples, comparing more than two independent samples, comparing differences in a paired sample, assessing associations between two variables)
2. Research question
3. Type of data (categorical, ordinal, continuous)

Details as to when to apply which test are shown in Chapter 2 of this book, and in the *Oxford Handbook of Medical Statistics*.

Once analysed, data are presented in the form of results. These can be discussed in relation to the original research questions set out at the beginning. Discovering findings in this way constitutes one of the most exciting parts of the research process. It is then important to have these findings reviewed by peers and share lessons learned with the rest of the world through journal publication and presentation. The importance of

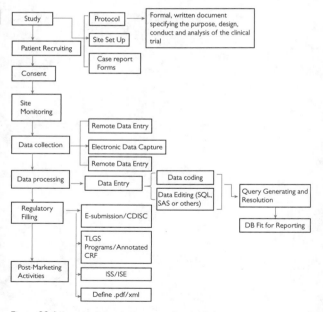

Figure 28.4 Steps leading to the reporting of research data.

finding the right journal; audience, and impact factor are all critical in being able to extend the legacy of any research and add to the evidence base in a given area. Other ways of dissemination (e.g. conferences and meetings) are an opportunity to not only showcase work but also develop new collaborations. Please refer to Chapter 27 for details of publication/ dissemination.

Continuing with a research career—steps to becoming an independent researcher

Once a Masters or doctorate has been completed, there are a number of options open to those who wish to continue research. This chapter describes these options, what is possible and what could be possible given a little gumption, confidence, and convincing.

An important element of the career development of an independent researcher is the readiness to move to a different country to pursue a specific research interest. This is likely to lay foundations of the future research area and contribute to the expansion of one's own research network. In the selection of the research group and institution, several key characteristics play a crucial role:

1. Expertise in the field
2. Achievements of the group and impact of its research on clinical or public health practice
3. Overall institutional reputation in academia.

The traditional career path

The traditional path for an aspiring academic is an undergraduate degree, followed by a PhD (or a Masters and then a PhD), postdoctoral research, and then academia (teaching, with research); in the UK this tends to be a lectureship, whereas in the US and Canada this will be a tenure-track position/assistant professor. Academics can establish themselves by achieving a successful programme of teaching, securing appropriate funding and publishing papers in peer-reviewed journals. Measurements such as impact factor, citation index and h-index (Chapter 27) can be used to assess a researcher's contribution to a field. In the UK, a periodic assessment called the Research Excellence Framework is carried out by impartial assessors who are experts in the field of study for each department being examined.

Other options

Research scientist at an Institute

In the UK and around the world there are a number of government-funded (Medical Research Council, MRC; National Physics Laboratory, NPL; National Institute of Health, NIH), or industry-funded research institutes (Novartis's Institutes of BioMedical Research, http://www.nibr.com/), which all aim to produce high standards of excellence in focused programmes of research. These institutes are generally very competitive and require high-quality outputs (publications, patents, governmental reports). They have internal funding available for their researchers, in addition to external grants (personal fellowships and research grants) which can be competed for on a national or international level.

Research fellowships (research-focused, with some teaching)

A number of governmental research councils and charities offer research fellowships for high-achieving young and experienced researchers. These may provide a researcher's salary initially for five years, and some start-up funds. Although the post is generally for five years in the first instance, this can be extended to eight or ten years, depending on the funding body/agency. Some universities will follow a fellowship with an offer of an academic position, such as a lectureship or a readership, to keep a high-performing fellow in the same institution once the fellowship has ended.

Career Development Awards/Fellowships (CDF)

The MRC offers five years of support to postdocs to help them make the transition to independent researcher. However, these awards are highly sought after, and only available to exceptional applicants. Applicants must have a PhD or DPhil and at least three years but not greater than six years of postdoctoral research experience. These awards allow one year's training outside the UK.

Traditional methods of finding postdoctoral research

Advertisement

Keep an eye on websites for appropriate openings (in the UK try ℘ www.jobs.ac.uk ℘ www.academicjobseu.com, Nature, Science, or New Scientist job sites), or in the jobs section on the website of the university of interest, and apply by submitting an application form, curriculum vitae (CV), cover letter, and normally, the names and contact details for three referees. There is often the opportunity to make casual inquires via e-mail with the principal investigator (PI) or head of department (HOD), and perhaps even a face-to-face meeting, if it is possible to travel there.

Referral

If there is the potential to continue a PhD project into a postdoc, or the PhD supervisor gets another grant that overlaps with the finishing of a PhD, a budding researcher might have the opportunity to stay in the same lab. Supervisors might be approached as they often know of similar work in other labs, at home or abroad. With enough notice, it is possible to apply for a couple of grants in labs of interest, and receive funding before the end of a PhD.

Other considerations

Other labs and institutions may be running projects of interest. Why not apply to these for any role available, and wait for the most appropriate role to become vacant.

Industry

Another way to continue research activities and use those skills honed during a PhD is to become a research scientist in industry. Major pharmaceutical companies, medical device manufacturers, engineering firms, or novel start-ups are all potential employers. Working in industry is very different to working elsewhere and this can present some challenges. Critical thinking, self-organization, and problem-solving skills may be 'key transferable skills' required, and the work may involve a great deal paperwork, adhering to strict industry standards, guidelines, and protocols. These companies are commercially driven, and achieving marketing authorization, profits, and company growth are the main focus, rather than carrying out fundamental research. Some people find work in industry immensely satisfying. Creating a product that will eventually be tested for use in patients, or some other applications, can make for a much more satisfying career than publishing the results, although in some situations publishing is also possible, where it does not conflict with IP and patent laws.

Bear in mind that industry can also fund academic research. Hiring a post-doc is a very cost-efficient way for industry to undertake research. In the UK, the Technology Strategy Board (TSB) often funds academic-industry partnerships, as does the Royal Society. In addition, the Royal Society offers an industry-linked fellowship scheme (the Industry Fellowship) which would be helpful to keep in mind during the exciting but grinding years of an industry-funded postdoc.

Importance of developing an early track record
The last 10 years has seen a large change to academic funding and as a consequence, competition and expectations in academia have grown such that the earlier one can establish a track record, in terms of lab experience and publications, the better in terms of career opportunities.

Funding independent research within a postdoc— what are the options?
Internal funding
Departments, colleges, and institutions may have some money available to fund a small project or pilot. Travel funding is also something that can be available from these sources.

Junior research fellowships
These are prestigious funding awards for early researchers, which either means those about to complete their PhDs or have not completed more than three to five years' postdoctoral research before applying. They fund membership of a college and all the benefits this brings, plus funding to cover living expenses for three years. Successful applicants may be required to run college tutorials and undertake examinations marking.

Further details of some of these can be found in the *Cambridge Reporter*, Cambridge Postdoc's guide to finding a postdoc (please see the link in the reference section), the *University of Oxford Gazette*, and Durham University also offers International Research Fellowships.

Travelling fellowships
Travelling fellowships are also worth considering. These funds are meant for researchers at any level to spend time in another lab, often abroad, to form collaborations, learn techniques, and create new projects, within or across disciplines.
- For example, the Royal Society offers an International Exchanges Scheme. The scheme offers funds to cover living expenses and a small amount of money for research expenses.
- The MRC offers a Partnership Scheme which '[a]ny UK-based researcher who can demonstrate that they will direct the proposed partnership activities and manage the funding on behalf of the MRC to ensure that progress is made against the aims.'
- The Engineering and Physical Sciences Research Council (EPSRC) funds Overseas Travel Grants. Although those at the postdoc level cannot

apply, a principal investigator (PI) can list co-applicants and PhD students on the application, and these individuals may be eligible for travel.

Society/Association-related bursaries
Consider joining a society These offer a range of opportunities, bulletins, and discounts for a relatively low membership fee. Bursaries for conference attendance are often available via these.

Industry bursaries
Investigate the availability of these. It may be that the company/industry contact will require the completion of some research in their interests in exchange for this support.

Making change happen
Talk to people!
Set up a mentoring scheme to help give individuals career advice, support, and possibly contacts and networking opportunities.

Networks
Joining a local, national, or international network may also be helpful and inspirational, and offer additional opportunities for making contacts who may at some point lead to funding or research opportunities. For women in science, engineering, or construction, a helpful network in the UK is Woman in Science, Engineering and Construction (WISE, ℘ http://wise-campaign.org.uk/about-us), which has local societies around the country. The aim of this network is to offer mentorships and provide support in, at times, a male-dominated field.

Initiate a fund for early researchers
Schemes are available and which are specifically for early-career researchers. Glaxo Smith Kline (GSK), for example, provides small amounts of funding for early-career researchers (less than five years' from PhD completion) to undertake dental research projects.

Approach encouraging colleagues/collaborators
Maintain a network of supportive individuals.

Now what? Doing early-career research with no money
Supervisor—releasing extra funds (i.e. begging and pleading)
Draw up a small proposal, give a small presentation to your supervisor, or maybe just have a chat over a coffee. Try your best and see what your supervisor can do for you. In exchange he or she may get an improved or additional publication, and a happier postdoc!

Collaborating with colleagues and other universities
Collaboration might be of great importance when doing early-career research with no money.

Equipment with bursaries attached
In the UK, funding bodies such as the EPSRC (EPSRC Access) will fund expensive pieces of equipment under an agreement where the lab hosting the equipment will give access and support other users from other institutions to this equipment, free of charge. In fact, sometimes the equipment

can be actually moved on a temporary basis to the external research lab, or costs for travel and accommodation might be reimbursed. It may be necessary to list scientists supporting the project as a co-author or acknowledge them in the acknowledgements section of any resulting publication.

Conclusion

This chapter has reviewed different ways of furthering a postdoc career and finding funding opportunities to support independent research initiatives. Further information and links are provided in the reference section. Do remember that the approval and support of the research supervisor/PI is essential to any endeavour beyond the original actual postdoc project.

The importance of clear goals and general enthusiasm: don't forget to sell your success!

One of the most important things to remember during the postdoc years is to have clear goals, approach any opportunity with enthusiasm and a willingness to undertake hard (sometimes monotonous) work. It is also important sometimes to step back and consider a career over the longer term. Where have you come from? Where are you going now?

Be sure to make the most of any successes during this time and to sell these.

Keep enthusiastic, persistent, and ambitious, and good luck!

Further reading

Isaac JL (2002). The Career Path to Research Fellow. ℘ http://sciencecareers.sciencemag.org/career_magazine/previous_issues/articles/2002_11_15/noDOI.13411641766596976648

MRC Fellowships ℘ www.mrc.ac.uk/Fundingopportunities/Fellowships

Innovate UK ℘ http://www.innovateuk.org/

The Cambridge Reporter ℘ http://www.admin.cam.ac.uk/reporter/

The Oxford Gazette ℘ http://www.ox.ac.uk/gazette/

Durham University ℘ http://www.dur.ac.uk/ias/diferens/junior/

The Royal Society ℘ http://royalsociety.org/grants/schemes/industry-fellowship

MRC Funding Opportunities ℘ www.mrc.ac.uk/Fundingopportunities/Grants/Partnershipgrant/MRC006414

The Engineering and Physical Sciences Research Council (EPSRC) fund Overseas Travel Grants ℘ https://www.epsrc.ac.uk/funding/howtoapply/routes/international/otgs/

The Clinical Research Network ℘ www.crn.nihr.ac.uk/researchers

Postdocs of Cambridge (PdOC): Guide to finding a Postdoc Job (includes some tips about funding and Junior Research Fellowships) ℘ http://groups.ds.cam.ac.uk/pdoc/docs/PdOC_how%20to%20find%20a%20postdoc%20guide.pdf

US-based National Postdoctoral Association's Career Planning Resources ℘ www.nationalpostdoc.org/careers/career-planning-resources

Vitae: A UK organization championing the personal, professional and career development of doctoral researchers and research staff in higher education institutions and research institutes. ℘ www.vitae.ac.uk/

Editorial (2004). Wanted: career path for postdocs *Nature* Materials 2004;3(1). ℘ www.nature.com/nmat/journal/v3/n1/full/nmat1055.html

Where do all the postdocs go? *Nature* 402:9–10. ℘ www.nature.com/nature/journal/v402/n6758supp/full/402a009a0.html

Index